Clinical Psychopharmacology

A PRACTICAL REFERENCE FOR NONMEDICAL PSYCHOTHERAPISTS

Contributors

Gary W. Lawson, Ph.D.

Craig A. Cooperrider, Ph.D.

Robert B. Cohen, Ph.D.

Carl B. Gacono, Ph.D.

Ann W. Lawson, M.A., M.F.C.C.

Gary R. Lewis, M.A., R.N.

John McCaig, M.A.

Michael J. Nanko, Ph.D.

M. Gene Ondrusek, Ph.D.

Delia Thrasher, M.A.

Jerry Williams, Ph.D.

Thomas J. Young, Ph.D.

Clinical Psychopharmacology

A PRACTICAL REFERENCE FOR NONMEDICAL PSYCHOTHERAPISTS

Edited by

Gary W. Lawson, Ph.D.
United States International University
San Diego, California

Craig A. Cooperrider, Ph.D.
Pioneer Mental Health Center
Seward, Nebraska

AN ASPEN PUBLICATION®
Aspen Publishers, Inc.

1988

Rockville, Maryland
Royal Tunbridge Wells

Library of Congress Cataloging-in-Publication Data

Clinical psychopharmacology: a practical reference for nonmedical
psychotherapists/edited by Gary W. Lawson, Craig Cooperrider.
p.   cm.
"An Aspen publication."
Includes bibliographies and index.
ISBN: 0-87189-751-2
1. Psychopharmacology. 2. Psychotropic drugs. I. Lawson, Gary.
II. Cooperrider, Craig.
[DNLM: 1. Psychopharmacology. 2. Psychotropic Drugs. QV 77
C6416]
RM315.C554   1988
615'.78—dc19
DNLM/DLC
for Library of Congress   87-33480
CIP

The authors have made every effort to ensure the accuracy of the information herein,
particularly with regard to drug selection and dose. However, appropriate information sources should be consulted, especially for new or unfamiliar drugs or procedures. It is the responsibility of every practitioner to evaluate the appropriateness of
a particular opinion in the context of actual clinical situations and with due consideration to new developments. Authors, editors, and the publisher cannot be held responsible for any typographical or other errors found in this book.

Editorial Services: Jane Coyle Garwood

Library of Congress Catalog Card Number: 87-33480
ISBN: 0-87189-751-2

Printed in the United States of America

2   3   4   5

Table of Contents

Preface

Each year for the past eight years the senior author of this book has taught a course in psychopharmacology for psychologists and other nonmedical mental health practitioners. The books available as texts for the course have fallen into two categories: undergraduate texts designed to teach the basic drugs, and practitioners' manuals written primarily for those in the medical profession who prescribe medication. Books in the first group are too basic and do not cover many of the areas that a course for nonmedical mental health practitioners should cover. For example, ways to identify and work with a trustworthy physician are not addressed. Books in the second group are too detailed and presume prior knowledge that few nonmedical therapists received during their training.

The original concept of this book was to provide the nonmedical practitioner with all the updated information regarding issues on psychopharmacology that would be useful for the practice of psychotherapy. It became painfully clear, however, that this was an impossible task. First of all, having written several books before, we were aware that it would be at least 6 months from the time we handed in a completed manuscript until the book became available on the market; it could be as long as a year. With new drugs and drug-related research appearing each day, the best we could hope for was to provide all the information available at the time we finished the manuscript. But as we wrote and completed each chapter, we found new material that needed to be included. Each day's mail brought a new batch of flyers on the latest books about psychopharmacology. We were beginning to go broke buying the latest books in the field, and there was no end in sight.

With the axiom ''it is better to teach people to fish than to give them a fish'' in mind, we changed the focus of the book. This is now a book that will teach readers to fish. That is, with the information provided in this book readers will be able to seek out, find, and understand the material on psychopharmacology and issues related to psychopharmacology that they will need to know to maximize their effectiveness as psychotherapists.

Thinking in terms of psychopharmacology can change the way in which a therapist looks at and responds to situations in everyday practice. For example, the senior author of this book was to teach a practicum in psychotherapy at a large Midwestern university. The practicum was taught through the university clinic, where clients from both the university and the community came for help with various problems. When the professor who had taught the course before was asked how many of the cases were drug or alcohol related, he said "very few, less than 10%." After providing the practicum students with some limited information about what to look for and what questions to ask related to drug problems, we discovered that 60% of our cases (essentially the same clients who were at the clinic the semester before) clearly had drug- or alcohol-related problems. Not all these cases were obvious, and some had to do with adults who grew up in alcoholic families and were having adjustment problems related to their childhood. Still others were patients who had histories of being medicated or overmedicated for problems that still existed. The point is that a working knowledge of psychopharmacology and related issues can provide the psychotherapist with tools that can make psychotherapy much more beneficial to the patient. This book is designed to help the therapist gain that information.

The sections of this book are designed to build on one another and at the same time can be used independently for reference material or for specific information. Some of the material presented in the beginning of the book may be very basic for those with experience in the field of mental health. Nevertheless, it would be impossible to present the material that follows without making sure that the reader has a clear understanding of the basics of psychopathology. The experienced reader might use this section for a review or, if the material is too basic, advance to the next section. The book provides an understandable explanation of how drugs work, major classifications of drugs, major psychological problems that respond to drugs, and potential problems with drugs including addiction and abuse. The book also provides advice for therapists about how to work with physicians and psychiatrists to improve patient care relative to the use of psychotropic medications.

The philosophy of the book is that nonmedical psychotherapists and medical practitioners can work more closely together for improved treatment of the patient. Often, patients will respond best to a course of therapy that includes both psychotherapy and psychotropic medications. This book provides the nonmedical practitioner with the background and motivation to improve relations with medical practitioners. It also provides other sources that can be useful in gaining information in the area of psychopharmacology. The question and answer section is a quick reference to the questions most frequently asked about psychopharmacology by nonmedical practitioners. Appendix D lists suggested readings for specific information not covered in the book. The glossary of terms is designed to assist in reading the *Physicians' Desk Reference* and other important works that assume a knowledge of medical terms.

We feel strongly that the psychologist, social worker, and others who provide counseling and psychotherapy should have a working knowledge of psychopharmacology. We have done our best to provide much of that information in this book. So, for the patients who will be helped because of your increased knowledge of psychopharmacology—GOOD FISHING!

Gary W. Lawson
Craig Cooperrider

Acknowledgments

We would like to express our appreciation to our students, teachers, colleagues, and clients who have taught and shown us so much about this ever-growing field. Also, thanks to our artist, Sandra Peters, and typists Linda Dannacher, Lorrie Brown, and Debbie Kidd for their diligence in this project. Most important, we express gratitude to our wives, husbands, and children for their never-ending support, assistance, and love.

Part I

Review of Psychopharmacology

Nonmedical psychotherapists and counselors come in all shapes and sizes and with a wide range of educational backgrounds. There are psychologists who have had courses in chemistry and neurophysiology, and there are addiction counselors who have had no formal education beyond high school. This section is designed to provide a background in psychopharmacology for those who have had little or no formal training in this area. Those who have a broad background may find this section simplistic, and those who have no background may find it difficult. Our goal, however, is to provide nonmedical psychotherapists with sufficient information to allow them to understand and make use of the information presented later in the book.

Chapter 1

The Brain and the Nervous System

Craig Cooperrider

Pharmaceutical agents are chemicals that interact with chemical processes within the body to produce changes. Psychiatric medications are no exception in that they interact with chemical processes in the brain and nervous system. In order to comprehend these processes, it is critical to have a basic understanding of the structures and functions of the brain and nervous system.

This chapter discusses the principles of neuroanatomy and physiology that are essential to the understanding of the functions of psychiatric medication. Reference will be made in later chapters to the specific areas discussed in this chapter related to the actions of various drugs. It should be noted, however, that this chapter in no way represents a compendium of the information regarding neuroanatomy or psychophysiology. There are numerous sources addressing these issues and all the related components critical to their understanding. For a further reference, see Gardner (1975), Gilman and Newman (1987), Kolb and Whishaw (1980), or Liebman and Tadmor (1986).

In considering the brain and nervous system, the discussion is focused on three areas. To begin, the anatomy and physiology of the brain, and specifically the core structures and the ways in which they are affected by the introduction of various psychiatric medications, are examined. The second area of emphasis is the spinal cord and peripheral nervous system. In addition to the anatomy and physiology of these systems, the discussion also includes the neuron, which is the basic unit of communication within the brain and nervous system. The interactions of the brain, spinal cord, and peripheral nervous system structures are explained. Finally, the processes of neural transmission within the brain and nervous system are described. These reactions within the nervous system form the basis of most theories of psychopharmacological action.

THE BRAIN

With the advent of transplants and artificial organs, it is clear that medical science has come a long way in understanding the structure and mechanics of the human body. Even with this fundamental understanding, however, knowledge of the brain is still in its infancy. New advances and theories regarding this frontier are being reported, but there still remains a void in the understanding of this vital organ, which lies at the root of all human behavior.

Levinthal (1983) describes the brain in terms of three fundamental areas—the hindbrain, the midbrain, and the forebrain. For the purposes of the present discussion, each area is considered separately. It is important to remember that the brain is more than the sum of its parts. There is a tremendous amount of overlap and interaction between each of its structures.

The Hindbrain

The hindbrain, also called the brain stem, is the lowest portion of the brain relative to the top of the head and is composed of three areas: the medulla, the pons, and the cerebellum (Figure 1-1). These three areas play an important role in the basic functioning of the body.

The medulla is the link between the brain and the spinal cord. Many of the basic life support functions, including maintenance of blood pressure, heartbeat, and breathing rate, are regulated at this point. A number of the cranial nerves discussed later in this chapter are found within these structures.

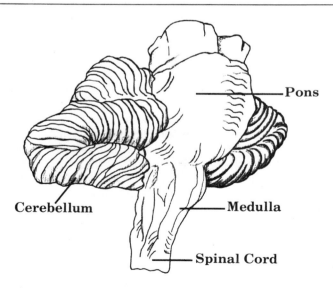

Figure 1-1 The Hindbrain (Brain Stem) and Its Component Parts

At the upper portion and in front of the medulla is the pons. It is here that various nerve fibers come together, linking different parts of the brain to other parts of the brain and to the nervous system.

Directly behind the medulla lies the cerebellum, which has the function of integrating body movement, position, and balance. Input comes to the cerebellum from receptors in the inner ear and the various joints within the body. When the cerebellum is coordinating body movement and position, the result is smooth integrated body motion.

Goldsmith (1977) points out that damage to the cerebellum results in clumsy, jerky movements. Alcohol is the drug that most affects the cerebellum, and its effects are seen in the drunken gait, slurred speech, impaired balance, and limited dexterity and motion of an intoxicated person. Barbiturates also have these effects.

The Midbrain

Surrounding the upper and lower portions of the medulla and the pons are the two structures that compose the midbrain: the tectum and the tegmentum. Figure 1-2 shows a medial view (view from the middle) of the brain and points out the location of these structures relative to some of the hindbrain structures discussed above.

The tectum contains two structures referred to as the superior colliculus and inferior colliculus, which mediate visual and auditory sensory data, respectively.

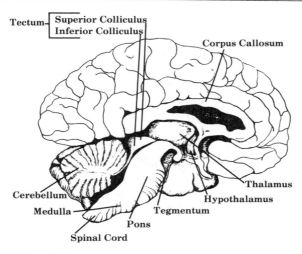

Figure 1-2 Medial View of the Brain Featuring Associated Forebrain, Midbrain, and Hindbrain Structures

They are particularly concerned with whole-body orientation to visual and auditory stimuli.

The tegmentum consists of a number of sensory and motor nerves. Also found there are the nuclei of the oculomotor and trochlear cranial nerves, which will be discussed later in this chapter.

One other important structure is the reticular formation or the reticular activating system, which runs from the thalamus (part of the forebrain) through the midbrain and extends into the brain stem. The reticular formation is directly involved in the maintenance of arousal and supplies information concerning this state to and from the cortex (part of the forebrain). It is also important in the study of psychopharmacology because some of the major body chemicals affected by psychiatric medications are actively present and used in this system.

The Forebrain

In terms of the study of psychopharmacology, the activity in the forebrain is of central importance. It is here that centers of emotion, memory, reasoning, and judgment are found. The forebrain involves structures surrounding the midbrain as well as the brain's outer layer, referred to as the cerebral cortex.

At the upper end of the medulla is the thalamus (see Figure 1-2). Its function within the brain and nervous system is extremely important in that it serves as a relay of sensory information to the different areas of the cerebral cortex. This information is received from various systems within the body and is passed to areas within the cortex. Some of the sensory data received include visual and auditory stimuli, tactile sensation, pressure, pain, and temperature.

Just beneath the thalamus is the hypothalamus. Its main functions are in the areas of motivational and emotional expression, feeding, drinking, sexual activity, and temperature regulation. Hypothalamus functions also extend to some control of the pituitary gland, which regulates many of the other endocrine glands within the body. This area will be examined in more detail in Chapter 2.

The limbic system (Figure 1-3) is composed of a number of subcortical structures that are closely related to the cortex and also the thalamus and hypothalamus. Three main areas in the limbic system are the amygdala, the septum, and the hippocampus. Gardner (1975) emphasizes that little is known about the physiology of the limbic system. Furthermore, it is difficult to make generalizations from research with animals; it seems that the limbic system has different functions in different animals. It is believed that the limbic system is one of the main structures involved in the expression of emotion in humans and has a number of links with endocrine functioning. It also plays a major role in memory. The limbic system and its component parts are discussed frequently in relation to various psychiatric illnesses and in regard to the action of various tranquilizers.

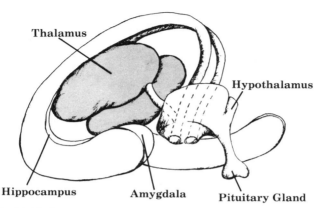

Figure 1-3 The Limbic System

In the area of the limbic system structures and around the thalamus are the basal ganglia (Figure 1-4). These are nuclei that are involved in muscular activities. The basal ganglia receive input from the cerebral cortex and pass it on to nerves within the brain stem. Included among the basal ganglia are the caudate nucleus and the lenticular nucleus, which is composed of the globus pallidus and the putamen. The lenticular nucleus is of particular importance because of its involvement with certain nervous system chemicals associated with schizophrenia and Parkinson's disease. Understanding of these structures is still very limited and speculative, however.

The final major area in the forebrain is the neocortex (Figure 1-5), which is a layer of tissue that covers the areas of the forebrain and midbrain discussed above. This tissue gives the brain its many convolutions.

The neocortex is divided into four areas, referred to as lobes: the frontal lobes, the temporal lobes, the parietal lobes, and the occipital lobes. The lobes consist of

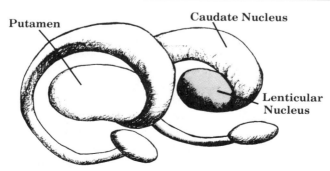

Figure 1-4 Basal Ganglia

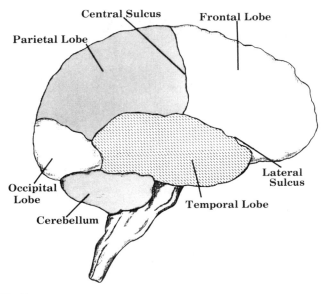

Figure 1-5 The Neocortex

large masses or bulges of tissue referred to as gyri, which are separated by grooves called sulci. One major sulcus, known as the central sulcus, runs from side to side and separates the frontal lobes from the parietal lobes. It is also referred to as the fissure of Rolando. The other major sulcus is the lateral sulcus, which runs from the frontal lobe to the occipital lobe and separates the parietal and temporal lobes. It is often referred to as the fissure of Sylvius.

The frontal lobes compose the area of the cerebral cortex from the forehead to the front of the central sulcus. It has been argued for many years that the human frontal lobe is special in that it houses the high mental processes not seen in other animals. Kolb and Whishaw (1980) dispute this idea, however, on the basis that there is no evidence that human frontal lobes have any special characteristics. It is difficult to pinpoint the functions of the frontal lobes. It seems to be true that the frontal lobes do have responsibility for various personality and emotional traits, planning and organizational skills, speech and language, and control of motor functioning.

Directly behind the frontal lobes are the parietal lobes, which share a number of functions with other areas of the brain. They have primary responsibility for receiving various somatic sensations and perceptions while at the same time integrating sensory data from a number of sources, including visual, auditory, and somatic sensations. The parietal lobes are also believed to play a role in gross motor functioning, in contrast to the frontal lobes, which are involved in fine motor functioning.

Immediately below the parietal lobes are the temporal lobes; these seem to be directly involved with auditory processing of information and long-term memory.

The occipital lobes are located at the back of the cortex, directly behind the parietal and temporal lobes. Their primary responsibility is in visual processing.

The cerebral cortex is divided down the middle from front to back into two hemispheres, the left brain and the right brain. Each side has one of the four corresponding lobes discussed above. Although the brain may look symmetrical, as shown in the view in Figure 1-6, the lobes on each side control different areas of functioning related to the functions noted previously. Also, just because the brain is separated into right and left hemispheres does not mean that the right brain does not know what the left brain is doing (and vice versa). The two sides are linked beneath the surface of the cortex by a system of nerve fibers referred to as the corpus callosum, which is located just above the midbrain structures.

THE SPINAL CORD AND PERIPHERAL NERVOUS SYSTEM

The brain is only half of what is called the central nervous system; the other half is the spinal cord. Beyond the nerves within the central nervous system are those

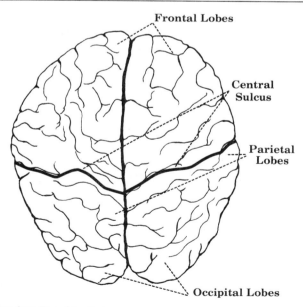

Figure 1-6 View from Top of the Brain

which extend to all parts of the body, referred to collectively as the peripheral nervous system.

The spinal cord extends from the brain stem downward through the vertebral column. It serves a dual function: it carries information from the brain to peripheral nerves in the body, and it transfers information from peripheral nerves from various places in the body to a number of sites in the brain. Thus the spinal cord contains both ascending (sensory) pathways and descending (motor) pathways.

The Peripheral Nervous System

For the purpose of discussion, this section focuses on motor nerves (i.e., those nerves that transfer information from the central nervous system to the various organs and muscles).

The motor nerves are either voluntary or involuntary (autonomic). Primarily, the function of voluntary motor nerves is to provide information from the central nervous system to the various muscles that are involved in voluntary movement. The autonomic nerves carry information to the organs and glands, where movement is involuntary. This information originates in either spinal or cranial nerves. Spinal nerves are those directly connected to the spinal cord. Their location is the point at which they leave the spinal cord and relates to the particular type of vertebra found at that point (i.e., cervical, thoracic, lumbar, or sacral). The cranial nerves comprise 12 pairs of nerves that originate in the brain (see Table 1-1).

Table 1-1 The Cranial Nerves

Cranial Nerve	Point of Origin	Function(s)
Olfactory	Olfactory cortex	Sense of smell
Optic	Thalamus and superior colliculus	Vision
Oculomotor	Midbrain	Eye movements; pupil size and accommodation
Trochlear	Midbrain	Eye movements
Trigeminal	Pons	Chewing movements
Abducens	Pons	Abduction of eyes
Facial	Pons	Facial expressions; saliva secretion
Auditory vestibular	Pons and medulla	Equilibrium; hearing
Glossopharyngeal	Medulla	Movements of tongue and pharynx
Vagus	Medulla	Movements of heart, blood vessels, viscera; voice production
Spinal accessory	Medulla	Neck muscle control
Hypoglossal	Medulla	Tongue muscle control

The autonomic nervous system also has two subdivisions: the sympathetic and parasympathetic nervous systems. The sympathetic nervous system is directly involved in producing changes in the body in reaction to a stressful event. These nerves originate at the spinal cord at the thoracic and lumbar levels (middle and lower back). Parasympathetic nerves are those involved in body functions that contribute to rest. These nerves originate as cranial nerves or at the cervical and sacral levels (neck and extreme upper and extreme lower back). Table 1-2 lists some of the more common sympathetic and parasympathetic functions.

In the spinal cord there are two pathways assumed by motor nerves: pyramidal and extrapyramidal pathways. Pyramidal nerve fibers control discrete motor movements and are thought to originate in particular locations in the neocortex. Extrapyramidal fibers allow for motor activity that is smooth and integrated. These nerve fibers have their origin in both cortical and subcortical regions of the brain. This is significant in that a number of the side effects in various psychiatric medications are said to be extrapyramidal.

THE NEURON AND NEUROTRANSMISSION

The basic unit of function in the nervous system is the nerve cell or neuron. The entire peripheral nervous system is composed of a vast network of these cells, which connect directly with similar cells in the spinal cord and ultimately in the brain.

Table 1-2 Sympathetic and Parasympathetic Nervous System Functions

Sympathetic	*Parasympathetic*
Pupil dilation	Pupil constriction
Salivary gland inhibition	Tear gland stimulation
Blood vessels and sweat glands of hands	Salivary gland stimulation
Sweat glands and blood vessels of upper limbs	Heart inhibition
Heart acceleration	Constriction of lungs and bronchi
Arteriole constriction	Intestinal tract stimulation
Dilation of lungs and bronchi	Liver stimulation
Esophageal motility	Gallbladder stimulation
Aorta constriction	Pancreas stimulation
Adrenal gland secretions	Colon stimulation
Kidney plexus	Urinary bladder contraction
Colon and rectum inhibition	
Pancreas inhibition	
Urinary bladder and genital inhibition	
Sweat glands of lower limbs	

Neurons all have essentially the same structure; Figure 1-7 shows a simplistic view of a neuron and its fundamental parts. Each neuron has a cell body, often referred to as the soma. The nucleus of the cell is located here, as well as a number of other structures involved in the passing of information through the cell. On the receiving end of the cell are processes known as dendrites that emerge from the cell body. It is here that information is received from other neurons. Extending from the cell body is a single shaft called the axon, which may be of various lengths and have numerous branches. Its function is to pass information on to other neurons.

At the end of an axon branch are small processes known as end feet. These are located fairly close to the processes of another neuron, usually the dendrites. It is here that chemicals are released between neurons, ultimately influencing behavior, thinking, and the like. The space between an axon end foot and another neuron, where this chemical activity occurs, is known as the synapse. The action of most psychopharmaceuticals occurs at the synapse of the neurons involved.

How do neurons go about passing information from one to another? First of all, "information" is in the form of chemical and electrical impulses that are sent from the joints, skin, muscles, and glands to the spinal cord and brain, and vice versa. An impulse, however, does not move from one neuron to another simply by touching or jumping to the next neuron. Instead, as the impulse travels through the cell, a chemical substance referred to as a neurotransmitter is first released to the synaptic area and serves as a bridge for the impulse to travel between two neurons. After its release, the neurotransmitter is either taken back into the sending neuron (or the receiving neuron) or is destroyed. Some of the major neurotransmitter sub-

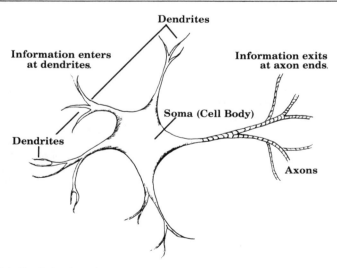

Figure 1-7 A Simplistic View of a Neuron

stances found in the brain include acetylcholine, norepinephrine, dopamine, serotonin, γ-aminobutyric acid (GABA), glycine, and substance P (Levinthal, 1983).

Neurotransmitters are formed in various parts of the body. Neurons synthesize precursors of neurotransmitters and then store the prepared neurotransmitter at the end feet. Generally, the synthesis of neurotransmitters involves the use of various enzymes in and around the cell.

All the processes involved in neurotransmission can be affected by the introduction of drugs and other substances. The major theories regarding the operation of psychiatric drugs seem to suggest that the changes the drugs make in certain neurotransmission processes lead to various alterations in the behavior and thinking of the person taking the drug.

REFERENCES

Gardner, E. (1975). *Fundamentals of neurology* (6th ed.). Philadelphia: W.B. Saunders.

Gilman, S., & Newman, S.W. (1987). *Manter and Gatz's essentials of clinical neuroanatomy and neurophysiology* (7th ed.). Philadelphia: F.A. Davis.

Goldsmith, W. (1977). *Psychiatric drugs for the non-medical mental health worker.* Springfield, IL: Charles C Thomas.

Kolb, B., & Whishaw, I.Q. (1980). *Fundamentals of human neuropsychology.* San Francisco: W.H. Freeman.

Levinthal, C.F. (1983). *Introduction to physiological psychology* (2nd ed.). Englewood Cliffs, NJ: Prentice-Hall.

Liebman, M., & Tadmor, R. (1986). *Neuroanatomy made easy and understandable* (3rd ed.). Rockville, MD: Aspen Publishers.

Chapter 2

The Endocrine System and the Body Metabolism

Craig Cooperrider

Chapter 1 focused on the brain, the nervous system, and the neuron as the primary influencers of behavior; however, the picture is not yet complete. Within the brain and throughout the body there are various structures that secrete chemicals into the bloodstream, which in turn also play a significant role in human behavior. This system of structures is referred to as the endocrine system. The structures are known as endocrine glands, and the chemicals secreted are hormones.

The purpose of this chapter is to discuss briefly the anatomy and physiology of the endocrine system; Levinthal (1983) and Anthony and Kolthoff (1971) provide extensive information about the functioning of the various components of the endocrine system. Emphasis here is placed on normal endocrine functioning; however, certain endocrine disorders are considered because of their tendency to produce symptoms similar to those seen in mental disorders. The discussion also includes effects seen in the administration of hormonal drugs.

ENDOCRINE SYSTEM FUNCTION

As mentioned above, endocrine glands secrete hormones directly into the bloodstream. These hormones exert their influence on various sites in the body, including cells, organs, and other glands.

The endocrine system is not an independently functioning system; like other body parts, it is controlled by the central nervous system. Its primary function, according to Levinthal (1983), is the maintenance of body homeostasis; that is, it is designed to keep all body organs and response mechanisms working together in a controlled manner. The endocrine system's function is primarily regulatory, as far as the body is concerned, but the various hormones serve to speed up or slow down various body processes in order to maintain homeostasis.

THE ENDOCRINE GLANDS

Table 2-1 lists the endocrine glands, together with the hormones secreted by each and a brief description of their function.

The Pituitary Gland

The pituitary gland is located just beneath the hypothalamus. It has a number of neuronal and vascular links with the hypothalamus and in fact receives direction from the hypothalamus. As various stimuli impinge on the hypothalamus, either neuronal or chemical signals are sent to the pituitary gland to direct the release of appropriate hormones to the bloodstream. These then influence other glands to release hormones or impinge on certain organs or cells in prescribed ways.

The pituitary gland is divided into three sections: posterior, intermediate, and anterior. The posterior section is responsible for the release of oxytocin and vasopressin. Oxytocin is secreted at the time that a pregnant female enters labor. This hormone stimulates uterine contractions and other physical changes so as to facilitate the birth process. It also has some responsibility in the expulsion of milk from the breasts as infants are sucking. Vasopressin is also known as antidiuretic hormone (ADH). This name basically describes its function, which is to stimulate the kidneys to produce a more concentrated urine, thereby ensuring that the body has sufficient fluids. Without a sufficient amount of vasopressin, too much water is eliminated in the urine and not adequately used by the body. This condition is referred to as diabetes insipidus, and its major symptom is an excessive thirst because the body cannot maintain adequate fluid levels.

The intermediate section of the pituitary gland has only one known function, which is primarily cellular in nature. The hormone it produces is known as melanocyte-stimulating hormone (MSH). Melanocytes are responsible for secreting melanin, which is a pigment found in the skin (Goldsmith, 1977); MSH activates melanocyte secretions.

The anterior section of the pituitary gland serves a number of different functions. The first of these has a direct effect on the thyroid gland. The thyroid gland secretes a hormone known as thyroxin, which must be maintained at an adequate level in the bloodstream. The hypothalamus detects any decrease in thyroxin levels and sends a stimulus to the anterior section of the pituitary gland to release a hormone known as thyrotropin, or thyroid-stimulating hormone (TSH). As TSH is released into blood circulation, the thyroid gland is eventually stimulated to produce more thyroxin. As thyroxin in the bloodstream increases, a corresponding reverse action is generated in the hypothalamus and anterior pituitary, thereby lowering the production rate of TSH.

Table 2-1 Endocrine Glands, Hormones, and Hormonal Functions

Gland	Hormone	Function(s)
Pituitary		
Posterior	Oxytocin	Uterine contractions; breast milk expulsion
	Vasopressin (antidiuretic hormone, ADH)	Maintenance of body fluid levels
Intermediate	Melanocyte-stimulating hormone (MSH)	Cell production of melanin (skin pigment)
Anterior	Thyrotropin (thyroid-stimulating hormone, TSH)	Production of thyroxin in thyroid gland
	Adrenocorticotropic hormone (ACTH)	Metabolism of two adrenal hormones in stress
	Somatotropin (growth hormone, GH)	Cellular growth regulation
	Follicle-stimulating hormone (FSH)	Females: secretion of estrogen and promotion of ovum development; males: promotion of sperm development
	Luteinizing hormone (LH)	Secretion of progesterone (females)
	Interstitial cell–stimulating hormone	Secretion of androgens (males)
	Prolactin	Stimulation of breast milk production
Thyroid	Thyroxin	Maintenance of body metabolism rates
Parathyroid	Parathormone (with vitamin D)	Maintenance of calcium levels in bloodstream
Pancreas		
α cells	Glycagon	Maintenance of glucose in bloodstream (increase)
β cells	Insulin	Maintenance of glucose in bloodstream (decrease)
Adrenal cortex	Mineral corticoids	Monitoring of levels of minerals
	Glucocorticoids	Conversion of proteins and fats to glucose
Adrenal medulla	Epinephrine	Sympathetic physical reactions to stress
	Norepinephrine	Stimulation of ACTH response
Gonads		
Ovaries	Estrogens	Female sexual development
	Progesterone	Female uterus development for pregnancy
Testes	Testosterone	Male sexual development and behavior

The second function served by the anterior pituitary is directed at the adrenal gland. This particular function becomes especially important at times of stress. In a moment of stress, the hypothalamus sends a stimulus to the anterior section of the pituitary gland to release adrenocorticotropic hormone (ACTH). As this hormone reaches the adrenal glands, two adrenal hormones are released; both these hormones serve a valuable function in terms of body maintenance. ACTH also has a reverse effect: it slows down the release of adrenal hormones when they are present in excess concentrations in the bloodstream.

A hormone known as somatotropin (often referred to as growth hormone, GH) is also secreted by the anterior pituitary. This hormone works directly on cells in the body, particularly those in the bones. The hypothalamus inhibits, rather than stimulates, the release of GH from the anterior pituitary. The function of this hormone is regulatory; that is, it ensures that physical growth occurs at an orderly rate, despite different rates of growth for separate parts of the body.

Two anterior pituitary hormones have direct bearing on the menstrual cycle, and their effect is on the ovaries. These are follicle-stimulating hormone (FSH) and luteinizing hormone (LH). Both of these hormones are secreted on stimulation from the hypothalamus. FSH is secreted during the first half of the average menstrual cycle and LH during the second half. When FSH reaches the ovaries through the bloodstream, the ovaries are stimulated to secrete another hormone, estrogen; as estrogen levels in the blood increase, the need for FSH diminishes. Toward the end of the first half of the menstrual cycle, FSH levels begin to decrease and LH levels increase dramatically. LH causes the ovaries to prepare to release an ovum (egg) and also stimulates the follicle cells to allow progesterone to be secreted.

In the male, FSH also serves a reproductive function by stimulating the creation of sperm. A male hormone corresponding to LH known as interstitial cell–stimulating hormone stimulates the release of male sex hormones called androgens.

One other hormone secreted by the anterior section of the pituitary gland is known as prolactin, which is responsible for stimulating the breasts to produce milk.

The Thyroid Gland

The thyroid gland is located in the neck, fairly close to the larynx, and is responsible for the secretion of the hormone thyroxin. Thyroxin secretion is involved with the rate at which food is metabolized (i.e., used for energy or eliminated as waste). When the body produces too little thyroxin, hypothyroidism occurs, which in young children can lead to the condition of cretinism. With hypothyroidism, the individual experiences slow, lethargic movements, poor maintenance of body temperature, and a less energetic disposition. When too much thyroxin is in the bloodstream, hyperthyroidism can occur. Symptoms of this condition include insomnia, limited concentration, and overexcitability. These two conditions, however, are fairly infrequent because of the regulatory function played by the hypothalamus and pituitary gland in monitoring the amount of thyroxin in the blood.

The Parathyroid Glands

The parathyroid glands are found in the same area as the thyroid gland. They secrete a substance known as parathormone, which works in various parts of the body to ensure that the body has sufficient calcium. In order for parathormone to function, vitamin D must be present.

Low amounts of calcium in the bloodstream will lead to overexcitability and possibly seizures. Calcium in excessive quantities may produce general sluggishness and lethargy.

The Pancreas

The pancreas is located in the area of the stomach and small intestine and secretes two important hormones: insulin, which is secreted by pancreatic β cells, and glycagon, which is secreted by pancreatic α cells. The main function of insulin is to promote the movement of glucose in the bloodstream to various cells so that it can be converted to energy. When there is an insufficient quantity of insulin for this purpose, some form of diabetes, especially diabetes mellitus, may eventually occur. When this condition develops, the diabetic person must take insulin and attempt to maintain an appropriate balance between the amount of insulin and the amount of glucose. If there is too much insulin and too little glucose, the disorder known as hypoglycemia occurs.

The role of glycagon is exactly the opposite of that of insulin. It maintains glucose levels within the bloodstream and works as an insulin antagonist (i.e., it blocks the action of insulin).

The Adrenal Gland

The adrenal gland is involved in maintaining body homeostasis in times of stress. This gland is located just above the kidneys and in essence has two sections: the cortex and the medulla. The adrenal cortex receives the hormone ACTH from the pituitary gland, which activates adrenal secretion of hormones known as corticoids.

Corticoids are classified as mineral corticoids and glucocorticoids. Mineral corticoids monitor the level of various minerals, such as sodium and potassium, in the body. Minerals have a great deal to do with the effective functioning of neurons and if they are not maintained at appropriate levels, various nervous system problems may arise.

Glucocorticoids are directly involved in the conversion of proteins and fats to glucose. Often under conditions of stress it is necessary for the body to produce additional quantities of energy, so that glucose metabolism must increase. The amount of one glucocorticoid known as 17-hydroxycorticosteroid (17-OHCS) seems to correlate with the amount of stress a person is experiencing. As stress increases, so also does the level of 17-OHCS. As 17-OHCS increases in the bloodstream, the level of ACTH decreases, thus demonstrating another feedback loop between the hypothalamus and pituitary gland and the adrenal cortex.

The adrenal medulla works independently of the pituitary gland but responds to stress through the secretion of epinephrine and norepinephrine (also known as adrenalin and noradrenalin, respectively). As these hormones are added to the bloodstream, the body then undergoes changes associated with stress reactions. Included among these are increased heart rate and muscle tone, constriction of blood vessels, and other sympathetic nervous system responses. These hormones also stimulate the pituitary gland to release ACTH, which affects the adrenal cortex and its hormones.

The Gonads

The gonads are also referred to as the sex glands. In females they are the ovaries and in males they are the testes. Each of these secrete different hormones that contribute to defining the individual's sexuality.

Female sexual hormones consist of estrogens and progesterone. Estrogens function in several ways. During childhood and adolescence, they affect the development of secondary sexual characteristics. They also stimulate the development of the ova that are released by the ovaries. Progesterone produces changes in the uterus so that it is better able to receive a fertilized egg. These changes include thickening of the uterus walls and the provision of nutrients for the developing fetus. If the egg is not fertilized, progesterone levels decrease and the thickened uterus wall is not maintained. This then leads to menstruation.

The testes in males are responsible for the production of sperm. The hormones they secrete are known as androgens, the most common of which is testosterone. This hormone is mainly responsible for the development of secondary sexual characteristics and sexual behavior.

PSYCHIATRIC SYMPTOMS RESULTING FROM
ENDOCRINE DYSFUNCTION

There are a number of medical conditions that result from endocrine deficiencies (DeLisi, 1984). Many of these illnesses have symptoms that are similar to symptoms associated with mental disorders; some of these are listed in Table 2-2. Other disturbances attributable to endocrine disorders that present with psychiatric symptoms include diabetes, hypoglycemia, and premenstrual syndrome. These clearly demonstrate the link between endocrine function and behavior.

HORMONES AS DRUGS

At times when an endocrine deficiency is suspected, hormones are prescribed as treatment. Generally, hormone therapy works well and without complication. There are some psychiatric complications that may emerge, however. Ross, Walker, Covington, and Cools (1984) discuss a number of hormonal medications and the psychiatric complications that may result; Table 2-3 lists a number of these concerns.

Psychiatric medications may trigger changes in endocrine activity (discussed in Section III). Hormonal drugs are also sometimes used in conjunction with certain psychoactive medications to obtain more satisfactory results.

There is no question about the role that is played by the structures and chemicals of the endocrine system in the formation of human behavior and emotions.

Table 2-2 Psychiatric Symptoms Resulting from Endocrine Disorders

Endocrine Disorder	Psychiatric Symptoms
Hyperthyroidism (Graves' disease)	Memory and judgment problems; disorientation; manic or schizophreniform behavior
Hypothyroidism	Lethargy; depression; psychomotor retardation;* delusions and hallucinations*
Adrenal cortical insufficiency (Addison's disease)	Apathy; irritability; fatigability; depression
Excessive cortisol excretion (Cushing's syndrome)	Insomnia; anxiety; depression
Parathyroid dysfunction	Anxiety; psychosis; severe depression
Adrenal medulla tumor (pheochromocytoma)	Diffuse psychiatric symptoms

*Severe cases only.

Table 2-3 Psychiatric Effects of Hormone Drugs

Drug	Psychiatric Effects
Corticosteroids (Prednisone, ACTH)	Delirium; manic psychosis
TSH	Anxiety
Oral contraceptives	Depression
Insulin	Confusion; headache

Nevertheless, this role must be recognized by nonmedical practitioners attempting to render diagnoses and make decisions regarding patient problems on the basis of symptoms that are psychiatric in nature. In some cases, what may seem to be a psychiatric disorder in the classical form is instead a manifestation of some other physiological concern. Certainly, the responsibility lies with the practitioner in considering and examining the role that may be played by either hormonal deficiencies or hormonal drugs, since they directly shape the problems being experienced by the patient.

REFERENCES

Anthony, C.P., & Kolthoff, N.J. (1971). *Textbook of anatomy and physiology* (8th ed.). St. Louis, MO: C.V. Mosby.

DeLisi, L.E. (1984). Use of the clinical laboratory. In J.L. Sullivan & P.D. Sullivan (Eds.), *Biomedical psychiatric therapeutics* (pp. 89–119). Boston: Butterworth.

Goldsmith, W. (1977). *Psychiatric drugs for the non-medical mental health worker*. Springfield, IL: Charles C Thomas.

Levinthal, C.F. (1983). *Introduction to physiological psychology* (2nd ed.). Englewood Cliffs, NJ: Prentice-Hall.

Ross, D.R., Walker, J.I., Covington, T., & Cools, J. (1984). Psychiatric complications of non-psychiatric drugs. In J.L. Sullivan & P.D. Sullivan (Eds.), *Biomedical psychiatric therapeutics* (pp. 207–218). Boston: Butterworth.

Chapter 3

The Basics of Pharmacology

Craig Cooperrider

The purpose of this chapter is to introduce certain basics pertaining to the administration and metabolism of drugs, in particular psychoactive medications (those that produce a direct effect in the brain), as well as a rudimentary system of classification for substances used in treating psychiatric disorders. Some of the basic sources of information about drugs are also provided.

THE ADMINISTRATION OF DRUGS

As an individual grows and experiences the typical illnesses associated with childhood, adolescence, and adulthood, it is usually the case that he or she will be exposed to drugs in their various forms and modes of administration. Drugs are commonly administered in the form of tablets, capsules, injections, or liquids. They generally enter the body through the mouth, the rectum, the muscles, blood vessels, or skin, or the lungs (Julien, 1985).

Administration through the Mouth

The mouth is the most common place by which drugs are administered. Tablets, capsules, or liquid forms of medications are all administered orally. Most drugs that gain entrance to the body through the mouth progress through the stomach, enter the intestines, and are absorbed into the bloodstream through the intestinal wall.

The major criticism of oral medication relates to the uncertainty of the dosage actually reaching the bloodstream. It cannot always be determined how much of a tablet or a capsule is dissolved and actually passes through the intestinal wall. Furthermore, some drugs are destroyed by digestive fluids in the stomach before

23

they are absorbed. Occasionally, the effectiveness of an orally administered drug may be less than that of its counterpart administered through other routes.

Administration through the Rectum

Drugs that enter the body through the rectum are usually in the form of suppositories. In general, drugs are administered through the rectum for two reasons: (1) for the treatment of infections or irritations in the rectal area, or (2) when the patient is unable to take medication orally because of excessive vomiting, unconsciousness, or inability to swallow. As is true of oral medications, drugs administered through the rectum are unpredictable in terms of the actual dosage rendered because of the uncertainty as to how much of the drug is absorbed from the rectum into the rest of the body.

Administration through the Muscles, Blood Vessels, and Skin

Drugs that enter the body through the muscles, blood vessels, and skin are given by way of injection. This is by far the fastest and most predictable way of administering a drug. The most common method of injecting medication into the body is intramuscularly because it is absorbed more slowly than other methods of injection. The drug is usually injected into the muscle tissue in the upper arm or the buttocks. Many psychotropic drugs, when not given orally, are administered in this manner.

Drugs are also injected directly into the bloodstream through a vein or an artery. All uncertainties concerning the amount of the drug entering the bloodstream are eliminated by this method. The medication takes effect rapidly in intravenous or intra-arterial injection, which can be either a positive or a negative quality; Julien (1985) notes some of the drawbacks of such injections, including the possibility of life-threatening events if the drug is administered too rapidly, allergic reactions, and the possibility of infection if the drug is not administered under sterile conditions. Many of these same concerns apply to intramuscular administrations as well.

Drugs can also be injected into the various layers of the skin; these are referred to as intradermal injections. Similarly, a subcutaneous injection is one that is made just under the layers of the skin (Goldsmith, 1977). Medication is rapidly absorbed by this method as well, although this can vary depending on the drug.

Administration by Inhalation

Drugs that are inhaled are absorbed through the lungs and the mucous linings of the respiratory system and enter the body through the nose or the mouth. Absorption of drugs through the lungs is generally quite effective because of the lungs' direct access to blood vessels. Marijuana, cocaine, nitrous oxide, and ether are all examples of drugs administered by inhalation. The major problem with the introduction of drugs to the body in this manner is the extreme irritability of the lungs in the presence of foreign substances.

DRUGS IN THE BODY

After administration via one of the routes described above, some or all of the drug enters the bloodstream through capillary walls at the point of entry and proceeds through the circulatory system. At any given time, only a small quantity of the drug is at the site of action (the area to be treated); the remainder is circulated throughout the body at a rate of about 5 liters per minute. Once a drug enters the bloodstream, then, it is only a matter of minutes before it reaches all parts of the body (Julien, 1985).

Drugs reach the brain and eventually interact with neurons in the following way. When a drug is dispersed throughout the circulatory system and reaches capillaries at a given location, its molecules are able to pass through pores in the capillary walls into nearby tissue. In the brain, there exists a special structure known as the blood-brain barrier, which provides the brain with additional protection compared with other tissue areas. It is much more difficult for molecules to pass through the capillary walls in the brain. The actual amount of a drug in the brain is usually small compared to that in the rest of the body.

Once a drug has entered the body, it is eliminated in the same manner as other substances. Depending on the location of the drug at the time of its termination, it may be eliminated through the urine, bile, sweat, tears, breast milk, lungs, or other body secretions and excretions.

CLASSIFICATION OF AND REFERENCES FOR DRUGS

Drugs are classified in a number of different ways. To begin, they are grouped together in terms of their function. Examples of these categories of drugs include anticoagulants, muscle relaxants, analgesics, and so forth. These categories are purely for grouping purposes, and each category is not mutually exclusive. Several drugs may be found in a number of different categories, thus demonstrating the multiple functioning capabilities of some drugs as well as the difficulty in developing a categorization system for the extensive variety of drugs currently in existence. The different categories of drugs of a psychoactive nature are discussed here briefly; the chapters that follow offer a more comprehensive examination.

Within each category of drugs are different products developed to serve the function designated by the category name. Each drug product carries with it a generic name and a trade name. The generic name is the accepted chemical name of the drug, and the trade name is the name under which the drug is sold. The trade name is usually created by the drug manufacturer.

Most people are fairly familiar with drugs classified as analgesics. Common illnesses are often treated in the home with some type of analgesic (such as aspirin). Within this category are a number of generic classifications, such as acetaminophen, aspirin, and codeine. Different manufacturers market each of these generic brands under different names. For example, acetaminophen is marketed as Tylenol, Datril, Tempra, and Comtrex, to name a few. Aspirin is marketed as Bayer, Bufferin, Excedrin, Midol, and so on. Within each of the categories, both trade and generic drugs are dispensed in the various forms discussed above: tablets, capsules, injections, suppositories, liquids, and the like.

There are a number of reference volumes on drugs and pharmaceutical products that are currently available. The universally accepted resource for the health practitioner seeking information on a particular drug, however, is the *Physicians' Desk Reference* (PDR; Medical Economics Company, 1987). The PDR is published annually and is intended to be the most thorough and up-to-date guide for physicians in the prescription of various pharmaceutical agents. During the year, as new information becomes available, supplements are produced for the PDR.

Within this volume are seven sections. Section 1 is the manufacturers' index, in which all manufacturers who have provided information about their products are listed together with their addresses and telephone numbers. Section 2 contains the product name index. Each drug referenced in the PDR is included in this list along with the manufacturer's name and the page numbers where reference is made to it later in the volume (sections 3 and 4 also provide this type of cross-referencing). In addition, section 2 contains an index of discontinued products. Section 3 is the product classification index, in which products are listed by category. This index is used to determine whether there are several drugs designed to produce similar results. Section 4 lists the trade names for each generic drug. Section 5 provides color photographs of many of the drugs grouped by manufacturing company. The photographs are generally actual size, so that, for example, an unknown tablet could be identified on the basis of its color, shape, and size. Section 6, the largest section, presents descriptions of the drugs in alphabetical order by manufacturing company. Each description contains information regarding composition, action and uses, administration and dosage, contraindications, precautions, side effects, and forms. Section 7 discusses products used for diagnostic purposes.

In addition to these seven sections, there are two smaller sections in the PDR. One of these lists the poison control centers across the United States and its territories. The other provides a guide to management of drug overdoses.

The practitioner involved in mental health care should have a PDR at his or her disposal. Not only is the information it contains regarding psychoactive drugs invaluable, but it is a definite asset for the practitioner to be aware of the ramifications of clients or patients taking other types of medication that may affect their response to psychotherapeutic or counseling interventions. A medical dictionary may at times be necessary to clarify the terminology used in the PDR.

THE LANGUAGE OF PRESCRIPTIONS

The abbreviations used in physicians' prescriptions and orders for medication in clinical and hospital records are a language unto themselves. Only doctors, nurses, pharmacists, and a few "privileged others" have been trained in this language. Some of the commonly used abbreviations are listed in Table 3-1.

PSYCHOACTIVE MEDICATIONS

In describing medications that directly affect the brain, it is helpful to utilize a classification system to categorize the drugs. There are numerous ways of doing this, but for the purposes of the present discussion the most reasonable classification system is as follows.

Table 3-1 Abbreviations Used in Prescriptions

Abbreviation	Latin Meaning	English Translation
b.i.d.	*bis in die*	two times per day
h.s.	*hora somni*	hour of sleep
I.M.		intramuscularly
I.V.		Intravenously
P.O.	*per os*	orally
p.r.n.	*pro re nata*	according as circumstances may require (as often as needed)
q.d.	*quaque die*	every day
q.h.	*quaque hora*	every hour
q.i.d.	*quater in die*	four times per day
q.s.	*quantum satis*	sufficient quantity
q.suff.	*quantum sufficit*	as much as suffices
t.i.d.	*ter in die*	three times per day

1. antipsychotics
2. antidepressants
3. central nervous system depressants, tranquilizers, and sedatives
4. stimulants
5. narcotics
6. hallucinogens

This text addresses each of these categories as described below.

Antipsychotics

Antipsychotic drugs, such as Thorazine, Haldol, and lithium, are used in the treatment of the various forms of psychosis and manic-depressive illness. Chapter 9 is devoted to the various antipsychotic agents, and Chapter 11 deals specifically with lithium.

Antidepressants

Antidepressants are the drugs generally used in the treatment of depression and its symptoms. These drugs are different from the stimulants in that they do not produce euphoria. Chapter 10 is devoted to these drugs and their effects.

Central Nervous System Depressants, Tranquilizers, and Sedatives

Drugs that are depressants to the central nervous system include alcohol, barbiturates such as phenobarbitol, hypnotics such as Quaalude, and anesthetic gases and liquids. Also included in this category are antianxiety agents such as Valium and Librium, which are frequently prescribed for a wide variety of concerns. Alcohol, barbiturates, and antianxiety agents are discussed in detail in Chapters 12, 13, and 17.

Stimulants

Certain drugs are utilized as stimulants to the central nervous system and overt behavior. Caffeine and nicotine are common substances that produce stimulant effects. Amphetamines such as Benzedrine, Dexedrine, and cocaine also fall into this category. Chapters 14, 19, and 23 address substances that act as stimulants.

Narcotics

Drugs categorized as narcotics include opium, heroin, morphine, and codeine. Codeine is frequently prescribed for management of pain. Some mention of these drugs is made in later chapters; Chapter 20 discusses heroin in the context of substance abuse.

Hallucinogens

Most of the drugs categorized as hallucinogens are illegal in the United States and have questionable medical value. Cannabis (marijuana) is the most widely known of these drugs. Lysergic acid diethylamide (LSD), mescaline, phencyclidine (PCP), and other ''mind-expanding'' drugs are included in this group. Generally, it is characteristic of these drugs to alter perception of reality, and their effects include hallucinations and psychotic behaviors. Not all hallucinogens work alike or to the same degree; in particular, the effects of cannabis are certainly not as striking as those of some of the other drugs in this category. PCP and marijuana are discussed in Chapters 18 and 21, respectively.

REFERENCES

Goldsmith, W. (1977). *Psychiatric drugs for the non-medical mental health worker*. Springfield, IL: Charles C Thomas.

Julien, R.M. (1985). *A primer of drug action* (4th ed.). New York: W.H. Freeman.

Medical Economics Company. (1987). *Physicians' desk reference* (39th ed.). Oradell, NJ: Author. (The PDR is updated annually.)

Part II

Mental Disorders That Respond to Drugs

Some background in psychopathology is important in the understanding of psychopharmacology. There are many professional degrees that allow individuals to practice as counselors or psychotherapists that do not presuppose a background in psychopathology. This section provides a review of psychopathologies necessary for a complete understanding of psychopharmacology.

Chapter 4

Psychoses and Schizophrenia

Craig Cooperrider

Mental illness and psychiatric difficulties, unlike some other medical concerns, do not have clear-cut criteria from which to obtain accurate diagnoses. For example, it is sometimes difficult to distinguish between certain forms of schizophrenia and some affective disorders. Much of the diagnostic information gathered is based solely on the subjective reporting of the patient. On the basis of this subjective reporting, however, diagnoses are rendered, treatments are planned, and medications are prescribed. Often these medications produce positive effects but at the same time are potentially harmful in terms of side effects, addiction possibilities, and mind-altering properties.

This and the following four chapters discuss the various diagnostic categories in terms of their symptoms and associated behaviors, their etiologies, and other information relevant to their understanding. The focus of this chapter is the psychotic and schizophrenic disorders. Even though diagnostic criteria are far from being precise or consistent, there are nevertheless some criteria that are applied in establishing the diagnosis of schizophrenia or other forms of psychosis. The standards most commonly applied are taken from *The Diagnostic and Statistical Manual of Mental Disorders* (Third Edition—Revised), otherwise known as DSM-III-R (American Psychiatric Association, 1987). Before considering these disorders, it is important to discuss some of the symptomatology common to all psychotic disorders, including schizophrenia.

COMMON SYMPTOMATOLOGY

The common symptoms of psychosis may be grouped as follows: (1) disorders of thought, (2) disorders of speech, (3) delusional activity, (4) hallucinations, (5) affect disorders, (6) impaired orientation, and (7) abnormal psychomotor activity.

Disorders of Thought

Disorders of thought are exactly that. The individual believes something about his or her thoughts that is discrepant from reality. For example, patients may believe that others can hear their thoughts (thought broadcasting) or that their thoughts are not their own but have been inserted by some person or force outside themselves (thought insertion). Some patients also experience the removal of thoughts from their minds (thought withdrawal); again, this is usually attributed to someone or something external.

Disorders of Speech

Speech problems (problems with the content of speech) are closely related to thought disorders because a person's speech often is a reflection of his or her mental activity. A common symptom related to speech disorders is referred to as loose associations, which is demonstrated by frequent changes in subjects or topics of conversation. A listener may experience difficulty in following a conversation because of tangential shifts or confabulations on the part of the patient.

Another disorder of speech is marked incoherence. Often sentences do not make sense either in grammar or syntax, so that it is often difficult to determine what is meant in statements made by the patient. There is also a problem with the actual content of what is being said. This is often referred to as poverty of speech and is manifested by the patient being unable to express a point with any sort of directness. There is often excessive rambling with little meaning and no conclusion.

Delusional Activity

Bockar (1976) describes delusions as firmly held beliefs that are not true or culturally accepted and cannot be modified by logical explanation. Generally, the delusion does not fully emerge from the patient's past or present experiences.

There are two types of delusional symptoms commonly reported: delusions of persecution and delusions of grandeur. In the case of delusions of persecution, the individual believes that some person or organization is "out to get" him or her. Patients perceive this as physical danger (bodily injury or death) or other forms of harm (threats to reputation). These perceptions are generally accompanied by the feeling that nothing has been done to deserve this.

Patients experiencing delusions of grandeur believe that they are, or will become, someone special. They feel that they are "God" or that they are different from the normal individual. They may believe that they have special powers, have been selected for a special cause, or are someone returned from the dead (usually someone famous).

Related to delusional phenomena is a special symptom referred to as ideas of reference. This is the belief that nearly any event, even one that is remote, may have a special relation to the individual. Patients may believe that the event was meant to happen to them or that there is at least an implicit message intended for them from that particular set of circumstances.

Hallucinations

Hallucinations are perceptions that have no basis in reality. They are generally auditory or visual but can be experienced through any of the senses. Auditory hallucinations may be experienced as voices speaking directly to the patient, speaking about the patient, or making statements regarding the patient's thoughts or actions. Visual hallucinations are occurring when the patient claims to see objects that do not exist or are not seen by others.

Affect Symptoms

A person's emotional makeup may be affected in three ways. Affect may be cut back or blunted; it may be inappropriate or incongruent with the subject being discussed; or it may be essentially nonexistent or flattened. Any of these terms, blunt, inappropriate, or flattened, may be used to describe the affect of those experiencing psychosis or schizophrenia.

Impaired Orientation

Often, psychoses affect the patient's orientation to time, place, and person. In other words, the patient is unaware of the approximate date and time; the patient does not know where he or she is; the patient has little or no idea as to the identities of familiar people in the immediate environment or to his or her own identity; the patient does not know why he or she is in any given place.

Abnormal Psychomotor Activity

The most severe psychomotor symptom is referred to as catatonia, the state in which there is little or no movement. Psychomotor disorders may also take the form of excessive agitation and acting out, or of very cautious, hesitant movements.

CLASSIFICATION OF PSYCHOTIC AND SCHIZOPHRENIC DISORDERS

The symptoms of the primary psychotic and schizophrenic disorders described below are paraphrased from DSM-III-R. Page numbers from DSM-III-R are listed at the end of each description.

Schizophrenia

One of the following three criteria must be present during the active phase of the disorder for at least one week for a diagnosis of schizophrenia to be appropriate.

1. Two of the following symptoms:
   a. delusions
   b. prominent hallucinations
   c. incoherence or marked loosening of associations
   d. catatonic behavior
   e. flat or grossly inappropriate affect
2. Bizarre delusions that are regarded as implausible
3. Prominent hallucinations that are
   a. generally auditory and have no relationship to depression or elation
   b. a running commentary on the person's behavior or thoughts
   c. two or more voices conversing

These symptoms cannot be attributed to schizoaffective disorder or a mood disorder with psychotic features. If a depressive or manic period does occur during the active phase of the disorder, it is relatively brief.

There must be deterioration from a previous level of functioning in such areas as work, social relations, and self-care. Further, there must be continuous signs of the illness for a period of at least 6 months at some point during the person's life, with some signs of the illness at the present time. This 6-month period must contain an active phase that includes any of the symptoms listed above, with or without a prodromal or residual phase. The prodromal phase is the period that precedes the active phase and consists of at least two of the symptoms noted below; the residual phase is the period that follows the active phase and consists of at least two of the symptoms listed below:

1. social isolation or withdrawal
2. marked impairment in role functioning
3. noted peculiar behavior
4. marked impairment in personal hygiene and grooming
5. blunted, flat, or inappropriate affect
6. speech peculiarities
7. odd or bizarre ideation
8. unusual perceptual experiences
9. apathy and lack of ambition

Any severe depressive or manic symptoms must have developed after the psychotic symptoms appeared or have been previously brief. Prodromal or active symptoms must have developed before age 45. These symptoms cannot be due to any organic mental disorder or mental retardation.

Schizophrenic disorders are often distinguished by different types. These are (1) disorganized, (2) catatonic, (3) paranoid, (4) undifferentiated, and (5) residual. Schizophrenic disorder, disorganized type is distinguished from others by the presence of frequent incoherence, loosening of associations, absence of delusional systems, and blunted, inappropriate, or silly affect. The catatonic type of schizophrenia is marked by any of the following symptoms: (1) decrease in response to external stimuli or decreased spontaneity, (2) resistance to instructions, (3) maintenance of a rigid posture, (4) excited and purposeless motor activity, or (5) the assumption of a bizarre posture. Paranoid schizophrenia is characterized by delusions of grandeur or persecution, jealousy, or hallucinations of a grandiose or persecutory nature. The criteria for schizophrenic disorder, undifferentiated type are the presence of schizophrenic symptoms (delusions, hallucinations, and so on) and the failure of the illness to meet the criteria of any of the other types. Finally, the term residual is used to describe symptoms in cases where there is a history of schizophrenia with prominent psychotic symptoms. There must also be a clinical picture without prominent psychotic symptoms and continued evidence of the illness with the presence of such symptoms as illogical thinking, social withdrawal, or blunted or inappropriate affect (pp. 194–198).

Schizophreniform Disorder

Schizophreniform disorder meets all the criteria of a schizophrenic disorder with the exception of the duration requirement (6 months). It must last more than 2 weeks but less than 6 months (p. 208).

Brief Reactive Psychosis

Brief reactive psychosis is characterized by the presence of a stressor that would probably be stressful for most individuals. There is emotional turmoil accompanied by any of the following symptoms: (1) incoherence or looseness of associations; (2) delusions; (3) hallucinations; or (4) disorganized or catatonic behavior. The symptoms must last more than a few hours but less than one month, with an eventual return to premorbid functioning. There is no period of increasing psychopathology before the appearance of the stressor. This disturbance cannot be due to any other mental disorder (pp. 206–207).

Schizoaffective Disorder

The criteria for schizoaffective disorder have not always been clear; DSM-III-R attempts to clarify them. This classification developed because in practice there are some individuals who experience a combination of symptoms from both the schizophrenia and mood disorders (discussed in Chapter 5).

A diagnosis of schizoaffective disorder is appropriate under the following conditions.

1. A mood disorder accompanies the first criterion for schizophrenia.
2. Delusions or hallucinations lasting at least two weeks and without mood symptoms are present.
3. Symptoms of the mood disorder are persistent (i.e., are not brief in comparison to the overall psychotic symptoms described in the criteria for schizophrenia).
4. No evidence of an organic factor that has caused or contributed to the disorder exists (pp. 208–210).

PERSPECTIVE ON ETIOLOGY AND TREATMENT OF PSYCHOSES AND SCHIZOPHRENIA

The topics of etiology and treatment of psychoses and schizophrenia have sparked controversy within the mental health profession for nearly a century. Much of the information provided in the present discussion is taken from literature on schizophrenia, because it is the most prevalent by far of the diagnoses described above and because all the disorders that were considered have similar symptoms, differing only in the duration and severity of the symptoms.

Bellack (1984) indicates that schizophrenia is a heterogenous phenomenon. It is still believed in certain circles that this disorder can only be attributed to a unitary source. Strong arguments are made for genetic causes, family dysfunction, biochemical problems, attention deficits, information-processing problems, and the lack of learning opportunities for the development of adequate problem-solving or social skills. Bellack maintains that, instead of viewing schizophrenia as resulting from a single factor, it is more appropriate to view it as a variable combination of genetic concerns, biochemical problems, and psychosocial stressors.

In support of this, Liberman et al. (1984) propose a multidimensional interactive model of schizophrenia. This model suggests that the symptoms can be attributed to vulnerability factors. As these factors are influenced, the likelihood of the manifestation of the symptoms of schizophrenia and psychosis increases. Vulnerability factors include environmental influences, individual behaviors, and genetic or biochemical factors. An individual's vulnerability increases with the introduction of overwhelming stressful events from the environment, the elimination or weakening of the individual's social support system, the introduction of stimuli for which no coping mechanisms or problem-solving skills have been developed, sensory overload and an inability to process information effectively, the presence of neurotransmission irregularities, and any genetic predisposition. As can be seen, all or any of these factors can work together to increase an individual's vulnerability to schizophrenic disorders.

One other issue that is now fairly certain regarding schizophrenia is that there is no single treatment or intervention that cures or remits the disorder (Bellack, 1984). In most cases a multidisciplinary approach is needed to deal with each of the functional deficiencies that may be present in the patient. Even with the success of pharmaceutical agents, it is still necessary to incorporate a comprehensive approach that includes social skills training, social support, family therapy, and vocational rehabilitation.

The group of medications commonly used in the treatment of schizophrenic disorders are the antipsychotics. Antidepressants, lithium, and antianxiety agents may also be used solely or in combination with the antipsychotics, depending on the nature of the disorder. Psychiatric medications, particularly the antipsychotics, may be used in the treatment of a number of other psychiatric disorders that have symptoms similar to those described above. These include paranoid disorders (e.g., paranoia, shared paranoid disorder, and acute paranoid disorder) and certain organic mental disorders due to substance abuse, dementia, or other organic brain syndromes.

Liberman et al. (1984) provide an interesting perspective regarding the use of antipsychotic medications. They indicate that these drugs will exert an influence on the biological vulnerability factors but that drugs cannot fully correct the possibility of relapse due to increasing numbers of stressors, breakdown of social systems, or the lack of problem-solving methods. This may help to explain the high relapse rate in this population despite the success of antipsychotic medications.

REFERENCES

American Psychiatric Association. (1987). *Diagnostic and statistical manual of mental disorders* (3rd ed.—revised). Washington, DC: Author.

Bellack, A.S. (Ed.). (1984). *Schizophrenia: Treatment, management and rehabilitation*. Orlando, FL: Grune & Stratton.

Bockar, J.A. (1976). *Primer for the nonmedical psychotherapist*. New York: Spectrum.

Liberman, R.P., Marshall, B.D., Marder, S.R., Dawson, M.E., Nuechterlein, K.H., & Doane, J.A. (1984). The nature and problem of schizophrenia. In A.S. Bellack (Ed.), *Schizophrenia: Treatment, management, and rehabilitation* (pp. 1–34). Orlando, FL: Grune & Stratton.

Chapter 5

Depression and Other Mood Disorders

Craig Cooperrider

Depression, unlike some of the other psychiatric disorders discussed in this book, has become a commonplace in the thoughts, vocabulary, and experiences of the general population. The term is used quite freely to express or describe an individual's feelings. Actually, the word connotes or describes conditions ranging from very short-term sadness, to grief associated with loss, to an overall pervasive feeling that may be present in a person's life for years. As Kline (1974) states: "Depression . . . is an inherent part of the human condition, a price we pay for those infinitely complicated physical mechanisms and emotional patterns that make us sensitive, intelligent, and aware. I assume that nearly everyone suffers from some degree of the condition at one time or another. It becomes an illness when this ordinary human reaction takes on severe symptoms and chronic form" (pp. 1–2). This being the case, it is not surprising that depression has become the most common condition treated by mental health care professionals.

The purpose of this chapter is to clarify what is clinically meant by the term depression and to provide a basic understanding of other mood disorders, with the eventual aim of discussing them in a psychopharmacological context. To begin, the discussion centers on classification issues related to depression and other mood disorders. Terms commonly associated with these diagnoses are defined according to common practice. The criteria for these diagnoses are described, as are issues surrounding etiology and treatment, particularly as they relate to the use of psychiatric medications.

CLASSIFICATION OF DEPRESSION AND MOOD DISORDERS

There is a great deal of unclarity about what depression and mood disorders are and about how they should be classified. Wetzel (1984) describes a number of the currently employed classification systems and begins by discussing the endogenous-exogenous dichotomy. Endogenous depression is caused by internal factors, whereas exogenous depression (sometimes called reactive depression) is caused by external factors. This classification is used quite frequently in discussions of depression. Also, as a rule of thumb, it serves as a guideline for treatment, with endogenous depression being treated with drugs and exogenous depression through other means such as psychotherapy.

The reactive-autonomous schema represents a second classification of mood disorders. In reactive depression, there is good patient response to an intervention, whereas with autonomous depression attempts at facilitating change are limited at best.

A third classification, which dates back to the *Diagnostic and Statistical Manual of Mental Disorders* (Second Edition) (DSM-II; American Psychiatric Association, 1968), is psychotic and neurotic depression. In this classification the major difference is based on the extent of the patient's contact with reality. With psychotic depression, severe symptoms accompanied by a loss of contact with reality, as well as other typical psychotic symptoms, are often noted.

There are also primary and secondary mood disorders. This classification is based on whether or not the patient has an existing history of other mental or physical disorders not including depression. Depression is considered a primary mood disorder if there is no previously existing mental illness other than depression. It is a secondary mood disorder when there is a history of a major mental or physical disorder not including depression.

A classification that is prevalent in contemporary psychiatry is the unipolar-bipolar dichotomy. A unipolar type of mood disorder is characterized by repeated bouts of depression, whereas a bipolar type manifests as mood swings that may vary from periods of severe mania, to normal reactions, to periods of severe depression.

DIAGNOSTIC CRITERIA OF MOOD DISORDERS

As was done in Chapter 4, the diagnostic criteria presented for mood disorders are as described in DSM-III-R (American Psychiatric Association, 1987), since these are the standard criteria commonly used in practice. Page numbers from DSM-III-R are given after each section. In the discussion that follows, mood disorders refer to mania or elation as well as depression.

Major Mood Disorders

The mood disorders are primarily of two types. These are: (1) bipolar disorders and (2) depressive disorders. The two are distinguished on the basis of whether there is an accompanying manic period or periods; bipolar disorders are accompanied by periods of mania.

Mood disorders are further characterized by the presence of various episodic conditions, i.e., manic episodes, major depressive episodes, or both. Before discussing the two types of disorders noted above, it is necessary to describe these episodic conditions.

Manic Episode

The diagnostic criteria for a manic episode begin with the presence of one or more distinct periods with a predominantly elevated, expansive, and irritable mood. This mood must be a major and persistent part of the illness, even though it may alternate with a depressed mood, and cause a marked impairment of occupational, social, or interpersonal functioning, or it must pose a threat to the patient or others. These symptoms must persist and at least three of the following symptoms (four if the mood is only irritable) must be present.

1. increase in activity or physical restlessness
2. greater talkativeness than usual or a sense of pressure to keep talking
3. flight of ideas or reports of racing thoughts
4. inflated self-esteem or grandiosity
5. decreased need for sleep
6. distractibility
7. excessive involvement in pleasurable activities that have a high potential for painful consequences that are not recognized (e.g., buying sprees, reckless driving)

Delusional thinking or hallucinations that occur in this disorder cannot last longer than 2 weeks without the manifestation of the prominent mood symptoms. The episode cannot be superimposed on schizophrenia, schizophreniform disorder, or delusional disorder, nor can it be due to any organic mental disorder (such as substance intoxication).

It is possible that a manic episode may occur with some psychotic features. These can either be mood congruent or incongruent. Mood-congruent psychotic symptoms are delusions or hallucinations that are in agreement with themes of inflated worth, power, knowledge, identity, or special relationship to a deity or famous person. Patients may also experience flight of ideas without an apparent awareness that their speech is not understandable and that their thoughts are not consistent as they speak.

Mood-incongruent psychotic features are delusions or hallucinations where the content does not involve the themes noted above but is more generally of a psychotic nature, such as delusions of persecution, thought disorders, delusions of being controlled, and so forth. In contrast, the content may be represented by catatonic symptoms such as stupor, mutism, negativism, or posturing (pp. 214–218).

Major Depressive Episode

A major depressive episode is characterized by a dysphoric mood or loss of interest or pleasure in nearly all activities. This mood manifests as sadness, hopelessness, irritability, and a feeling of being "down in the dumps." This disturbance in mood must be prominent but not necessarily the most dominant symptom.

At least five of the following symptoms must have been present nearly every day for at least 2 weeks.

1. depressed mood, as noted by the patient or others
2. poor appetite or significant weight loss, or increased appetite or significant weight gain
3. insomnia or hypersomnia
4. psychomotor agitation or retardation
5. loss of interest or pleasure in usual activities, or decrease in sexual drive not limited to a period when delusions or hallucinations are present
6. loss of energy or fatigue
7. feeling of worthlessness, self-reproach, or excessive or inappropriate guilt (either may be delusional)
8. complaints or evidence of diminished ability to think or concentrate (such as slowed thinking), or indecisiveness not associated with marked loosening of associations or incoherence
9. recurrent thoughts of death, suicidal ideation, wishes to be dead, or suicide plans or attempts

As is the case with a manic episode, in a major depressive episode there must be delusional thinking or hallucinations lasting longer than 2 weeks without the prominent mood symptoms. This episode cannot be superimposed on schizophrenia, schizophreniform disorder, or a delusional disorder, nor can it be due to any organic mental disorder or uncomplicated bereavement. Finally, it cannot be accompanied by any manic episode (p. 218).

A major depressive episode can occur with psychotic features, which can be either mood congruent or incongruent. Psychotic features of a major depressive episode that are mood congruent include delusions or hallucinations that are consistent with themes of personal inadequacy, guilt, disease, death, nihilism, or deserved punishment. Mood-incongruent psychotic features include typical psychotic symptoms not involving these themes.

Melancholia is also possible with a major depressive episode. When this occurs there is a loss of pleasure in almost all usual activities, lack of response to usually pleasurable stimuli, and at least five of the following.

1. loss of pleasure in almost all usual activities
2. lack of response to usually pleasurable stimuli
3. regular worsening of depression in the morning
4. early morning awakening
5. marked psychomotor retardation or agitation
6. significant anorexia or weight loss
7. no significant personality disturbance prior to initial depressive episode
8. one or more previous major depressive episodes followed by good recovery
9. previous good response to somatic antidepressant therapy (pp. 222–224)

Having described these episodic conditions, the major mood disorders can be considered.

Bipolar Disorders

There are two general types of bipolar disorders that are generally used diagnostically. These are: (1) bipolar disorder and (2) cyclothymia.

Mixed Type

This diagnosis is appropriate when the current or most recent episode involves the full symptomatic scheme of manic and major depressive episodes intermixed or alternating every few days. Depressive symptoms must be prominent and last at least 1 day (p. 226).

Manic Type

This diagnosis is appropriate when there is currently or most recently has been a manic episode (p. 226).

Depressed Type

This diagnosis is appropriate when the patient has had one or more manic episodes and is currently in a major depressive episode (p. 226).

Cyclothymia

In order for a diagnosis of cyclothymia to be rendered, its symptoms must be present for at least two years. During this time, the individual experiences hypomanic episodes as well as periods of depressed mood. Hypomanic episodes are defined as manic episodes in which the individual does not experience marked impairment in social or occupational functioning and is not a threat to self or others. The periods of depressed mood do not meet all of the criteria for a major depressive episode.

The person experiencing cyclothymia is never without hypomanic or depressive symptoms for more than two months at a time. There is no sign of a manic episode or a major depressive episode during the first two years of the disorder. It is not superimposed on any psychotic disorder and cannot be tied to an organic factor (pp. 227–228).

Depressive Disorders

There are two depressive disorders: (1) major depression and (2) dysthymia.

Major depression can be either a single episode or recurrent. The criterion is very simple: the individual must have had one (single) or more (recurrent) major depressive episodes but never a manic or hypomanic episode (pp. 229–230).

During the disorder, the individual is constantly depressed for longer than two months at a time. There is no history of a manic or hypomanic disorder and no underlying psychotic disorder. Neither is the condition tied to any organic factor (pp. 232–233).

Dysthymia was originally referred to as depressive neurosis. For this diagnosis to be rendered, the individual must have experienced symptoms of depression for at least two years. While the individual is depressed at least two of the following symptoms must be present:

1. insomnia or hypersomnia
2. low energy level or chronic tiredness
3. poor appetite or overeating
4. feelings of inadequacy, loss of self-esteem, or self-deprecation
5. decreased attention, decreased concentration, or difficulty making decisions

ETIOLOGY AND TREATMENT

Just as there is no single etiology of psychosis and schizophrenia (as discussed in Chapter 4), there is no single etiology of depression and other mood disorders.

Treatment issues are likewise imperfectly understood, and research has not been particularly helpful in providing clarification. It is widely held, however, that endogenous depressions (which are largely due to dysfunctions in neurotransmission mechanisms) respond best to drug therapy and that exogenous depressions are probably best treated by some form of psychotherapy (Rush, 1984; Extein, Pottash, Gold, Goggans, & Lydiard, 1984). This difference is not "black and white"; research by Beck, Rush, Shaw, and Emery (1979) indicates that there is a number of cases in which there is merit for both drug therapy and psychotherapy in the treatment of depression.

It is fairly safe to assume that depression can be both endogenous and exogenous, but the etiology of either condition alone is complicated. Levitt, Lubin, and Brooks (1983) describe causal factors in five different areas that are related to exogenous depression: learning, development, social skills, thought processes (cognitive distortions), and social class. Causal factors in any one of these areas can give rise to depression, but it is more likely that a combination of factors is responsible.

The same types of causal factors can be referred to when discussing other mood disorders, such as mania. With mania or bipolar illness, however, in many cases there seems to be a more definitive link to physiological causes (discussed in Chapter 11).

Gilbert (1984) espouses a view that summarizes a number of the positions noted above, both endogenous and exogenous, using the analogy of the interaction between computer software (external events) and computer hardware (internal makeup). In the same way that both these aspects must be taken into account when operating a computer, Gilbert states, ". . . illness and distress reside in influences from our own life histories meeting the biological history of our past" (p. 222).

PSYCHOPHARMACOLOGY OF MOOD DISORDERS

A number of different drugs are frequently used in treating the mood disorders. Primarily, antidepressant medication is used in the treatment of depression, and lithium compounds are used in treating bipolar disorders and mania. There is nothing "hard and fast" about this separation, however; antipsychotics and antianxiety agents may often be used, depending on the nature of the disorder (see Chapters 10 and 11).

REFERENCES

American Psychiatric Association. (1968). *Diagnostic and statistical manual of mental disorders* (2nd ed.). Washington, DC: Author.

American Psychiatric Association. (1987). *Diagnostic and statistical manual of mental disorders* (3rd ed.). Washington, DC: Author.

Beck, A.T., Rush, A.J., Shaw, B.F., & Emery, G. (1979). *Cognitive therapy of depression.* New York: Guilford.

Extein, I., Pottash, A.L.C., Gold, M.S., Goggans, R., & Lydiard, R.B. (1984). Antidepressants: Predicting response/maximizing efficacy. In M.S. Gold, R.B. Lydiard, & J.S. Carman (Eds.), *Advances in psychopharmacology. Predicting and improving treatment response* (pp. 83–106). Boca Raton, FL: CRC.

Gilbert, P. (1984). *Depression: From psychology to brain state.* London: Lawrence Erlbaum.

Kline, N.S. (1974). *From sad to glad.* New York: Ballantine.

Levitt, E.E., Lubin, B., & Brooks, J.M. (1983). *Depression: Concepts, controversies, and some new facts* (2nd ed.). Hillsdale, NJ: Lawrence Erlbaum.

Rush, A.J. (1984). Cognitive therapy in combination with antidepressant medication. In B.D. Beitman & G.L. Klerman (Eds.), *Combining psychotherapy and drug therapy in clinical practice* (pp. 149–165). New York: Spectrum.

Wetzel, J.W. (1984). *Clinical handbook of depression.* New York: Gardner.

Chapter 6

Anxiety Disorders

Craig Cooperrider

The present times have been described by many as the "Age of Anxiety." Anxiety and associated terms such as stress and tension have become common vocabulary and are used frequently. Furthermore, individuals are attempting to reduce the effects of anxiety and stress in their lives by attending stress-management courses; exercising; using biofeedback; learning meditation, imaging, and relaxation techniques; and, of course, receiving mental health therapy from various sources. In many parts of the world, anxiety is very much a part of contemporary life.

Kelly (1980) defines anxiety as the "subjective experience of apprehension or tension, imposed by the expectation of danger or distress or the need for a special effort" (p. 3). For most people, anxiety plays a useful role. It provides protection by cueing an individual to events that should be feared, and it promotes self-enhancement by stimulating individuals to comply with certain norms, rules, and guidelines for which they will be rewarded. In this sense, anxiety may be regarded as a healthy response that serves a valuable function in guiding human behavior.

This kind of "normal" anxiety is different from "pathological" anxiety, however. Normal anxiety is what is experienced as a result of everyday stressors within an individual's experience. This anxiety is commonly seen in persons preparing for or anticipating events, such as a test, a major change, or a crucial decision. But there comes a point at which anxiety is no longer healthy. In fact, reactions resulting from pathological anxiety are unproductive and at times even damaging to the individual. Functioning becomes impaired to the point where the person is no longer capable of performing in what is considered an appropriate manner. This chapter primarily addresses this type of anxiety.

ANXIETY AND RELATED TERMS

Terms such as anxiety and fear are often used interchangeably. The discussion that follows draws distinctions between these and other terms and provides definitions of terms commonly used when speaking of anxiety disorders. Some of the terms considered are anxiety, fear, phobia, panic, free-floating anxiety, obsessions, and compulsions.

Beck and Emery (1985) distinguish anxiety from fear by defining fear as a cognitive assessment of a threatening stimulus, whereas anxiety is the emotional reaction to that assessment. Fear is future-directed and occurs as an individual considers an event. Anxiety is a present-oriented occurrence in that it is experienced at the time of a stressful event. As anxiety is experienced, a number of physiological reactions may occur simultaneously.

These authors define a phobia as a fear of a specific object or event. Individuals with phobias fear the phobic object by perceiving it as dangerous or threatening and experience anxiety when in the presence of the object or when they picture themselves in its presence. Phobic objects include heights, closed spaces, deep water, social situations, and public speaking. Physical symptoms associated with anxiety may also be manifested in an individual when in the presence of a phobic object.

Panic, according to Beck and Emery, is a sudden and intense attack of anxiety usually associated with some particular event. During a panic reaction, individuals believe that something catastrophic is about to occur and that they must either escape or find help. Generally, a panic reaction is an extreme case of anxiety. A great deal of recent research provides evidence for a physiological component in panic disorders. Furthermore, there is some evidence that some antianxiety agents, especially alprazolam, are effective in the treatment of panic disorders.

A concept discussed frequently in relation to anxiety disorders is free-floating anxiety, which is defined as the manifestation of anxious symptoms at a time when no significant threat or danger is present. It has been questioned whether this phenomenon truly exists. Beck and Emery suggest that it is impossible to be aware of all that is going on within an individual's life and thereby to assume that there is no source of threat or danger. Their conclusion is that no one except the individual can determine the presence or absence of a threat.

Obsessions are continuous and repetitive thoughts that cause an individual to be preoccupied with the contents of the thoughts. Compulsions are repetitive, ritualistic behaviors that are usually carried out to excess with the thought of preventing some anxiety-producing problem that possibly, but not probably, could occur.

CLASSIFICATION OF ANXIETY DISORDERS

Anxiety disorders usually involve anxiety, avoidance behavior, or both. These components exist within each of the disorders to be discussed. As for Chapters 4 and 5, in the following discussion DSM-III-R (American Psychiatric Association, 1987) is used as the guide to the classification of these disorders. Diagnostic criteria are paraphrased, and the appropriate page numbers from DSM-III-R are given after each section.

Agoraphobia without History of Panic Disorder

The diagnosis of agoraphobia is appropriate when an individual has a marked fear of being alone in public places where (1) there may be a possibility of sudden incapacitation, (2) escape is not possible, (3) help is not available, and (4) acute embarrassment is possible. Symptoms include dizziness, loss of bladder or bowel control, or cardiac distress. Typical sites include crowds, tunnels, and bridges. Fear causes the person to reduce normal activities, and it becomes the basis on which life decisions are made. Agoraphobia is not due to a major depressive episode, obsessive compulsive disorder, paranoid personality disorder, or schizophrenia. Furthermore, there is no history of panic disorder (p. 241).

Social Phobia

A social phobia is diagnosed when the individual has an irrational fear of situations in which he or she may be under the scrutiny of others. There is also the fear that he or she may behave in a way that is humiliating or embarrassing. The individual experiences significant distress because of these fears and recognizes that they are excessive or unreasonable. Although other disorders may be present, this fear is unrelated. This disorder is not due to another mental disorder, such as major depression or avoidant personality disorder (p. 243).

Simple Phobia

Simple phobia is characterized by a persistent, irrational fear and a compelling desire to avoid certain events or objects (other than those noted above for agoraphobia or social phobia). Phobic objects are often animals, and phobic situations often involve heights or closed spaces. The disorder produces significant distress, and the individual recognizes that the fear is excessive or unreasonable. Simple phobia is not due to another mental disorder, such as schizophrenia, posttraumatic stress disorder, or obsessive compulsive disorder (pp. 244–245).

Panic Disorder

In the case of panic disorder, the individual has had one or more unexpected panic attacks not caused by being in situations where he or she was the focus of attention. Either four of these attacks must have occurred within a 4-week period or one or more attacks has been followed by at least a month of fear of another attack. A minimum of four of these symptoms must have occurred during at least one of the attacks.

1. dyspnea (shortness of breath)
2. dizziness or faintness
3. palpitations or tachycardia
4. trembling or shaking
5. sweating
6. choking
7. nausea
8. depersonalization or derealization
9. numbness or tingling sensations
10. hot flashes or chills
11. chest pain
12. fear of dying
13. fear of losing control or going crazy

These symptoms cannot be tied to a specific organic condition.

There are two specific types of panic disorder: (1) panic disorder with agoraphobia and (2) panic disorder without agoraphobia. Both of these meet the conditions for a panic disorder, but they are distinguished by the presence or absence of agoraphobic symptoms (pp. 237–239).

Generalized Anxiety Disorder

A generalized anxiety disorder is said to occur when there is unrealistic and excessive anxiety about two or more life circumstances for at least six months during which the person has been bothered more days than not by the concern. The anxiety is not related to another mental disorder. It does not occur during the presence of a mood disorder or a psychotic disorder and cannot be linked to any organic factors.

At least six of the following eighteen symptoms are present when anxious.

1. trembling and shakiness
2. muscle tension and aches
3. restlessness
4. easy fatigability
5. shortness of breath
6. palpitations or tachycardia

7. sweating or cold clammy hands
8. dry mouth
9. dizziness
10. nausea or diarrhea
11. hot flashes or chills
12. frequent urination
13. difficulty in swallowing
14. feeling keyed up
15. exaggerated startle response
16. difficulty in concentrating
17. difficulty in falling or staying asleep
18. irritability (pp. 252–253)

Obsessive Compulsive Disorder

The diagnostic criterion for obsessive compulsive disorder is the presence of either obsessions or compulsions. Obsessions are described as recurrent, persistent ideas, thoughts, images, or impulses that are not experienced as voluntarily produced but rather as thoughts deemed senseless by the individual. The individual does make attempts at ignoring these thoughts.

Compulsions are repetitive, purposeful behaviors that are performed according to rules, norms, or ritual. The behavior is designed to produce or prevent a future event. The activity does not logically connect with activities that actually need to be done, however, or it is clearly excessive. Initially, the individual may desire to resist the compulsion. The purposelessness of the behavior is usually recognized, but carrying out the behavior ultimately releases tension on a short-term basis.

The obsessions or compulsions distress the individual and may interfere with appropriate social functioning. They cannot be due to another mental disorder such as schizophrenia, major depression, or organic mental disorder (p. 247).

Posttraumatic Stress Disorder

The criteria for this disorder include the existence of a recognizable stressor that would produce symptoms of distress in nearly anyone. There must be a re-experiencing of the trauma as evidenced by at least one of the following: (1) repeated recollections of the event, (2) frequent dreams of the event, (3) sudden feelings that the event is about to happen again, or (4) intense psychological distress during exposure to events symbolic of the traumatic event, including anniversaries. The individual seems to lack responsiveness or involvement in the external environment, as evidenced in at least three of the following ways:

(1) declining interest in usually significant activities, (2) feelings of detachment or separation from others, (3) constricted affect, (4) efforts to avoid thoughts or feelings associated with the trauma, (5) efforts to avoid activities that may arouse memories of the trauma, (6) inability to remember some part of the trauma, or (7) sense of a foreshortened future.

At least two of the following symptoms reflect increased arousal and were not manifest before the trauma: (1) exaggerated startle response, (2) difficulty falling or staying asleep, (3) anger outbursts, (4) difficulty in concentrating, (5) hypervigilance, or (6) increase in physical symptoms when the individual is exposed to events that symbolize or resemble the traumatic event (pp. 250–251).

TREATMENT AND PSYCHOPHARMACOLOGY OF ANXIETY DISORDERS

As with previously discussed disorders, there are a number of theories attempting to explain the anxiety disorders (Klein & Rabkin, 1980; Hallam, 1985). It is perhaps more helpful to look at anxiety and associated disorders as related to certain predisposing factors (Beck & Emery, 1985). These factors include hereditary concerns, physical diseases, developmental traumas, inadequate personal and learning experiences, and inappropriate and counterproductive cognitions and belief systems. The course of anxiety disorders is most appropriately seen as the interrelation or interaction of genetic, developmental, environmental, and psychological factors.

There are also various medical and psychological approaches used in treating the anxiety disorders and stress. The psychotherapeutic interventions range from supportive therapy, to psychoanalytic approaches, to relaxation training, to cognitive behavior modification, to desensitization. A major problem, however, is that the circumstances where one approach, or a combination of approaches, is the most appropriate to use are difficult to identify accurately and completely.

Regarding the psychopharmacology of these disorders, there are also a number of uncertainties. Certain drugs such as Valium and Librium are clearly antianxiety agents; in particular, drugs categorized as benzodiazepines are frequently used. In certain cases, some antidepressants are also recommended in the treatment of certain anxiety disorders (see Chapters 10 and 12).

REFERENCES

American Psychiatric Association. (1987). *Diagnostic and statistical manual of mental disorders* (3rd ed.). Washington, DC: Author.

Beck, A.T., & Emery, G. (1985). *Anxiety disorders and phobias*. New York: Basic Books.

Hallam, R.S. (1985). *Anxiety: Psychological perspectives on panic and agoraphobia.* London: Academic Press.

Kelly, D. (1980). *Anxiety and emotions.* Springfield, IL: Charles C Thomas.

Klein, D.F., & Rabkin, J.G. (Eds.). (1980). *Anxiety: New research and changing concepts.* New York: Raven.

Chapter 7

Neurological Disorders

Craig Cooperrider

There are a number of disorders that directly affect the brain and nervous system, and certain medications of a psychoactive nature are often used to reduce the effects of these disorders. The purpose of this chapter is to examine some of the more common of these disorders: epilepsy and convulsive disorders, Parkinson's disease, Huntington's chorea, Korsakoff's psychosis, multiple sclerosis, and migraine headaches. Attention is given to symptomatology, etiology, particular idiosyncrasies regarding each of the conditions, and general pharmacological treatment methods. For a more thorough discussion of various neurological disorders, see Mohr (1984), Leech and Shuman (1982), and Matthews and Miller (1975).

EPILEPSY

Epilepsy is not a singular disorder but a number of different disorders all manifested by seizures that directly affect the consciousness and awareness of the individual. There is a great deal of variance among the seizures of each of the different forms of epilepsy. Generally, a seizure is characterized by an irregular firing of neurons (brain cells) in the cerebrum. This definition, however, is not completely accurate in that all individuals experiencing seizures or cerebral abnormalities (as measured by electroencephalography) do not necessarily have epilepsy.

Classification of Epileptic Seizures

There are two major classifications of epileptic seizures: generalized and partial. Generalized seizures occur bilaterally (on both sides of the brain) and have

57

no particular location of origin. In contrast, partial seizures have a particular point of origin and spread to other parts of the brain.

The grand mal seizure is one form of a generalized seizure, characterized by an intense stiffening of the body followed by the sharp, jerky movements that are commonly associated with seizure activity. Subsequently there is a period of unconsciousness, from which the individual awakens in a confused and disoriented state. Generally, the individual cannot recall events immediately preceding the seizure. The entire seizure normally lasts approximately 20 minutes, but it can last longer. The early phases of rigidity and jerky movements last only a few minutes, and the unconscious period lasts at least 15 minutes. Other related problems may involve tongue biting or tongue swallowing, bodily injury, excessive fatigue, and urinary incontinence.

Petit mal seizures are another form of the generalized seizures. These are approximately 5 to 10 seconds in length, during which time the individual loses awareness of activities around him or her. There is little to no movement, limited facial expression, and only occasionally eye movements. The severity of petit mal seizures is not as great as that of grand mal seizures; the individual usually does not fall, and there may or may not be a state of confusion at the time of return to consciousness.

A third type of generalized seizure is referred to as myoclonic seizure. This consists of sudden jerkiness and contractions in the body. The individual does not typically lose consciousness.

Partial seizures, as noted above, generally have a point of origin within the brain and then spread to other locations. These are typically caused by some type of localized pathology, such as a traumatic head injury, tumors, abscesses, or cerebrovascular accidents (Lueders, 1984).

The most common type of partial seizures are known as the jacksonian seizures. They can be either motor or sensory depending on their point of origin. Motor seizures take the form of muscular contractions in a certain area, such as the mouth, fingers, or toes. The contractions then spread to other muscle groups. They may stop or eventually result in a grand mal seizure. The origin in the brain is generally the frontal lobe.

Sensory seizures have their origin in the parts of the cerebrum involved in sensory processing and generally cause sensory distortions, illusions, or hallucinations. The individual may experience tingling, coldness, flashing lights, or visual hallucinations.

A third type of partial seizure generally originates from the temporal lobes of the cerebrum. The most common symptoms are inappropriate movements and behaviors such as lip smacking, chewing, shuffling papers, and the like. The jerky muscle movements common in other forms are not as likely to be present. Movement is usually coordinated and organized but not appropriate for the given situation. There are subjective reports of déjà vu, repetitive thoughts, or hallucinations. The individual's consciousness, as described by Matthews and Miller (1975), is "clouded" rather than lost. There may be a period of time when the individual behaves as an automaton, carrying on normal activities without being aware of what he or she is doing or remembering what he or she has done.

Epileptic seizures can be brought on by a number of different factors, including stress, sleep deprivation, flashing lights, coughing, trauma, menses, or puberty (Kolb & Whishaw, 1980). A number of the drugs discussed in later chapters may also induce seizures in an individual with epilepsy; phenothiazines and other antipsychotics, tricyclic antidepressants, alcohol, and excessive anticonvulsants are all examples.

Some seizures may be preceded by a warning sign, referred to as an aura. Various sensations of odors, noises, or lights, or simply the impression that a seizure may occur, are all types of auras experienced by individuals with epilepsy.

Pharmacological Treatment

The preferred treatment in epilepsy, as in other medical disorders, is to address the cause. This may be possible for some forms of epilepsy, such as those caused by tumors, cerebral injuries, or diseases. Direct treatment of the cause is not always possible particularly with generalized epilepsy, in which a cause may not be identified, or in situations where there is brain damage of a more permanent nature. Therefore, in order to reduce the possibility of seizures, drugs are utilized.

Anticonvulsant medications are currently the treatment of choice for individuals with epilepsy. Medications such as diphenylhydantoin (Dilantin) and phenobarbital are the most frequently used, and new anticonvulsant medications are continually being developed and tested (see Chapter 13). Medications enable most individuals to lead fairly productive lives, but it is critical that certain cautions be routinely observed, such as avoiding high places and not operating dangerous machinery. Further information about epilepsy is provided in Sands (1982).

PARKINSON'S DISEASE

Parkinson's disease is a progressive illness caused by degeneration of neurons in upper parts of the brain stem and corresponding locations in the basal ganglia. The disease is characterized by a dopamine (a neurotransmitter) deficiency in these brain areas. Typically, Parkinson's disease occurs in individuals between the ages of 40 and 65.

Symptomatology and Etiology

The symptoms of the disease, which manifest as impaired motor functioning, fall into four categories (Kase, 1984): hypokinesia, tremor, rigidity, and dementia. Hypokinesia involves slower initiation of normal voluntary movements. Tremors are typically the first symptom to appear and normally occur while the individual is at rest; as various limbs are active, the tremor is not as apparent. The third symptom of rigidity affects muscles in the limbs, trunk, and face.

Kolb and Whishaw (1980) report a number of additional symptoms. There is difficulty in maintaining certain body parts in their normal position relative to other parts. Impaired equilibrium makes it difficult for the individual to maintain an erect position without support or to take steps. Because of rigidity, the individual has trouble speaking. There is little expression in the face and even akinesia at times. The individual may experience difficulty in chewing and swallowing.

All the symptoms of Parkinson's disease on occasion appear, disappear, and appear again. When placed in situations requiring activity and attention, the individual may appear to be in remission. Symptoms generally return when activity and attention are no longer required, however. Dementia is also a frequent occurrence in Parkinson's disease.

In terms of etiology, it is speculated that somehow certain structures in the brain stem and the basal ganglia are destroyed or that dopamine neurotransmission is blocked in the neurons in these areas. Beyond this, however, little is known because of the current incomplete knowledge of the functioning of these brain structures.

Pharmacological Treatment

Parkinson's disease cannot be cured, so that treatment is oriented toward reducing the effects of its symptoms. A number of drug agents are used to attempt to increase dopamine activity. Perhaps most widely used is a drug known as L-dopa, which is a precursor of dopamine (meaning that in the body this substance becomes chemically changed to dopamine). Antiparkinsonian medications, such as benzotropine (Cogentin) and trihexylphenidyl (Artane), are also used. Kolb and Whishaw (1980) also recommend counseling to aid the individual in coping with the disability. It is important that individuals come to understand the disease and its implications at an early point.

HUNTINGTON'S CHOREA

Huntington's chorea is a genetically transmitted disease that prompts the degeneration of structures in the basal ganglia and parts of the cerebral cortex.

Even though the disease is passed on genetically, its onset does not typically become apparent until the individual reaches his or her thirties. Death usually follows approximately 15 to 20 years after the initial appearance of symptoms.

Symptomatology

The disorder is characterized by a number of symptoms, which vary widely among individuals. As a result of its progressive nature, the initial symptoms are generally not noticeable. Mild personality and behavioral changes, including withdrawal and a falling off of usual interests, are the first signs. Involuntary and restless movements then begin to appear, eventually becoming more frequent and most apparent in the limbs, mouth, and face. Intellectual and cognitive functioning, including memory, also deteriorate. As the disease progresses psychiatric difficulties begin to develop; these may include bizarre behaviors and psychotic manifestations.

Psychopharmacological Treatment

In treatments for Huntington's chorea, a number of drugs are frequently prescribed. None of these drugs was specifically designed for the disease, but they show some degree of effectiveness. The most widely used medications for treating the movement and behavioral problems of the disorder are some of the antipsychotic medications, including haloperidol (Haldol), chlorpromazine (Thorazine), and other phenothiazines. Current drug treatments, however, at best provide only some symptom relief.

KORSAKOFF'S PSYCHOSIS

Korsakoff's psychosis, also called chronic alcoholic delirium, is actually a neurological impairment that is the direct result of the use of a psychoactive drug (alcohol). The disorder results from a thiamine (vitamin B_1) deficiency due to excessive use of alcohol. It is regarded as a syndrome that directly affects the individual's memory. Talland (1969) indicates some of the direct symptoms related to neurological functioning. These include:

1. inability to learn and retain newly presented material
2. loss of long-term memory or the ability to recall previous events (or both)
3. fabrication of stories when past information cannot be recalled (it is easier to do this than to admit to memory difficulties)
4. reduction in conversation skills due to inability to recall information

5. lack of insight regarding and knowledge of memory difficulties
6. general apathy and lack of interest in current activities

There is a great deal of uncertainty regarding the actual cause of these problems. It is believed that the thalamus and hypothalamus are the affected brain areas, but the reasons for the effects produced by the thiamine deficiency are highly speculative.

Korsakoff's psychosis is generally treated by large doses of vitamin B_1. The successful outcome of this method is doubtful, however, and only limited numbers of patients actually benefit, even after considerable periods of treatment.

MULTIPLE SCLEROSIS

Multiple sclerosis is the result of multiple lesions in various places in the nervous system, particularly in the upper levels of the spinal cord, the pons, the midbrain, and the optic nerve. After prolonged exposure to the lesions, affected neurons begin to undergo myelin degeneration or deterioration. Myelin is a "sheath" material that covers, protects, and insulates neurons. As these myelin sheaths are destroyed, they are replaced by scar tissue known as plaques. This eventually produces problems in the transmission of nerve impulses, thus leading to the symptoms of multiple sclerosis. The cause for the lesions and the eventual myelin degeneration is not known.

Symptomatology

The symptoms of multiple sclerosis are many and varied. Their occurrence is dependent on the location of the lesions, the number of lesions, and the duration of the illness. Many individuals initially experience sporadic visual problems. These may include either a blurring sensation or double vision. As the disease continues there are variable periods of remission, but eventually the symptoms begin to take the form of spasticity, tremor, fatigue, and falling. Problems with urinary initiation and retention generally occur. The individual's mental state becomes confused, and speech problems typically develop. Depression and other mood disorders are likely. Many individuals cannot function well in hot weather and tire very easily, and they may experience extreme frustration in simply attempting to plan a day because of many of these symptoms.

Multiple sclerosis is a progressive illness. Its manifestation is almost mysterious, in that an individual may have an attack or an exacerbation of symptoms and then not be bothered for a number of years. Kraft (1981) states ". . . prognostic indicators that can determine which patients are likely to show rapid disease progression and which will only show slow progression have yet to be determined'' (p. 112). Furthermore, there are a number of complications that result from the disease, including decubitus ulcers, urinary tract infections, and spasticity. Multiple sclerosis does not directly cause death, but these and other complications can all contribute to the death of the individual (Kraft, 1981).

Pharmacological Treatment

The pharmacological treatment for multiple sclerosis is generally through steroids. Adrenocorticotropic hormone (ACTH) is also used to reduce inflammation of lesions and to minimize periods of exacerbation. A number of other medications are used to reduce the effects of the various complications. Although these medications provide relief, they do nothing to prevent the progression of the illness.

MIGRAINE HEADACHES

The last disorder of the nervous system to be discussed is the migraine headache. The typical migraine begins with a visual sensation, described as a fluttering in certain places within the visual field and thought to be caused by a dilation of blood vessels within the eyes. After about 15-20 minutes the visual flutter begins to fade. As it diminishes, the headache begins.

The pain can be centralized on one side of the head, toward the back of the head, or over the total head. As the headache continues the patient may experience nausea and even vomiting. Other symptoms may include a numbness of the arms and extremities. There are often feelings of extreme weakness. However, as one symptom increases, others subside. Generally, the symptoms do not cease until the individual has slept.

The actual cause of a headache incident is difficult to determine. This is bewildering to the individual, who is attempting to determine what prompted the headache. Some precipitating events include the sudden appearance of a bright light, a change in surrounding temperature, changing physical activity, limited food consumption, and eating certain foods high in grease, sugar, or tyramine (e.g., cheese, chocolate, or alcohol).

Pharmacological treatment takes a variety of forms, including the use of analgesics, antianxiety agents, and muscle relaxants. Some medications are given at the onset of the headache and others can be taken prophylactically.

Another method of treatment involves the use of biofeedback, in which the patient is taught to recognize physical cues and eliminate the dilation of blood vessels, thereby reducing the likelihood of a headache.

REFERENCES

Kase, C.S. (1984). Parkinson's disease. In J.P. Mohr (Ed.), *Manual of clinical problems in neurology* (pp. 43–47). Boston: Little, Brown & Co.

Kolb, B., & Whishaw, I.Q. (1980). *Fundamentals of human neuropsychology*. San Francisco: W.H. Freeman.

Kraft, G.H. (1981). Multiple sclerosis. In W.C. Stolov & M.R. Clowers (Eds.), *Handbook of severe disability* (pp. 111–118). Washington, DC: U.S. Department of Education.

Leech, R.W., & Shuman, R.M. (1982). *Neuropathology*. Philadelphia: Harper & Row.

Lueders, H.O. (1984). Epilepsy. In J.P. Mohr (Ed.), *Manual of clinical problems in neurology* (pp. 11–15). Boston: Little, Brown & Co.

Matthews, W.B., & Miller, H. (1975). *Diseases of the nervous system* (2nd ed.). Oxford: Blackwell.

Mohr, J.P. (Ed.). (1984). *Manual of clinical problems in neurology*. Boston: Little, Brown & Co.

Sands, H. (Ed.). (1982). *Epilepsy: A handbook for the mental health professional*. New York: Brunner/Mazel.

Talland, G.A. (1969). *The pathology of memory*. New York: Academic Press.

Chapter 8

Addictive Processes

Gary R. Lewis and Gary W. Lawson

An agent to counteract the negative effects of the addictive process has been sought for centuries. The Old Testament book of Proverbs, dating from the tenth century B.C., gives advice about the evils of drinking alcohol to excess. The ancient Greeks believed that the color violet had the power to prevent intoxication, and the fragrant violet *Viola odorata* appears to have been frequently used to decorate the tables at their parties as a method to prevent the guests from becoming drunk. The purple semiprecious stone amethyst was also believed to have the power to prevent intoxication; in fact, the Greek word *amethustos* means literally "anti-intoxicant." In some specialties today the term "amethystic agent" is used instead of "sobering agent" as the search for a pharmacological cure continues.

TWO PERSPECTIVES FOR THE TREATMENT OF ADDICTION

Current modalities employed in the treatment of addictive processes are of two types, medical (pharmacological) and self-help or abstinence programs. An example of the latter is Alcoholics Anonymous, which emphasizes individual vulnerability to drugs and provides group settings in which common experiences are shared and abstinence is reinforced. Pharmacological interventions are completely rejected in self-help programs of this kind.

The medical approach, in contrast, is founded on a disease paradigm and focuses on the physiological effects of withdrawal from an addictive substance. For example, the withdrawal syndrome associated with narcotics is usually directly related to the individual narcotic involved, the dosages used, and the duration of the drug's effects. In its mildest form the first symptoms of withdrawal include lacrimation, rhinorrhea, diaphoresis, yawning, restlessness, and insomnia. In moderate form the withdrawal may progress to dilation of the pupils, muscle twitching, myalgia, arthralgia, severe restlessness, diarrhea, vomiting, dehydration, and hypotension. Withdrawal associated with narcotic drugs does not cause seizures or hallucinations. Even without treatment, complete withdrawal will not take more than 10 days. Complete recuperation may take up to 6 months and is not always dependent on the physical presence of the narcotic in the body.

For other kinds of drugs, including alcohol, the symptoms can be more severe and include both auditory and visual hallucinations with and without paranoia. The condition will continue to disintegrate until seizure activity develops. This can begin from 48 hours to 17 days after the beginning of abstinence depending on the type of drug taken, the time since it was last ingested, the tolerance that the individual has developed, and the mode of administration of the drug.

The scientific search for means to aid individuals in withdrawal from various drugs has been eclectic if nothing else. Vitamins, carbohydrates, hormones, amino acids, amphetamines and other stimulants, antihistamines, cholinergics, antianxiety and antidepressant drugs, as well as potassium and calcium, have all been seriously considered and evaluated. The presumed mode of action of all these substances varies greatly. Some, such as carbohydrates and certain hormones, seemed promising in treating alcohol withdrawal because they facilitated the body's ability to metabolize ethanol. Others, such as the stimulant drugs, offered hope because they appeared to counteract alcohol's depressant effect on the central nervous system.

MAJOR DRUGS USED IN THE TREATMENT OF ADDICTION

Advocates of medical programs feel that drugs are useful in the treatment of addiction in two ways: (1) alleviating or partially suppressing withdrawal symptoms, thereby enabling the addict to focus on other treatments that are offered at the same time (i.e., group therapy, occupation and recreational therapies, and nutritional counseling), and (2) providing a maintenance program for those people who seem unable to carry on their lives completely drug free.

Alcohol

Disulfiram, or Antabuse as it is more generally known, is used relatively infrequently today. This drug was accidentally developed in the late 1940s by a group of Danish scientists, who discovered that when a person ingested disulfiram and came in contact with alcohol a marked reaction took place. Disulfiram interferes with alcohol metabolism through its effect on the breakdown of acetaldehyde, an intermediate product of alcohol metabolism. Although acetaldehyde is normally present in the body, when it is combined with disulfiram toxic levels form. The symptoms associated with these toxic levels can be life threatening in some people, particularly those with heart disease, cirrhosis, diabetes, or any debilitating medical condition. The first noticeable symptom of toxicity is a sensation of heat, usually in the face. Additional reactions are throbbing in the head and neck, breathing difficulty, nausea, vomiting, sweating, tachycardia, weakness, and vertigo. These symptoms usually occur within 30 minutes after ingestion. In some cases even seizure activity is noted. Since alcohol in all forms produces a reaction, individuals must be instructed to avoid all disguised forms of alcohol, including preparations containing alcohol that can be absorbed through the skin (such as aftershave or skin preparation for an injection) and cough medicines and liquid cold preparations sold over the counter or any prescription that contains alcohol.

Metronidazole, or Flagyl, is used predominately to treat trichomonal infection, although it also affects alcohol metabolism and for this reason is used to manage withdrawal. When alcohol is used in association with metronidazole, an autonomic nervous system response is produced that is generally less violent than that with disulfiram. The most severe adverse reactions include convulsive seizures and peripheral neuropathy. More common reactions are simple gastrointestinal tract disturbances such as nausea and vomiting or constipation. Symptoms of overdose include nausea, vomiting, and ataxia. At this time there is no specific treatment or antidote for an overdose of metronidazole.

Psychotropic drugs, especially mild tranquilizers and antidepressants, are commonly used to treat various withdrawal symptoms, particularly anxiety and depression. Alcohol has a potentiating effect on the minor tranquilizers (e.g., diazepam and chlordiazepoxide) and on the phenothiazine and barbiturate sedatives. Individuals taking these types of drugs for withdrawal symptoms must be observed carefully to ensure their continued abstinence from alcohol. The effect of combining alcohol and antidepressants is still not known, but monoamine oxidase actions are inhibited (see Chapter 10).*

Opiate Drugs

Opiates are generally divided into categories on the basis of their chemical composition or their action. There are the organic alkaloids, such as morphine and codeine; synthetic derivatives of morphine, such as diacetylmorphine (heroin); synthetic derivatives of opiates other than morphine that have actions similar to morphine, such as meperidine (Demerol) and methadone (Dolaphine); and com-

---

*Monoamine oxidase is an enzyme normally found in the presynaptic membrane that degrades norepinephrine (and also serotonin and dopamine) when it is reabsorbed after a postsynaptic potential occurs (Seiden & Dykstra, 1977).

pounds that contain only small amounts of an opiate, such as paregoric (4% tincture of opium). To date, the major method of treatment for opiate addiction withdrawal has been either ''cold turkey'' or weaning the addict with the same or a similarly acting drug in decreasing dosages. A new technique is the use of narcotic blocking agents to prevent the craving associated with this type of addiction.

Methadone has been used both to wean and to maintain narcotic addicts. When used to wean the addict, a dosage of methadone determined by the amount of the addict's habit is administered on a daily basis. Once the amount has been constant for approximately 48 hours, the dosage is reduced, usually in the amount of 5 to 10 mg per day until the individual is completely withdrawn. In a methadone maintenance program the individual's minimum requirement for the drug is determined, and the dosage is no longer reduced. This type of program has many advocates as well as detractors. On the positive side, methadone does not produce the mood swings associated with heroin. Moreover, the maintained individual cannot achieve the ''rush'' usually obtained by ''mainlining'' the drug. The theory is that the individual can thereby avoid the temptation to return to the use of the narcotic. On the negative side, some addicts use methadone maintenance only to kick the expensive habit temporarily. By going through withdrawal, they reduce their tolerance level and then can begin using the illicit drug again at a lower dosage, and therefore at less cost. Others ''chip,'' which means that they take enough of the methadone to stop the withdrawal symptoms and then continue to use the illicit drug to obtain the ''high'' that they seek. Finally, methadone maintenance leaves the addict completely dependent on continued use of a drug, with all the attendant risks.

Cyclazocine is a potent, long-acting narcotic antagonist that also produces a certain amount of analgesia. When cyclazocine is administered, most of the same subjective effects as those of opiates are felt by the addict; the major difference is that cyclazocine usually produces a feeling of dysphoria rather than euphoria. Cyclazocine is used in much the same way and for the same reason as methadone. The usual program is one of maintenance, not withdrawal support. Side effects of cyclazocine are anxiety, agitation, dysphoria, racing thoughts, and hallucinations. These are believed to be the result of the agonist properties of cyclazocine. In the event of an overdose, naloxone is given to block the action of this drug.

Naloxone is considered a pure narcotic antagonist with few side effects and no agonist properties of its own. It does not produce respiratory depression, euphoria, or the other symptoms associated with opiate use even when taken at high dosages. After intravenous injection the onset of action is noticeable in 3 minutes. The major adverse reaction is that, when administered to addicts, it can produce the abstinence syndrome discussed earlier.

Naltrexone has recently been utilized in much the same way as naloxone. It also has no discernible agonist activity and provides a longer-lasting opiate blockage than cyclazocine or naloxone. Naltrexone is still being researched and is not yet available for clinical use.

Central Nervous System Depressants

Although there are concerns about geriatric dependence on "sleeping pills," the group that most often seeks treatment for depressant addiction comprises adolescents and young adults. It seems that this group uses both short- and intermediate-acting barbiturates and sedative-hypnotics to vary their moods. These "downers" are sometimes taken as part of a potpourri of drugs that includes amphetamines and opiates. Depressants are commonly called "yellow jackets," "red birds," "red devils," "rainbows," and "blue heavens."

Barbiturates can be divided into four categories in relation to the duration of their action. The ultrashort-action group includes sodium methohexital and sodium thiopental, which are used primarily as intravenous anesthetics. Drugs in the short- to intermediate-action group, including amobarbital, sodium pentobarbital, and secobarbital, are used chiefly for their sedative-hypnotic properties. The long-action drugs such as phenobarbital are sometimes used as sedative-hypnotics but usually are prescribed to control epilepsy. Within the past few years they have been used in the treatment of withdrawal from other sedative-hypnotic agents. Overdose of these drugs produces a depressant withdrawal syndrome, the severity of which varies with its concentration in the blood when its usage is discontinued. This syndrome is life threatening and requires the immediate attention of a professional to provide the physiological support that may become necessary.

Sedative-hypnotic drugs depress the central nervous system functioning. They are characterized according to chemical structure and pharmacological properties. Some of the drugs in this category are chloral hydrate, paraldehyde, methaqualone, and antianxiety agents such as the benzodiazepines and carbamates. Withdrawal from central nervous system depressants can lead to death; for this reason, detoxification should only be undertaken in a setting where the appropriate supportive medical care is available. The onset of withdrawal depends on the action of the drug taken, and its severity is in direct proportion to the magnitude of the physical addiction. Symptoms of withdrawal from the short-action barbiturates become noticeable 12 to 16 hours after the last dosage. The longer-action sedative-hypnotics may not produce withdrawal symptoms for up to 7 days after the last dosage.

Central Nervous System Stimulants

There is a wide variety of substances currently available that stimulate the central nervous system. Only three have been abused to any great extent: amphetamines, methamphetamines, and cocaine.

Amphetamines and methamphetamines produce their effect by stimulating sympathetic nerve endings. They excite some of the smooth muscle groups and inhibit some others. A major effect is the temporary excitation of the cardiac muscles. These drugs are occasionally useful in the treatment of withdrawal because in controlled dosages they produce increased mental alertness, a sense of initiative and confidence, and an increased ability to concentrate on simple tasks. At high dosages, dysphoria, dizziness, confusion, and headache are produced. The long-term dosage required to produce withdrawal varies and depends on the tolerance of the addict and the route used to administer the drug. Signs of withdrawal are headache, chills, an increase in body temperature, diarrhea, dryness of the mouth, and sweating. If the withdrawal is severe, seizure activity may occur. It is not uncommon for individuals in withdrawal to experience life-threatening symptoms; for this reason most addicts must undergo detoxification in a setting where appropriate professional help can be obtained.

For a complete discussion of cocaine addiction, see Chapter 19.

IMPLICATIONS FOR PSYCHOPHARMACOLOGICAL TREATMENT

Drugs have an appropriate place in the treatment of addictive process, but the results of research on the effectiveness of these drugs are inexact, perplexing, and dissatisfying. The research is autonomous in nature, which makes it difficult if not impossible to compare the results. Additionally even the criteria for the diagnosis of addiction are not standardized, so that various symptoms are used in the studies to determine the success of the agent used. Reviews by Azrin, Bisson, Meyers, and Godley (1982); McMillan (1981); and Ciraulo and Jaffe (1981) are pessimistic about all categories of agents currently used in the treatment of addiction.

Although there are significant chemical aids to the treatment of withdrawal from addiction, it must be stressed that no one of these represents a complete treatment of the addictive process itself. The area of greatest success seems to be the opiates, where antagonists take the ''kick'' out of the drug and minimize the addict's craving. Still, addicted individuals must be motivated to maintain their sobriety.

Habituated barbiturate and amphetamine abuse seem to be problems without much promise of resolution. The best that can be hoped for at this time is increased education and steps to curb the distribution of drugs.

Alcohol abuse is perhaps the most extensive of all the addictive processes that the professional must treat. Because of the wide acceptance and accessibility of alcohol, it is not possible to curb the source of supply. With alcohol use being such an established part of our cultural life, those who do not abuse alcohol might have great difficulty in tolerating the attempt to restrict its distribution. For the alcoholic, treatment with drugs (except for Antabuse) holds little promise of help.

Even with pharmacologic intervention, only the most motivated alcoholics will succeed in maintaining their sobriety for any great length of time.

REFERENCES

Azrin, N.H., Bisson, R.W., Meyers, S.B., & Godley, M. (1982). Alcoholism treatment by disulfiram and community reinforcement therapy. *Journal of Behavior Therapy and Experimental Psychiatry, 13*(2), 105–121.

Ciraulo, D.A., & Jaffe, J.H. (1981). Tricyclic antidepressants in the treatment of depression associated with alcoholism. *Journal of Clinical Psychopharmacology, 1*(3), 146–156.

McMillan, T.M. (1981). Lithium and the treatment of alcoholism: A critical review. *British Journal of Addiction, 76*(3), 245–258.

Seiden, L.S., & Dykstra, L.A. (1977). *Psychopharmacology: A biochemical and behavioral approach.* New York: Van Nostrand Reinhold.

Chapter 9

Antipsychotic Medications

Craig Cooperrider

Antipsychotic medications, also known as major tranquilizers and neuroleptics, are drugs administered for the purpose of counteracting the symptoms of a number of psychotic disorders, such as those described in Chapter 6 on psychoses and schizophrenia. These drugs do not cure psychoses or schizophrenia but only bring relief to some of the symptoms of the disorder.

The development of this class of drugs has perhaps played one of the most significant roles in the history of the provision of various mental health services. It has probably made the largest contribution to the deinstitutionalization of mental patients over the last 25 years.

HISTORY

The first antipsychotic drug to be widely used was chlorpromazine (Thorazine). The discovery of its use as an antipsychotic was quite by accident. It was theorized in the late 1940s and early 1950s that certain neurotransmitters, especially histamine, were involved in the development of postsurgical shock. If a drug could be developed to block the action of these neurotransmitters, the effects of shock would be reduced. Chlorpromazine was one of the drugs tested for this purpose. Its effects, including its sleep-inducing action, sedating qualities, and safety, drew the attention of psychiatric investigators. In 1952, Jean Delay and Pierre Deniker, two French psychiatrists, began to promote chlorpromazine as a treatment for individuals experiencing psychiatric difficulties (Spiegel & Aebi, 1984).

Since that time, a number of antipsychotics have been developed. Some are similar to chlorpromazine, and others have somewhat different effects. Caldwell (1978) provides a detailed account of the development of antipsychotic medications.

CLASSIFICATION

Antipsychotic medications have a number of different forms and are classified into five major groups: phenothiazines, butyrophenones, thioxanthenes, dibenzoxazepines, and dihydroindolones (Table 9-1). Within the phenothiazine group there are three subgroups: aliphatics, piperidines, and piperazines.

THE USE OF ANTIPSYCHOTIC MEDICATIONS

Despite the success that has been obtained with the various antipsychotics, there still exists some controversy as to their merits. Many professionals are critical of these drugs because of the adverse side effects that are often witnessed in patients using antipsychotics. Even though they are widely used by various mental health services, it is important that consideration be given to identifying which individuals should and should not receive these types of medications.

When Should Antipsychotic Medications Be Considered?

A number of sources list presenting symptoms appropriate for treatment with antipsychotic medication. Denber (1979) and Levenson (1981) provide lists that

Table 9-1 Common Antipsychotic Medications

Group	Generic Name	Trade Name
Phenothiazines		
Aliphatics	Chlorpromazine *H*	Thorazine
	Trifluopromazine *M*	Vesprin
Piperidines	Thioridazine *H*	Mellaril
	Mesoridazine *H*	Serentil
Piperazines	Fluphenazine hydrochloride *L*	Prolixin Hydrochloride
	Fluphenazine enanthate *L*	Prolixin Enanthate
	Fluphenazine decanoate *L*	Prolixin Decanoate
	Perphenazine *L*	Trilafon
	Trifluoperazine *L*	Stelazine
Butyrophenones	Haloperidol *L*	Haldol
Thioxanthenes	Thiothixene *low*	Navane
	Chlorprothixene *high*	Taractan
Dibenzoxazepines	Loxapine *M*	Loxitane
Dihydroindolones	Molindone *M*	Moban

are fairly comprehensive and representative of the indications for antipsychotic therapy. Their conclusions are summarized as follows.

1. acute and chronic schizophrenia
2. delusional thinking or hallucinations (or both)
3. involutional and senile psychosis
4. childhood schizophrenia
5. moderate to severe anxiety*
6. agitated and manic states*
7. acute alcoholic psychosis
8. bipolar disorder*
9. epileptic psychoses or psychoses due to organic brain disorders
10. agitated or anxious depression*
11. psychotic acting out with a psychopathic personality
12. paranoid thinking or severe thought disorder

Obviously, these symptoms and disorders are not mutually exclusive. What is important is that the manifestation of these symptoms are indications that antipsychotic medications may be appropriate.

When Should Antipsychotic Medications Not Be Considered?

Again, Levenson (1981) and Denber (1979) are excellent resources regarding contraindications for the use of antipsychotic medications. Such medications should be avoided if any of the following symptoms or conditions is present.

1. allergic reaction to previous antipsychotic medications
2. declining central nervous system consciousness due to internal brain injury, trauma, pressure, or extracerebral causes
3. previous liver disorders
4. hypertension
5. senile deterioration with related organic disorders

Furthermore, in referrals made to medical personnel, it may be helpful to call any one of these to their attention to ensure that an appropriate medication is selected.

---

*Other psychiatric medication may be considered in combination with or in place of antipsychotics.

Which Antipsychotic Should Be Used?

As a rule, most antipsychotic medications are equally effective in their actions; that is, they reduce the debilitating effects of the symptoms of various forms of psychoses. There are, however, some rules-of-thumb to consider in the choice of an antipsychotic.

To begin, consideration should be given to what has worked and not worked in the past. If a drug has been successful in the remission of symptoms, it should be considered for use again. Likewise, where little success has been achieved, the drug should probably not be used.

The next factor concerns the patient's primary symptoms. These can be separated into two categories: thought disorders and agitation. If the main symptom group centers around disorders of thinking, paranoid ideation, looseness of association, and the like, the medication of choice should probably be one that is less sedating in nature. Examples of these are trifluoperazine, thiothixene, fluphenazine, and haloperidol. On the other hand, if the primary symptomatology is marked by anxiety and psychomotor agitation, a more sedating medication is in order. Drugs of this type are chlorpromazine, thioridazine, and trifluopromazine. Table 9-2 lists the medications given in Table 9-1, showing where each of them falls in terms of their sedative and other properties.

Another issue in choosing the appropriate antipsychotic medication is the age of the patient. With elderly individuals, a less sedating medication is generally recommended. Haloperidol has been found to be effective with older patients (Goldsmith, 1977).

Medication compliance is another important consideration. Often, for various reasons, including the prescription of multiple medications, knowledge and experience of side effects, and the feeling of remission after long periods of taking the drug, the individual discontinues use of the prescribed medication (Kane, 1983). In the case where noncompliance may be a factor, long-acting injectable medication should be considered. There are two such antipsychotic medications currently in use: fluphenazine decanoate and fluphenazine enanthate. These can be given by injection once per week or once per month, depending on the dosage administered.

Finally, the patient's reaction to the medication in terms of side effects must be considered in selecting an antipsychotic medication. One drug may produce more adverse side effects than another. This problem may be alleviated by changing the medication to one less prone to cause side effects. Table 9-2 demonstrates how the various antipsychotics fall in terms of the development of side effects.

Dosage Considerations

Obviously, in considering the use of these types of drugs, dosage is an important variable. Davidson, Sullivan, Sullivan, and Letterie (1984) stress this by stating,

Table 9-2 Characteristics of Antipsychotic Medications

Drug	Common Daily Oral Dosage (milligrams)	Sedation/ Autonomic	Extra-Pyramidal
Taractan (Chlorprothixene)	50–600	High	Moderate
Thorazine (Chlorpromazine)	100–2000	High	Moderate
Mellaril (Thioridazine)	200–600	High	Low
Serentil (Mesoridazine)	50–400	High	Low
Moban (Molindone)	50–225	Moderate	Moderate
Vesprin (Trifluopromazine)	30–200	Moderate	Moderate
Trilafon (Perphenazine)	4–64	Low	High
Loxitane (Loxapine)	50–250	Moderate	Moderate
Stelazine (Trifluoperazine)	4–80	Low	High
Prolixin Hydrochloride (Fluphenazine hydrochloride)	2–20	Low	High
Prolixin Enanthate (Fluphenazine enanthate)	12.5–25*	Low	High
Prolixin Decanoate (Fluphenazine decanoate)	12.5–25†	Low	High
Navane (Thiothixene)	2–60	Low	High
Haldol (Haloperidol)	2–100	Low	High

*Every 1 to 2 weeks. †Every 1 to 4 weeks.

''Effective treatment requires avoiding suboptimal doses as well as an overly aggressive approach'' (p. 56).

Commonly administered dosages for each medication discussed in this chapter are presented in Table 9-2, from which it is easy to see that the dosage for one drug is different from the dosage for another. Often 100 mg of chlorpromazine is used as the standard, and other medications are measured as a ratio to this standard. Furthermore, there is a large difference in dosage for drugs given orally compared to those given intramuscularly. Levenson (1981) indicates that intramuscular administrations of antipsychotics are three to four times more potent than the same dosages given orally.

Age is also an important factor in making decisions about dosage. Levenson (1981) indicates that, if the patient is less than 18 years of age or older than 60 years of age, the dosage should be one fourth to one third the normal dosage. This is due to the inadequate and undeveloped metabolic activity for those younger than 18 and the reduction in metabolic activity in elderly individuals. Other physical factors of the patient will also determine differences in the dosage related to his or her age.

The patient's physique should also be taken into account. Levenson (1981) suggests that one fourth to one third the normal dosage be administered to those of small frame. No increase is recommended for those of larger stature, however.

The time of administration is also critical for those whose condition is being maintained without severe symptoms. With these patients, consideration should be given to having the drug taken at bedtime. In this way, the sedating effects do not interfere with normal daily activities.

A final consideration is the phase of the individual's condition. During the early phase (discussed below) large dosages are administered, which are then tapered off as symptoms are reduced.

Phases of Action

It is generally agreed that antipsychotic drug treatment occurs in three phases. Denber (1979) describes these as the acute phase, the stabilization phase, and the maintenance phase. During the acute phase of treatment, it is often necessary to administer large dosages intramuscularly in order to reduce symptoms that are disruptive and harmful.

As the acute, initial symptoms diminish, treatment moves to the stabilization phase. Once symptoms are controlled or no longer present, dosages are reduced further to a maintenance level that seems to be suitable for the eventual daily routines of the patient. Time frames for these three phases are difficult to predict and are determined largely on the basis of individual response to the medication. It is critical, however, that the patient be monitored closely during the initial period so that adjustments in dosage can be made as necessary.

Antipsychotics in Combination and with Other Types of Drugs

Most over-the-counter drugs can be used safely with antipsychotics. Bockar (1976) recommends that certain drugs be avoided, however. These include alcohol, cold medications containing narcotics, and sleeping aids.

In the case where there is acute mania or hypomania accompanied by agitation and psychotic symptoms, Levenson (1981) recommends the use of antipsychotics in association with lithium. Antidepressants may also be used in conjunction with antipsychotics. This is common in the treatment of schizoaffective disorder, where there are both schizophrenic and affective symptoms. Antidepressants are also used in the treatment of postpsychotic depression. This is often done when psychotic symptoms have been reduced and an overwhelming depression becomes the major symptom (Davis & Gierl, 1984). In such cases, it is recommended that the patient be monitored closely because symptoms of depression often resemble withdrawal behaviors seen in individuals diagnosed with some form of psychosis.

Prien and Caffey (1975) make some recommendations for the combined use of antipsychotics. Their first is to avoid polypharmacy unless there is evidence that a particular drug combination would be useful. Some psychiatrists and physicians follow this advice, primarily in hopes of reducing the side effects of certain antipsychotics while increasing the actual antipsychotic effect.

Antiparkinsonism medications (drugs used in the treatment of Parkinson's disease) are often used in combination with antipsychotic medications. This is done primarily to reduce the common side effects.

What Is Gained through the Use of Antipsychotic Medications?

The primary symptoms of psychosis are reduced or lowered in intensity through the use of these medicatons. Hallucinations are eliminated, and the amount of delusional thinking and agitation is reduced. Thinking and thought processes are improved, and anxiety is decreased to a more manageable level. Delusions may persist, but the individual is not as preoccupied with them (Bockar, 1976).

MECHANISMS OF ACTION OF ANTIPSYCHOTIC MEDICATIONS

Antipsychotics, as with most psychiatric medications, have provided investigators with only clues as to how they produce their effects. There exist several commonly accepted theories that provide an explanatory account as to the effects of antipsychotics. Three of these are thoroughly discussed by Spiegel and Aebi (1984). In current practice, however, the dopamine hypothesis has emerged as the most widely accepted explanation.

The basic premise of the dopamine hypothesis states that common symptoms of various psychoses are the result of excessive levels of and activity in dopamine neurotransmission in the limbic system and various cortical areas in the brain. Antipsychotics supposedly inhibit or prevent dopamine neurotransmission in these locations. Major support for this position comes from many of the observable side effects that resemble symptoms of Parkinson's disease. Since Parkinson's disease is the result of a deficiency in dopamine in various locations in the brain, it is believed that antipsychotic medications have similar effects, that is, that they inhibit or block dopamine activity. Furthermore, the side effects associated with the use of antipsychotic medications are relieved or reduced through the use of additional medication designed to counteract the effects of Parkinson's disease. It is also known that substances that produce dopaminergic activity, when given in large dosages also produce psychotic (especially schizophrenic) symptoms. Various stimulants including amphetamines, methylphenidate, and cocaine are known to have this effect (Davis & Gierl, 1984). Even though the evidence appears to be convincing, it is far from conclusive; there are still a number of studies that show the uncertainty of this hypothesis.

As was stated earlier, numerous other theories and hypotheses exist explaining the etiology of psychosis, and especially schizophrenia, and the mechanism of action of antipsychotic medication. Some emphasize other neurotransmitters such as serotonin (Trulson & Jacobs, 1979); others suggest that antipsychotic action occurs in structures larger than the neuron. The reticular activating system, the limbic system, and the basal ganglia are implicated in these various theories (Levenson, 1981). Nevertheless, the dopamine hypothesis still seems to be the most prevalent position.

SIDE EFFECTS OF ANTIPSYCHOTIC MEDICATIONS

One of the most frequently criticized aspects of antipsychotics is the side effects that they often produce in patients (Leavitt, 1982). There is often a great deal of confusion and uncertainty regarding these side effects, which can lead to patient noncompliance with medication usage as well as ultimate relapses. Often non-medical personnel are uncertain about what to tell patients regarding side effects they are experiencing or decisions to terminate the use of medication.

Spiegel and Aebi (1984) distinguish two major classifications of side effects: vegetative and extrapyramidal.

Vegetative Side Effects

Vegetative side effects are most commonly found with medications that have potent sedating effects (see Table 9-2); sedation, drowsiness, and hindered alertness are the most common side effects of antipsychotic drugs. These particular side effects should be somewhat lessened within 2 to 3 weeks after the initiation of the medication. If a tolerance is not developed within a reasonably short period of time, this should be reported to the physician. It may be necessary to decrease the dosage or change the medication to one that is less sedating. Other vegetative side effects include the following.

Orthostatic Hypotension and Other Hypotensive Effects

A common side effect is a lowering of blood pressure; perhaps most typical is orthostatic hypotension. This phenomenon occurs when the patient moves from a seated or prone position to a standing position and experiences a corresponding decrease in blood pressure. This causes feelings of dizziness and instability due to a short-term lack of blood in the brain. Orthostatic hypotension episodes are usually of limited duration, and the patient should return to normal functioning within a short period of time.

On occasion, according to Goldsmith (1977), antipsychotic medications produce a drop in blood pressure that could be potentially fatal. When this occurs, the patient may go into shock. Epinephrine is most often used in the treatment of shock; however, it should not be used for shock caused by antipsychotics because the combination causes blood vessels to dilate, thus creating a further decrease in blood pressure. Instead, a medication such as Neo-Synephrine should be used, which tends to have a solely constricting effect on blood vessels. Generally, this type of shock may be treated by laying the patient on his or her back and elevating the legs. Goldsmith summarizes by saying simply, "Since epinephrine is often one of the first drugs resorted to in treating shock, the attending physician must be aware of the reversed epinephrine effect. If he is not aware of it (and no physician knows everything), a word from the non-medical practitioner may not only be appreciated but lifesaving" (p. 86).

Cardiac Effects

There is a great deal of controversy as to the effects of antipsychotic medications on heart functioning. Research does suggest that death due to cardiac dysfunction occurs more often in individuals receiving antipsychotic medications than in those not receiving them (Levenson, Beard, & Murphy, 1980). This occurs infrequently, however. What is known is that antipsychotics produce changes in electrocardiogram readings. Pulse rates have been known to both rise and become depressed, and various dysrhythmias have been reported. Therefore, these drugs must be used with a great deal of caution with individuals who have a history of cardiac problems.

Dry Mouth

The use of antipsychotic medications often causes the normal secretion of saliva to be reduced. This side effect usually disappears after continual use of the medication. When patients complain of this, they should be encouraged to drink water often or to chew gum.

Constipation

Antipsychotic medications reduce muscular activity within the intestinal tract. This results in constipation and may ultimately cause bowel obstruction. Bulk foods are recommended when this occurs. This side effect also should end after these medications have been used for a while.

Sexual Dysfunction

The main side effect associated with sexual dysfunction is male impotence. Goldsmith (1977) reports that this occurs most frequently with Mellaril. There may be problems with developing an erection or in the ability to ejaculate.

Extrapyramidal Side Effects

Table 9-2 lists the antipsychotic medications that have strong extrapyramidal effects. As the potency of the medication increases, so also does the likelihood of extrapyramidal side effects.

As was indicated earlier, these side effects resemble a number of the symptoms of Parkinson's disease. It is this similarity that provides some of the evidence in support of the dopamine hypothesis. It is suspected that these side effects are the result of the restriction of dopamine activity within the caudate nucleus of the brain. Antiparkinson drugs (discussed later) are particularly useful in bringing some relief to extrapyramidal side effects. The effects may also be reduced by decreasing the dosage of the antipsychotic medication.

The early administration of antipsychotic medication is marked by a number of these effects, which include rotational movements of the upper extremities (head, neck, and shoulders), tongue movements, visual spasms, and grimacing. As the length of treatment increases, so does the severity of extrapyramidal side effects. Some of the more common of these are as follows.

Akathisia

Akathisia is excessive restlessness. Often the patient cannot remain seated or in one place for any period of time. There is definitely the appearance of a great amount of anxiety. This side effect is often confused with an increase in symptoms associated with the psychosis being treated. To counter this increase in symptomatology, more medication is often prescribed, and the side effects are made worse.

Akinesia

Another extrapyramidal side effect is manifested as akinesia, which is a lack of motor activity, limited spontaneity, and seeming apathy. These symptoms generally apply to all activities of the patient.

Dystonias

The dystonias can occur at any point during the administration of antipsychotics but usually arise early in the process. They are spasms of the facial, neck, back, and ocular muscles that can be very painful.

Three types of dystonias are commonly experienced. The first is known as opisthotonus, in which the head and heels are bent backward and the body is bowed forward. Oculogyric crisis is the most common dystonia associated with the use of antipsychotic medications. This is where the muscles of the eyes force a painful stare in an upward direction. It is generally very alarming and uncomfortable to the patient. A third type of dystonia is called torticollis. In this situation, the patient's head is forced to lean and turn to one side. This can result in problems in swallowing.

Tardive Dyskinesia

The final and most severe side effect of antipsychotic medication is known as tardive dyskinesia, which is generally the result of actual brain tissue damage and as a rule is irreversible. It is usually seen in patients who have taken antipsychotics for an extended period of time, but it has been found on rare occasions in individuals who have taken the medication for a fairly short period of time. The condition is caused supposedly by overly sensitive dopamine receptors that have increased in number as a result of the long-term blockage of dopamine receptors by antipsychotics (Lemberger & Crabtree, 1979). Irreparable harm occurs at the synaptic membrane, which leads to uncontrolled firing of the neurons involved.

The symptoms begin with abnormal movements of the mouth and tongue. The tongue is often protruded, perhaps with a twisting, thrusting movement. There is also the tendency to make chewing motions. In addition, restless body movements occur in the arms and legs, with the possible presence of rocking motion.

Little is known about treatment for tardive dyskinesia. In fact, in some patients it is difficult to detect because the extreme manifestations of its symptoms are not revealed until the patient stops taking the drug for a short period of time. Often, since relief is obtained through the use of the medication, dosages are increased. This is only a short-term solution, however; usually when the dosage is increased the symptoms eventually reappear. Other drugs that affect dopamine activity, including antiparkinson medications, have been tried but with little success.

Probably the best treatment is prevention. Patients taking antipsychotic medications need to be monitored on a regular basis, and physicians should watch for some of the early signs that were noted above. Dosages must be continually adjusted to ensure that the patient is receiving the minimum medication needed to maintain stability. Occasionally, "drug holidays" are recommended to prevent the damage caused by constant antipsychotic use.

Spiegel and Aebi (1984) point out a number of the unanswered questions surrounding the problem of tardive dyskinesia. These include the following.

1. The criteria are unclear as to what actually constitutes tardive dyskinesia.
2. It is uncertain as to when tardive dyskinesia arises; it could be at any point from the time of treatment initiation to several years after discontinuation.

3. It is not certain whether these motor impairments are the result of the usual motor problems experienced in advanced age or whether they are the result of tardive dyskinesia.
4. It is not known whether tardive dyskinesia eventually remits.
5. It is not known whether certain antipsychotics are more prone to cause tardive dyskinesia than others.

Allergic Reactions

Allergic reactions are different from standard side effects. When an individual has an allergic reaction, it is caused by the immune system's attempt to counteract the introduction of a foreign substance, or antigen. As a result, the immune system produces antibodies to combat this antigen. When the antigen and the antibody combine, the cell membrane, at the point of their interaction, becomes disturbed, thereby resulting in the release of some type of cellular compound that produces the allergic reaction. Perhaps the most common of these cellular compounds is histamine. Those who suffer from hay fever or other respiratory allergies are certainly familiar with the allergic effects produced by histamine, which include itchy and watery eyes, dilatation of blood vessels, and respiratory irritation.

There are a number of skin allergies that may be produced through the use of antipsychotic medication. Rashes and hives are common. Another is referred to as exfoliative dermatitis, which is manifested by a scaling or peeling of the skin accompanied by itching and fever. If this occurs, the patient should be checked immediately by a physician (Goldsmith, 1977).

Other Effects

A common effect found with the use of antipsychotics is known as photosensitivity, which becomes evident through the development of a severe sunburn. Not only is the burn more severe in nature, but it generally occurs at a much more rapid rate than sunburn in individuals not taking antipsychotics. Mellaril does not seem to produce this effect to the extent seen with other antipsychotics. Patients should avoid excessive exposure to direct sunlight. At a minimum it is recommended that some type of sunscreen be used if long periods in direct sunlight are being considered (Mason & Granacher, 1980).

There are two endocrine disorders seen with the administration of antipsychotics. They are referred to as lactation and amenorrhea. Lactation can occur in both males and females and is manifested through enlargement of the breasts and in some cases, an actual lactation response. Amenorrhea refers to menstrual irregularities and usually the cessation of menstruation. When this occurs, pregnancy must also be ruled out. By making changes in dosage, this problem is usually corrected.

There is a greater possibility of seizure activity in individuals with convulsive disorders taking antipsychotic medication. This can be controlled to some extent through careful monitoring of the antipsychotic dosage while at the same time determining whether an appropriate amount of an anticonvulsant medication is being used. Haloperidol and molindone are not as apt to cause this sort of problem (Baldessarini, 1977).

Another effect experienced by those taking antipsychotics is an alteration in blood sugar level. Individuals who are diabetic or borderline diabetic need to be monitored closely because of the possibility of increasing the severity of the diabetes.

Changes in the eyes have also been reported. Occasionally small granules or particles develop on the corneas and lenses of patients taking antipsychotic medication. These reportedly do not hamper vision. The retina has been known to become darker, resulting in decreased night vision. Annual eye examinations should be performed for these patients.

Appetite may also be affected. Generally, patients taking antipsychotic medication report weight gain due to the fact that their appetites are increased. It is not clear that this is directly attributable to the medication on all occasions, however.

Very rarely, death may occur as a result of antipsychotic medication. The most likely situation where this could be seen is when patients undergo surgery. Surgeons, anesthetists, and other medical personnel, if they do not already know, should be alerted to the fact that the patient is taking an antipsychotic medication. Adjustments in dosage may need to be made before the surgery.

THE USE OF ANTIPARKINSON DRUGS

As was noted earlier, antiparkinson drugs are used to counteract many of the extrapyramidal side effects that arise from the use of antipsychotic medications. The most commonly used antiparkinson medications are shown in Table 9-3.

Table 9-3 Common Antiparkinson Medications

Generic Name	Name	Common Daily Dosage (milligrams)
Benztropine	Cogentin	1–5
Trihexyphenidyl	Artane	5–15
Biperiden	Akineton	2–4
Diphenhydramine hydrochloride	Benadryl	25–100

There is debate among practitioners as to how antiparkinson drugs should be used (Lydiard, Carman, & Gold, 1984). Some suggest that they should be used with nearly all patients receiving antipsychotics for preventive purposes; others suggest that they should only be used on an as-needed basis. Those who support their universal usage contend that it would increase the likelihood of compliance in taking antipsychotics if the painful and adverse side effects could be reduced or rendered nonexistent. On the other hand, it is felt that antiparkinson drugs may in effect reduce the therapeutic benefit of the antipsychotic and should be administered only when Parkinsonian symptoms arise.

In most cases, antiparkinson medications need not be used on a regular basis. Many of the extrapyramidal side effects tend to diminish as dosages are adjusted to an appropriate level for the patient. Where these side effects are problematic, physicians often prescribe an antiparkinson medication at a low dosage on an as-needed basis. It is critical that the nonmedical practitioner be aware of the extrapyramidal side effects so that, if they occur, they can be called to the attention of the physician and an antiparkinson medication can be prescribed, if appropriate.

IMPLICATIONS FOR THE NONMEDICAL PRACTITIONER

It is obvious from the preceding discussion that the use of antipsychotic medications is a complex process in the stabilization, treatment, and rehabilitation of the individual diagnosed as psychotic or schizophrenic. Nevertheless, this part of treatment cannot be ignored by nonmedical practitioners providing services to these individuals.

The Importance of Education

Perhaps the most important service related to psychopharmacology that can be provided by nonmedical staff is education. Simply providing information to patients regarding their medication can work to avoid costly interruptions in services and even possible relapses.

Antipsychotic medications have received a great deal of "negative press." When a patient is placed in a situation where he or she must take these medications, it is quite natural that fears may develop. Fears are often based on not having all the information regarding the subject, so patient education can alleviate a number of fears by simply providing facts about the drug being administered.

Specifically, patient fears are often directed toward side effects. They may have begun to experience these, or they may have been told that they exist. It is the mental health practitioner's responsibility to deal with these questions as they come up. Information about side effects can be obtained through consulting the

Physicians' Desk Reference or other publications on specific drugs, through reading pamphlets concerning the various medications that should be available from a pharmacist, or through consulting a physician, preferably a psychiatrist. Nonmedical practitioners may be able to intervene with some of the minor side effects, for example by suggesting that the patient chew gum for a dry mouth.

Patient education must also be directed at how the medication should be used. It may be helpful to explain procedures of self-administration (that is, following the directions on the prescription). Information can be provided as to why antipsychotics are prescribed and what benefits can be expected. Furthermore, it is often necessary to explain the importance of continuing to take the medication, even after discharge from an inpatient facility or when the patient begins to feel better.

The education of patients regarding dealing with their physicians is extremely important. A twofold approach is helpful here. On the one hand, it is critical that patients be aware of possible side effects and other symptoms so that they can report these to their physicians. On the other hand, patients need to be aware that as they have specific questions regarding their medications they should bring them up to their physicians during their routine medication checkups. For whatever reason, patients are often intimidated by physicians and other professionals and may not feel comfortable asking these questions. In educating patients, it may even be necessary for the nonmedical practitioner to role play and rehearse these patient-physician interactions to establish these behaviors.

Finally, it may also be helpful to educate the patient's family or residential support system. Often, family members and significant others share many of the same concerns as the patient. These close supportive networks cannot be disregarded when it comes to education regarding medication. In all likelihood, family and friends are in the best possible position to reinforce continual compliance with drug regimens. If their fears, concerns, and lack of information can be dealt with as the patient is entering or re-entering a psychopharmacological program, it could result in more support for appropriate self-administration of medication and ultimate compliance.

Questions To Ask

Many nonmedical practitioners often do not see a patient until long after the patient has been stabilized with medication. In providing effective outpatient treatment planning, however, it is crucial that certain questions be considered that are related to the individual's antipsychotic drug use. These include the following.

1. What medication(s) is the patient taking?
2. What are the dosages of each of the medications? How is the medication administered (periodic injection, orally)?

3. What are the subjective effects (good and bad)? What does the patient experience as a result of these medications?
4. Who is the prescribing physician?
5. Does the patient take any antiparkinson medication? What are the dosages? Is this on an "as-needed" basis?
6. How does the medication affect the patient's current functioning?
7. What implications will these medications have for future functioning?
8. How long has the patient taken the medication? Were there medications previous to the one being currently used?
9. Does the patient take any type of medication other than antipsychotic(s)?
10. How does the patient feel about continued compliance? Does the patient take medication responsibly?
11. How often does the patient see the prescribing physician?
12. Are Parkinsonian side effects so devastating that the patient should be considered for antiparkinson medication?
13. Are there any concerns related to the medications that should be reported to the prescribing physician?
14. Can the patient afford the medication?

These questions are intended to serve only as a guide in interviews with patients. It is only through asking and exploring these areas with patients that this information may surface and ultimately contribute to the effectiveness of treatment.

The Problem of Noncompliance

As mentioned earlier, noncompliance can be addressed through the use of injectable long-acting medication as well as through patient education. Diamond (1983) states that this problem is not always one of resistance or mistaken dosages but may be the result of the patient desiring to gain further control of his or her life.

In order to deal effectively with this issue, practitioners must personalize the use of medication. The emphasis must be placed not on right and wrong but on the individual having a part in decisions made regarding medication. Primarily this may take the form of the educational strategies discussed above, but it may also simply involve some behavioral contracting so that patients agree to continue the use of the medication until their next visit with the psychiatrist. At that time, they should be encouraged to "make their case" regarding their concerns about their medication.

CONCLUSIONS

Even though the use of antipsychotic medication is primarily a medical responsibility, the nonmedical practitioner must be aware of the implications of their clients or patients being treated with these drugs. Effective services require that the practitioner be aware of how these medications are used and what to expect in the behavior of patients taking these drugs. Furthermore, the nonmedical practitioner can play a key role in the education of patients or clients in the use of antipsychotics. This then becomes a major part of the patient's achievement of success in his or her treatment.

REFERENCES

Baldessarini, R.J. (1977). *Chemotherapy in psychiatry.* Cambridge, MA: Harvard University Press.

Bockar, J.A. (1976). *Primer for the nonmedical psychotherapist.* New York: Spectrum.

Caldwell, A.E. (1978). History of psychopharmacology. In W.G. Clark & J. DelGiudice (Eds.), *Principles of psychopharmacology* (pp. 9–40). New York: Academic Press.

Davidson, J., Sullivan, J.L., Sullivan, P.D., & Letterie, M.M. (1984). Chemotherapy of schizophrenia. In J.L. Sullivan & P.D. Sullivan (Eds.), *Biomedical psychiatric therapeutics* (pp. 55-70). Boston: Butterworth.

Davis, J.M., & Gierl, B. (1984). Pharmacological treatment in the care of schizophrenic patients. In A.S. Bellack (Ed.), *Schizophrenia: Treatment, management, and rehabilitation* (pp. 133–173). Orlando, FL: Grune & Stratton.

Denber, H.C.B. (1979). *Textbook of clinical psychopharmacology.* New York: Stratton.

Diamond, R.J. (1983). Enhancing medication use in schizophrenic patients. *Journal of Clinical Psychiatry, 44*, 7–14.

Goldsmith, W. (1977). *Psychiatric drugs for the non-medical mental health worker.* Springfield, IL: Charles C Thomas.

Kane, J.M. (1983). Problems of compliance in the outpatient treatment of schizophrenia. *Journal of Clinical Psychiatry, 44*, 3–6.

Leavitt, F. (1982). *Drugs and behavior.* New York: Wiley.

Lemberger, L., & Crabtree, R.E. (1979). Pharmacologic effects in man of a potent, long-acting dopamine receptor agonist. *Science, 205.*

Levenson, A.J. (1981). *Basic psychopharmacology.* New York: Springer.

Levenson, A.J., Beard, O.W., & Murphy, M.L. (1980). Major tranquilizers and heart disease: To use or not use. *Geriatrics, 35*, 55–61.

Lydiard, R.B., Carman, J.S., & Gold, M.S. (1984). Antipsychotics: Predicting response/maximizing efficacy. In M.S. Gold, R.B. Lydiard, & J.S. Carman (Eds.), *Advances in psychopharmacology: Predicting and improving treatment response* (pp. 179–224). Boca Raton, FL: CRC Press.

Mason, A.S., & Granacher, R.P. (1980). *Clinical handbook of antipsychotic drug therapy.* New York: Brunner/Mazel.

Prien, R., & Caffey, E. (1975). Guidelines for antipsychotic drug use. *Resident Staff Physician, 9*, 165–172.

Spiegel, R., & Aebi, H.J. (1984). *Psychopharmacology.* Chichester: Wiley.

Trulson, M.E., & Jacobs, B.L. (1979). Long-term amphetamine treatment decreases brain serotonin metabolism: Implications for theories of schizophrenia. *Science, 205*, 1295–1297.

Chapter 10

Antidepressants

Craig Cooperrider

Despite the controversy and debate that have gone on for many years regarding the treatment of depression, it cannot be denied that the use of antidepressant medication has shown successful results. The positive response of depressed patients, particularly those experiencing an endogenous (chronic, nonreactive, and internally caused) depression, to these drugs cannot be disregarded. As was pointed out previously, the extensive research of Beck, Rush, Shaw, and Emery (1979) indicates that there is the need for both drug therapy and psychotherapy in the treatment of different forms of depression. In many cases, treatment is enhanced by making both therapies available.

The purpose of this chapter is to explore the common practices of physicians and psychiatrists in the pharmacological treatment of depression. The information presented encompasses a broad range of topics related to antidepressant medications. To provide some perspective, the history of the development of antidepressants is considered. Factors affecting the use of these drugs and their classification then follow. A special section dealing with electroconvulsive therapy is included because this approach is often used in conjunction with antidepressant therapy in the treatment of depressive disorders. Finally, consideration is given to the implications of these drugs for the nonmedical practitioner.

HISTORY

Before the discovery of antidepressant medications, few drugs were used to treat depression. Stimulants were employed to some extent but were never found to be significantly effective, especially in treating cases of endogenous depression. It was not until 1952 that progress in the development of antidepressant medication began to be made (Spiegel & Aebi, 1984). At that time, a compound known as iproniazid was used in the treatment of tuberculosis; it was noted that patients taking this compound experienced changes in mood and disposition that were not congruent with their symptoms. Eventually, this compound was tried with certain psychiatric disorders such as schizophrenia, but it had limited success. As trials with this drug continued it was found to have a stimulating effect but also dangerous side effects. Iproniazid, as well as other compounds similar to it, was eventually withdrawn from testing in the United States because of its harmful effects but was continued in other countries as a treatment for depression.

At about the same time, Roland Kuhn, a Swiss psychiatrist, began testing a group of drugs known as thymoleptics for their sedating and calming effects. It was found that these drugs did reduce some agitation, delusions, and hallucinations in schizophrenic patients. The similarities between the results obtained with these compounds and those obtained with chlorpromazine were further examined in the hope of finding a less expensive medication that produced results similar to those of chlorpromazine. Although the outcomes showed chlorpromazine to be most effective in the treatment of schizophrenic symptoms, it was discovered in 1957 that one of these thymoleptics, which was later named imipramine, had remarkable effects on the classical symptoms of endogenous depression. In some cases the drug produced these effects within days or weeks, and the investigators determined that if therapy was discontinued too soon there was a possibility of relapse (Spiegel & Aebi, 1984). Thus the development of antidepressant treatment began.

CLASSIFICATION OF ANTIDEPRESSANTS

Antidepressants similar to iproniazid are known as monoamine oxidase inhibitors (MAOIs) because of their supposed method of action within the brain. Medications similar to imipramine are referred to as tricyclic antidepressants. The tricyclics are the most widely used today, particularly in the United States, but MAOIs are available and are sometimes used in treatment. It should be noted at the outset of discussion that antidepressants work in a manner different from stimulants, in that stimulants produce a euphoric disposition that does not typically occur with the antidepressants.

Tricyclic Antidepressants

The chemical structure of tricyclics is similar to that of the phenothiazines, which are antipsychotics, but their effects are very different. The commonly used tricyclic antidepressants are listed in Table 10-1.

Table 10-1 Common Tricyclic* Antidepressants and Their Therapeutic Dosages

Generic Name	Trade Name(s)	Dosage (mg/day)
Imipramine	Tofranil	100– 300
	Janimine	
	SK-Pramine	
	Presamine	
Amitriptyline	Elavil	100– 300
	Endep	
Amoxapine**	Asendin	200–1400
Desipramine	Norpramin	100– 300
	Pertofrane	
Doxepin	Adapin	100– 400
	Sinequan	
Maprotiline**	Ludiomil	75– 150
Nortriptyline	Aventyl	50– 150
	Pamelor	
Protriptyline	Vivactil	15– 60
Trazodone**	Desyrel	100– 300

*Not all these drugs are truly tricyclic; it is perhaps more appropriate to refer to them as "heterocyclic."
**Heterocyclic.

When Should Tricyclic Antidepressants Be Considered?

Tricyclic antidepressants are effective in the treatment of endogenous depression and its corresponding symptoms. Denber (1979) notes that they should be considered especially when the depression is marked by motor retardation. They have been found to be useful in cases of involutional melancholia, senile depression, and psychotic depression where delusional thinking is not prominant. Many of the classic depressive symptoms including withdrawal, rumination, sleep disturbance, agitation, and anxiety can be relieved through the use of tricyclics.

When Should Tricyclics Not Be Used?

Levenson (1981) suggests that tricyclics should not be considered if the patient has experienced a previous allergic reaction to these or similar drugs. They should also not be used if the patient is losing consciousness as a result of physical difficulties. Denber (1979) also adds that they should not be used with individuals experiencing borderline disorders, schizophrenia in remission, cardiac disorders, and psychotic depression with severe delusional thinking.

Which Tricyclic Should Be Used?

In considering the merits of one drug over another it is commonly accepted that the tricyclics are all equally effective. Some minor differences should be mentioned, however. Some tricyclics are more likely to cause drowsiness, and others may produce greater anticholinergic effects (such as dry mouth, blurred vision, or constipation).

Concerning the issue of their soporific qualities, in patients demonstrating a sleep disturbance or even possible agitation, it may be necessary to use a drug such as imipramine or amitriptyline, both of which have been shown to be sedating. In cases where the patient has difficulty remaining alert, however, a less sedating drug such as protriptyline or nortriptyline should be considered.

Individuals experiencing anticholinergic effects may need to be prescribed a drug with less anticholinergic potential. Doxepin and amitriptyline tend to produce greater anticholinergic effects, whereas desipramine produces the least.

Dosage Considerations

There are fairly wide ranges among some of the tricyclics in terms of the dosage that can be administered (see Table 10-1). There are several items to consider when selecting the appropriate dosage to be administered.

First, all these drugs come in oral (tablet or capsule) form; only a small number of them are also available in liquid or injectable form. Furthermore, it is not at all uncommon for 2 weeks or more to elapse before there is a noticeable reduction in symptoms. It is critical that the appropriate dosage be chosen, because less than desired results will be obtained if too little or too much of the drug is administered.

Sullivan, Taska, Wise, and Goldstein (1984) offer a number of helpful guidelines regarding the selection of appropriate dosages in the administration of tricyclics. They begin by recommending an initial dosage of the chosen drug of 50 mg/day. The dosage is then increased every other day in intervals of 50 mg until approximately 150 to 200 mg (or a normal therapeutic dosage) is being administered per day. The patient is then maintained at this dosage for 2 to 3 weeks. The dosage is then increased as necessary up to the maximum amount noted in Table 10-1 (it is not increased once therapeutic gain is detected). These authors also recommend that the medication be given at night to ensure patient compliance and to avoid problems associated with sedation.

Recently a great deal of research has been done in the area of monitoring the blood plasma levels of these drugs in patients. It is believed that a range of the amount of the drug in the bloodstream can be determined that would constitute a therapeutically effective dosage. This range is referred to as a therapeutic window. This range has only been found to exist for a few of the tricyclic antidepressants such as nortriptyline and desipramine, however. Ideally, then, in determining the amount of an antidepressant to prescribe or whether to increase or decrease the dosage, the blood would be assayed to measure the amount of the drug present. If that amount was within the therapeutic window, it would be likely that the correct dosage was being administered. If the concentration was outside this range, however, the dosage would probably be too high or too low for optimum therapeutic benefit. The ability to perform this type of measurement is far from perfected, but investigators are obtaining positive results with some of these drugs (Risch, Janowsky, & Huey, 1981). Blood levels for the other antidepressants seem to be more linear in nature; that is, there is an exact therapeutic level. So long as the blood level is above this amount, but not at the toxic level, a therapeutic response will be obtained.

DeLisi (1984) indicates that blood plasma levels should be checked closely when patients are not responding to the medication after several weeks at conventional dosages in order to determine whether the patient is complying and to prevent the possibility of an overdose. Blood levels should also be monitored in elderly patients and in those who have had cardiovascular illnesses.

The age and stature of the patient must also be taken into account. Levenson (1981) suggests that patients younger than 18 years of age and those older than 60 receive one-fourth to one-third the normal dosage. These differences are attributed to immature metabolic functioning in young patients and to a lowering of metabolic activity in elderly patients. Persons of small stature should receive one-fourth to one-third the commonly administered amounts; for those of large stature the dosage should not be increased but remain consistent with normal prescribing practices.

Tricyclic antidepressants should never be withdrawn abruptly; the effects can be severe and include nausea, headache, chills, fatigue, akathisia, and muscle pains (Denber, 1979). Instead, as the patient enters remission and maintains at that level, the drug should be withdrawn at a rate of 25 to 50 mg/week until the smallest therapeutic dosage for maintenance is determined. The amount of the maintenance dosage and the length of time for which the patient receives it is an individual choice determined by the patient's long-term response to the medication.

Tricyclic Antidepressants in Combination with Other Drugs

As was the case with antipsychotic medications, tricyclics can usually be taken safely in combination with most over-the-counter medications. Nevertheless, drugs such as alcohol, sleeping aids, narcotics, and some cough preparations should be avoided. Patients who are receiving medication for blood pressure or other cardiovascular disorders should bring this to the attention of the prescribing physician. Interactions of these drugs could at least reduce the effects of both and at most be seriously dangerous.

Denber (1979) states that combining an antipsychotic with a tricyclic antidepressant is "not particularly effective in the treatment of anxious depression"

(p. 120). Drugs have been developed that combine an antipsychotic with a tricyclic antidepressant (Bockar, 1976), but the effectiveness of these agents is questionable. On the other hand, Denber does suggest the use of a tricyclic with an antianxiety medication if the anxiety is significant and present from the beginning of treatment.

Denber (1979) reports that certain tricyclics have been tried in combination with other tricyclics. The results have been fairly positive with such symptoms as hypochondriasis, apathy, insomnia, flattened affects, and depression, and minimal side effects have been reported. The tricyclics have also been administered in combination with the thyroid hormone known as T3. This is particularly recommended for those who do not respond to a tricyclic alone.

How Do Tricyclic Antidepressants Work?

Knowledge regarding the mechanisms of antidepressant action is limited, and the results of research in the area are conflicting. Two hypotheses are widely accepted: the catecholamine hypothesis and the serotonin hypothesis (see Spiegel & Aebi, 1984).

The catecholamine hypothesis, proposed by Schildkraut (1965), maintains that depression is caused by a deficiency in the amount of catecholamines at various neuron receptor sites in the brain. Catecholamine substances are one group of neurotransmitters, and norepinephrine is the major catecholamine neurotransmitter that is deficient according to this hypothesis. Drugs such as imipramine and other tricyclics are thought to prevent the uptake of norepinephrine back into the firing neuron once it has been released into the synapse. In other words, tricyclics maintain greater concentrations of norepinephrine in the synaptic cleft after the firing of a neuron.

What precipitated these studies was the observation that antihypertensive drugs such as reserpine reduced brain concentrations of norepinephrine, which in turn produced effects resembling depression. When imipramine was administered after reserpine, it ultimately had an antidepressant effect. Thus it is thought that the action of tricyclic antidepressants is largely due to the maintenance of norepinephrine levels in the synapse. It is believed that this occurs within the areas of the midbrain dealing with reward and arousal, namely the amygdala and the reticular formation (Goldsmith, 1977).

The serotonin hypothesis, first proposed by Coppen (1967), maintains that some forms of depression are due to a lack of serotonin, another neurotransmitter, in the brain stem. Spiegel and Aebi (1984) list a number of research findings supporting not only this hypothesis but also the catecholamine hypothesis. Serotonin and chemicals involved in its metabolism have been found to be reduced in cerebrospinal fluid of individuals experiencing depression. Precursors of serotonin and inhibitors of its uptake have been found to have antidepressant effects. Tricyclics, such as imipramine, prevent the uptake of serotonin from the synaptic cleft to the firing neuron, as is the case with the catecholamine norepinephrine.

Although these hypotheses have some support from research, there is still considerable controversy as to whether they adequately describe all the causal factors related to depression and the effects obtained with antidepressants. As Goldsmith (1977) states,

> The fact is that theories of action of all the psychotropic drugs are based on our present incomplete knowledge of normal brain function, especially with respect to neurotransmitters. The theories are useful models, but, will probably be proven wrong or, at best, only approximately correct. (p. 110)

Perhaps a more integrated approach is necessary. One criticism of these two positions is that they do not consider the balance between neurotransmission systems in the brain. Neurotransmitters work in conjunction with each other, and one cannot be changed without modifying another. In view of this, it has been proposed that depression is not only due to serotonin and norepinephrine deficiency but also to increased acetylcholine transmission. This position not only accounts for the previous two but also considers the anticholinergic effects of antidepressants. Thus it represents a more plausible position emphasizing the interaction of the various neurotransmitters.

Side Effects of Tricyclic Antidepressants

As noted above, the most prominent and frequently occurring side effects of tricyclic antidepressants are anticholinergic in nature. Goldsmith (1977) and Sullivan et al. (1984) recommend a drug known as bethanecol chloride for relief of anticholinergic side effects such as dry mouth, constipation, and urinary retention.

The most severe and dangerous side effects related to tricyclic use are cardiovascular problems. Orthostatic hypotension is common among users of tricyclic medication. Other cardiovascular effects can be much more serious; these include the potential for myocardial infarction and disruption in the heart beat, even to the point of cardiac arrest in the case of an overdose. Tofranil and Elavil produce cardiac problems more often than some of the other tricyclics. Sinequan has been found to be not as potentially dangerous as far as cardiac problems are concerned and is more frequently prescribed for elderly patients for this reason (Goldsmith, 1977).

Currently, there is still much controversy and discussion regarding tricyclic antidepressants and their effects on cardiovascular functioning. Orthostatic hypotension is a well-documented symptom, but the relation of these drugs to other cardiac symptoms is uncertain. Sullivan and co-workers (1984) even document research demonstrating cardiovascular improvement in patients taking tricyclics who have previously experienced heart conditions. At this point, it is probably safe to conclude that various cardiac irregularities should be watched for in patients receiving tricyclic antidepressants.

A number of other side effects have been noted with the use of tricyclics. Occasionally, patients will report hallucinations, delusions, or other psychotic symptoms. These are believed to be due primarily to the imbalance in neurotransmitters caused by changes in acetylcholine activity in the brain. It is rare that patients experience extrapyramidal side effects, which are common with antipsychotic medication, even though tricyclics are structurally similar to many of the antipsychotics. Generally, when extrapyramidal effects do occur it is only after the patient has been taking tricyclics for a considerable length of time. Tremors, dizziness, ataxia, and a lower seizure threshold are other neurological side effects that are reported on rare occasions.

Goldsmith (1977) also discusses the possibility of overdose, which cannot be discounted given the nature of depression. Some symptoms of a tricyclic overdose include disorientation, delusions, hallucinations, anxiety, confusion, and possible seizures. There is a rapid heart rate, dilatation of the pupils, increased body temperature, decreased salivation, urinary retention, and possible cardiac dysrhythmias. This type of overdose can be treated with a drug known as physostigmine, which counteracts the enzyme that destroys acetylcholine, thereby allowing it to begin building up again.

Monoamine Oxidase Inhibitors

The MAOI antidepressants were discovered before the tricyclics, but they were not seriously considered for use in the United States because of some of their more serious effects. The debate has gone on for several years regarding the use of MAOIs. Some research results suggest that MAOIs are little better than placebos, while others indicate that they have been misrepresented and underused.

The MAOIs are of two different types: hydrazine and nonhydrazine derivatives. Both types have certain drawbacks. Those derived from hydrazine are known to produce toxic effects on the liver. The nonhydrazine derivatives are similar to stimulants such as amphetamines; besides their typical antidepressant effects, they may produce some excitement, agitation, and even euphoria. Table 10-2 lists the commonly used MAOIs.

When Should MAOIs Be Considered?

Moreines and Gold (1984) review a number of studies attempting to determine whether there are particular symptoms or disorders for which MAOIs are

Table 10-2 Common MAOI Antidepressants and Their Therapeutic Dosages

Generic Name	Trade Name	Dosage (mg/day)
Hydrazine Type		
Isocarboxazid	Marplan	10–50
Phenelzine	Nardil	45–75
Nonhydrazine Type		
Tranylcypromine	Parnate	10–30

especially effective. This is not always easy to assess because of imprecise diagnostic standards, but some conclusions have been formed.

MAOIs are indicated in the treatment of endogenous depression only after tricyclics and tricyclics with other medications (thyroid hormones or central nervous system stimulants, for example) have been used with no response following normal prescribing practices. They are considered a second line of treatment and have demonstrated some effectiveness. The MAOIs have been shown to be considerably effective in treating atypical depression, which is depression accompanied by a major anxiety component or a lack of vegetative symptoms. They are sometimes used in the treatment of bipolar depression and may be used in conjunction with lithium. They have been used successfully in treating some of the depressive symptoms seen in borderline personality disorders. Panic disorders, narcolepsy, depression associated with schizophrenia, schizoaffective disorders (when treated together with neuroleptics), and other depressive disorders not responding to tricyclics represent additional conditions that may be treatable with MAOIs. The evidence is not strong related to these last conditions, however.

Obviously, there are a number of conditions that do lend themselves fairly well to treatment with MAOIs. In considering the use of MAOIs, Nies and Robinson (1982) state

> The last decade has seen a reawakening of interest in the MAO inhibitors and they are now known to be extraordinarily effective in the treatment of several neurotic syndromes, showing both anti-anxiety and anti-depressant effects. Their reputation for lack of efficacy is no longer warranted and with proper precautions they can be used with safety. Their most appropriate use is in agoraphobia and in chronic atypical and non-endogenous depressions. (p. 259)

When Should MAOIs Not Be Used?

MAOIs should not be administered to individuals with chronic alcoholism. Individuals with liver disorders, serious allergies to drugs, severe headaches or migraines, pheochromocytoma, or epilepsy should not be prescribed MAOIs. They are also contraindicated for persons with cardiovascular or cerebrovascular disorders (Denber, 1979).

Which MAOI Should Be Used?

In the past, a number of hydrazine derivatives were removed from the market in the United States because of their potentially toxic effects (Nies & Robinson, 1982). Those listed in Table 10-2, however, are still available and are currently in use.

It is questionable whether one MAOI is more effective than another; most research concludes that all MAOIs are equivalent in their effects. If one has failed, it is unlikely that another will succeed (Bockar, 1976). Nevertheless, a 2-week interval should separate the use of different medications. Moreines and Gold (1984) recommend starting with phenelzine and then moving eventually to tranylcypromine in the event of a partial or limited response to phenelzine. These circumstances require close monitoring because of the dangers associated with these drugs. Certainly, knowledge of the activity of MAOIs is limited and speculative at this time.

Dosage Considerations

The therapeutic dosage ranges for the commonly prescribed MAOIs are listed in Table 10-2. As with any medication, the appropriate dosage is critically important; in fact, one of the major criticisms of research comparing tricyclics with MAOIs is that adequate dosages were not used.

The primary activity of MAOIs is to inhibit the action of an enzyme known as monoamine oxidase. In order for a MAOI to be effective, it must be administered in a dosage that will inhibit 80% to 90% of monoamine oxidase activity (Raft, Davidson, Wasik, & Mattox, 1981). This is measured through assays of blood platelets, which is possible to do with the hydrazine MAOIs but not as effective with the nonhydrazine types.

The use of MAOIs in therapy is an extremely complicated, and in many respects, an experimental process. In selecting an appropriate dosage, Moreines and Gold (1984) suggest a number of prescribing instructions. To begin, phenelzine should be administered at 15 mg two times per day. This should be increased by 15 mg/day every 5 days up to a maximum of 60 mg/day at the end of 2 weeks. This dosage should be maintained for 2 weeks, at which time platelets should be assayed. The dosage should be adjusted to obtain an 80% to 90% inhibition of monoamine oxidase activity. That dosage is then maintained for an additional 2 weeks. It may be necessary to increase the dosage to as much as 90 mg/day, but the physician must be cautious so as to avoid complete inhibition of monoamine oxidase. In the case of a partial response, drugs such as lithium carbonate or L-tryptophan may be used as adjuncts to the MAOI therapy; tryptophan should be used only on a limited basis because monoamine oxidase activity should not be completely inhibited. The medication should be discontinued if there is no response within 2 weeks, and then no medication should be given for an additional 2 weeks. The physician may then wish to try a tricyclic antidepressant, a tricyclic plus a MAOI, or tranylcypromine, depending on the patient's previous response to treatment with MAOIs and tricyclics.

MAOIs in Combination with Other Drugs

Aside from liver toxicity, which was mentioned above, the major drawback to the use of MAOIs is related to their interaction with other drugs. Originally it was considered extremely dangerous to mix tricyclics with MAOIs, but it is now believed that such a combination can be appropriate as long as the drugs are prescribed judiciously in recommended dosages. Side effects are often greater than those reported when the drugs are used alone. This combination is one to consider if single use of either of the drugs has been only partial. It is usually necessary to wait 2 weeks before proceeding with a combination of this type.

MAOIs do not interact favorably with a number of other drugs, both prescription and over-the-counter, including antihistamines, decongestants, and hay fever or allergy medications (see Table 10-3). As a rule of thumb, anyone taking MAOIs should consult his or her physician before taking any other medications.

Table 10-3 Drugs That Should Not Be Used in Combination with MAOIs

Amphetamines and other sympathomimetics
Other MAOIs*
Tricyclic antidepressants*
L-Tryptophan*
Antihistamines
Decongestants (Ephedrine)
Cold, allergy, and hay fever medications
Cocaine, LSD, PCP
Alcohol
Antiparkinsonism medications and L-dopa (dopamine)
Neo-Synephrine (phenylephrine)
Insulin
Demerol (meperidine)
Antihypertensive drugs (guanethidine, α-methyldopa, reserpine)
Caffeine
Psychotropic medications
Diet medications

*These drugs can be administered in combination with MAOIs only if certain designated procedures are followed.

Furthermore, patients should be instructed to alert other physicians and dentists to the fact that they are being treated with MAOIs.

How Do MAOIs Work?

The activity of MAOIs is comparable to that of tricyclics. Monoamine oxidase is an enzyme responsible for the metabolism of a number of neurotransmitters, including norepinephrine and serotonin. Its activity generally occurs within the neuron. MAOIs actively work to prevent this action, thus enabling high concentrations of the neurotransmitters to accumulate within the neuron. It is believed that this leads to additional amounts of these substances in the area of the synapse at the time of actual neurotransmission.

Side Effects of MAOIs

The major side effects of MAOIs relate to medication restrictions, as noted above (see Table 10-3), and dietary restrictions. Table 10-4 lists many of the foods that should not be eaten while taking MAOIs; patient education and encouragement along these lines are critical.

The problematic substance in many of the foods noted in Table 10-4 is tyramine, which upon entering the body is eventually metabolized by monoamine oxidase in the liver or the intestine. Because of the inhibition of monoamine oxidase activity caused by MAOIs, tyramine continues to circulate and is not metabolized appropriately. When this occurs norepinephrine concentrations increase, leading eventually to blood vessel constriction, increased heart rate, and increased blood pressure. There is the potential that a blood vessel in the brain

---

Table 10-4 Foods That Should Not Be Consumed While Taking a MAOI

Most cheeses (excluding cream cheese and cottage cheese)
Aged and tenderized meats
Beer, wine (excluding white), and other alcoholic beverages
Liver
Yeast (except as used in breads and baked products)
Broad bean pods
Bananas
Chocolate
Beverages containing caffeine (coffee, tea, and colas)
Sour cream
Canned figs
Raisins
Herring
Soy sauce
Avocados

could rupture, resulting in stroke. This effect is also seen when sympathomimetic drugs (those simulating the sympathetic nervous system responses) are taken, producing a hypertensive reaction since the drug is not being effectively metabolized because of the MAOI (Goldsmith, 1977). If a patient complains of headache, dizziness, or rapid pulse while taking a MAOI, his or her blood pressure should be measured. If it is high, phentolamine should be administered, which counteracts the effects noted above by blocking the action of norepinephrine.

Not only should patients not consume certain foods and drugs while taking the MAOI, but they should wait at least 2 weeks after discontinuing treatment before again partaking of these substances. The reason is that it takes approximately 2 weeks to begin building up new supplies of monoamine oxidase.

Beyond food and drug ingestion as possible causes of side effects, the problem of liver toxicity must also be considered. Hydrazine MAOIs have been found to produce harmful effects to the liver, even though the incidence is relatively infrequent. The liver's functioning therefore should be routinely checked.

A number of patients experience some form of sleep disorder. This may include either insomnia or waking from sleep more often. Sleep disorders are often corrected by a change in the time that the medication is given.

Anticholinergic side effects, as discussed with the tricyclics, are not as apparent with MAOIs. Dry mouth, urinary retention, constipation, blurred vision, and sexual dysfunction are all possibilities, but their frequency is not as high as with the tricyclics. Many of the same remedies, with support and reassurance, can be used to alleviate some of these difficulties.

The primary cardiovascular side effect is orthostatic hypotension; the other cardiovascular irregularities discussed in relation to the tricyclics do not seem to arise with MAOIs. The absence of these effects makes this a more suitable antidepressant medication for patients who have a history of cardiac problems.

There may be a tendency in some patients toward an increase in appetite and a corresponding gain in weight. This problem can often be resolved by simply removing high-caloric foods from the patient's living situation or by lowering the dosage of the drug or discontinuing it if necessary.

Finally, the possibility of overdose is a serious problem. Moreines and Gold (1984) report that the lethal dosage is a 1-week supply of the normal therapeutic amount (which is not much). They indicate that symptoms of an overdose include agitation, hallucinations, hyperreflexia, hyperpyrexia, confusion, and convulsions. These symptoms all demand immediate medical treatment.

Other Antidepressants

It was pointed out in Table 10-1 that there are a number of antidepressants that produce effects similar to those of tricyclics but, because of their chemical structure, technically should be referred to as heterocyclics. There are some other medications that do not fall into the categories of the tricyclics (or heterocyclics) or the MAOIs but have been found to produce antidepressant effects. These include iprindole, mianserin, trazodone, bupropion, and alprazolam (Sullivan et al., 1984). These drugs do not seem to work in the same manner as the other antidepressants discussed above. Alprazolam (Xanax) has traditionally been used as an antianxiety agent, but some evidence suggests its effectiveness as an antidepressant as well, particularly in cases where depression and anxiety are both present and in reported moderate depression (Feighner, Aden, Fabre, Rickels, & Smith, 1983).

There is still a great deal of uncertainty surrounding the use of drugs that are not traditional antidepressants. The main reason for their use over the more common types relates to the idea, yet to be conclusively verified, that they may produce fewer undesirable side effects, especially anticholinergic and cardiovascular side effects.

ELECTROCONVULSIVE THERAPY AND THE USE OF ANTIDEPRESSANTS

The use of electroconvulsive therapy (ECT) or shock therapy has undergone a resurgence over the last decade. It was originally developed as a way to treat schizophrenic disorders on the basis of the theory that schizophrenia and epilepsy were "mutually antagonistic" (Kiloh, 1982). Originally, convulsant medications were used to induce convulsions because it was thought that if epilepsy-like convulsions could be created schizophrenic symptoms could be reduced. This mode of treatment, via drug-induced or electrically produced convulsions, was used until the 1950s, when the psychoactive drugs began to be used for treatment of mental and emotional disorders.

ECT does have some demonstrated effectiveness, primarily in the treatment of depression. According to Weiner (1984): "ECT is clearly the most effective treatment for major depressive episodes available to psychiatry at the current time" (p. 72). It appears that its effectiveness diminishes with less severe forms of depression. Its use as a first choice of treatment is in cases where prolonged drug trials could be detrimental to the patient; examples of this include actively suicidal individuals, those experiencing active delusions and hallucinations, and those for whom drug therapy may be contraindicated because of certain physical restrictions.

Weiner (1984) emphasizes the fact that ECT does not cure depression or any of the other disorders treated by it but instead brings about a remission, as do psychotropic drugs including antidepressants. Maintenance of remission is typically achieved through a gradual tapering of ECT treatments. The use of antidepressant medications after treatment by ECT has been found to be effective in preventing relapse and in maintaining gains (Seager & Bird, 1962). It is questionable, however, as to whether providing ECT and antidepressants simultaneously works to decrease the number of necessary treatments. For additional information regarding the clinical use and application of ECT, see Fink (1979), Palmer (1981), and Abrams and Essman (1982).

IMPLICATIONS FOR THE NONMEDICAL PRACTITIONER

Much of the discussion from the previous chapter about the implications of using antipsychotic medication applies to those working with patients who are using antidepressants, particularly with regard to patient education. It cannot be emphasized enough that the nonmedical practitioner should assume the responsibility of providing information to patients. Such educative efforts can indeed serve to prevent interruptions in treatment, increase the likelihood of patient stabilization, and prevent possible relapses. Providing information and dealing with patients' concerns regarding side effects are both extremely important. The nonmedical practitioner can obtain this information from various sources, so that as these concerns arise the practitioner will be in a position to address them.

When antidepressants, in particular the MAOIs, are in use it is especially important that the therapist support and reinforce the warnings that patients may have received from their pharmacist or physician about avoiding certain foods and drugs. As a precautionary measure, it certainly does not hurt to ask patients receiving MAOIs whether they are aware of the various food and drug items that they should not consume.

Other questions regarding antidepressants that frequently come up relate to their effects. Patients may anticipate effects comparable to those of "uppers" because of the misconception that antidepressants produce a "high" or euphoria. They may also anticipate results in a short period of time, and they may need to be informed or reminded that it often takes a minimum of 2 weeks for antidepressants to begin working. Some initial education may prevent noncompliance due to frustration from a lack of expected or immediate results. It is also important to teach patients to communicate their experiences with the antidepressants they are using to their physicians or psychiatrists. If they experience problems that they feel are related to their medication, they should discuss these concerns with their physicians.

Family members and other supportive individuals should also be educated about the therapeutic process. Education for these close individuals must be along the lines of providing reinforcement to the patient for compliance and of dealing with the patient's fears and misconceptions regarding the use of antidepressants.

Questions To Ask

In order to be completely effective, the nonmedical practitioner should inquire about the following.

1. What medication is the patient taking?
   What type of antidepressant is it?
2. What are the dosages of each medication?
3. What effects is the patient reporting? (These include positive, curative, and side effects.)
4. Who is the prescribing physician?
5. Does the patient have any other health impairments that could be complicated by using an antidepressant medication (e.g., cardiac conditions or liver problems)?
6. If the patient is taking a MAOI, have all food and drug warnings been issued? Is the patient following these instructions?
7. Is the patient taking any other medication?
8. How does the medication affect the patient's current functioning?
9. What implications will these medications have for the patient's future functioning?
10. Does the patient have a history of suicide attempts or ideation?
11. How long has the patient taken the medication? Were other antidepressants used before the one currently being used?
12. How does the patient feel about continued compliance?
    Does the patient take his or her medication responsibly?
13. How often does the patient see the prescribing physician?
14. Are there any concerns related to the prescribed medications that should be reported to the prescribing physician?
15. Can the patient afford the medication?

The Possibility of Suicide

Regardless of what type of therapeutic activity the depressed patient is undergoing, service providers must be continually aware of the possibility of suicide. Often when patients avail themselves of services, the severity of their depression is such that they may not be capable of reasoning out an effective suicide strategy. With the use of an antidepressant, however, they may become ''well enough'' to mobilize their abilities in such a way as to make an actual attempt.

All individuals involved in working with those experiencing depression must be aware of the possibility of suicide and be on guard for signs from their patients. Beck and colleagues (1979) stress that this issue should be confronted and questioned when suspected. They indicate from their experience that it is more helpful to discuss suicidal ideation rather than avoid it. It may give the patient a more realistic view of the situation and offer some comfort to the patient in being able to talk about it.

The Problem of Noncompliance

The nonmedical therapist certainly can play an important role in providing support and education to patients so as to encourage them to continue taking their medication. Beck and colleagues (1979) discuss possible cognitions that may prevent patients from taking their medication; their cognitive therapeutic strategies also suggest ways of approaching these cognitions. Some of these counterproductive ideas are as follows.

1. The medication is addicting. I'll never get off it.
2. I am a "stronger or better" person if I don't take the medication.
3. It won't work for me.
4. If I have to take medication, it means I am crazy.
5. The medication is only necessary when I feel bad.
6. The medication is not working since I am not perfectly well after _____ days or weeks. I should feel good right away.
7. The medication will solve all my problems.
8. I feel like a zombie when I take it.
9. I can't stand the dizziness or the side effects.

Many of these concerns result from misinformation or a lack of information; others may arise from an inappropriate dosage or medication. Whatever the case, the nonmedical practitioner should support the patient's adherence and continued involvement with the physician to ensure that he or she is getting appropriate treatment.

CONCLUSIONS

Depression and affective disorders are widespread concerns. Medication and other therapeutic forms have demonstrated their effectiveness in treating these conditions. On behalf of the patient, it is critical that nonmedical personnel become aware of the implications of the medications the patient is taking, because these medications can certainly influence therapeutic outcome. Thus the importance of being aware of what to expect in using antidepressants is critical. The educative and supportive functions of the nonmedical practitioner are vital.

REFERENCES

Abrams, R., & Essman, W.B. (Eds.). (1982). *Electroconvulsive therapies: Biological foundations and clinical application*. New York: SP Books.

Beck, A.T., Rush, A.J., Shaw, B.F., & Emery, G. (1979). *Cognitive therapy of depression*. New York: Guilford Press.

Bockar, J.A. (1976). *Primer for the nonmedical psychotherapist*. New York: Spectrum.

Coppen, A. (1967). Biochemistry of affective disorders. *British Journal of Psychiatry, 113*, 1237–1264.

DeLisi, L.E. (1984). Use of the clinical laboratory. In J.L. Sullivan & P.D. Sullivan (Eds.), *Biomedical psychiatric therapeutics* (pp. 89–119). Boston: Butterworth.

Denber, H.C.B. (1979). *Textbook of clinical psychopharmacology*. New York: Grune & Stratton.

Feighner, J.P., Aden, G.C., Fabre, L.F., Rickels, K., & Smith, W.T. (1983). Comparison of alprazolam, imipramine, and placebo in the treatment of depression. *Journal of the American Medical Association, 249*, 3057–3064.

Fink, M. (1979). *Convulsive therapy—Theory and practice*. New York: Raven.

Goldsmith, W. (1977). *Psychiatric drugs for the non-medical mental health worker*. Springfield, IL: Charles C Thomas.

Kiloh, L.G. (1982). Electroconvulsive therapy. In E.S. Paykel (Ed.), *Handbook of affective disorders* (pp. 262–275). New York: Guilford Press.

Levenson, A.J. (1981). *Basic psychopharmacology*. New York: Springer.

Moreines, R., & Gold, M.S. (1984). MAO inhibitors: Predicting response/maximizing efficacy. In M.S. Gold, R.B. Lydiard, & J.S. Carman (Eds.), *Advances in psychopharmacology: Predicting and improving treatment response* (pp. 157–178). Boca Raton, FL: CRC Press.

Nies, A., & Robinson, D.S. (1982). Monoamine oxidase inhibitors. In E.S. Paykel (Ed.), *Handbook of affective disorders* (pp. 246–261). New York: Guilford Press.

Palmer, R.L. (Ed.). (1981). *Electroconvulsive therapy: An appraisal*. Oxford: Oxford Univ. Press.

Raft, D., Davidson, J., Wasik, J., & Mattox, A. (1981). Relationship between response to phenelzine and MAO inhibition in a clinical trial of phenelzine, amitriptyline, and placebo. *Neuropsychobiology, 7*, 122.

Risch, S.C., Janowsky, D.S., & Huey, L.Y. (1981). Plasma levels of tricyclic antidepressants and clinical efficacy. In S.J. Enna, J.B. Malick, & E. Richelson (Eds.), *Antidepressants: Neurochemical, behavioral, and clinical perspectives* (pp. 183–217). New York: Raven.

Schildkraut, J.J. (1965). The catecholamine hypothesis of affective disorders: A review of supporting evidence. *American Journal of Psychiatry, 122*, 509–522.

Seager, C.P., & Bird, R.L. (1962). Imipramine with electrical treatment and depression—A controlled trial. *Journal of Mental Science, 108*, 704–707.

Spiegel, R., & Aebi, H.-J. (1984). *Psychopharmacology*. Chichester: Wiley.

Sullivan, J.L., Taska, R.J., Wise, T.N., & Goldstein, D.M. (1984). Chemotherapy of affective disorders. In J.L. Sullivan & P.D. Sullivan (Eds.), *Biomedical psychiatric therapeutics* (pp. 25–54). Boston: Butterworth.

Weiner, R.D. (1984). Electroconvulsive therapy. In J.L. Sullivan & P.D. Sullivan (Eds.), *Biomedical psychiatric therapeutics* (pp. 71–88). Boston: Butterworth.

Chapter 11

Lithium

Delia Thrasher and Gary W. Lawson

Lithium has been used to treat various disorders, including gout and arthritis. Currently its principal use is in the treatment of manic-depressive illness. Some research and application of lithium for other disorders also have shown promise. This chapter examines the history of this unique psychoactive drug and describes its pharmacology, metabolism, and hypothesized mechanisms of action. Emphasis is placed on treatment considerations for bipolar and other affective illnesses. Side effects, toxicity, drug interactions, and contraindications for treatment are also discussed.

HISTORY

Lithium was discovered as an element by the Swedish chemist Johan August Afvedson in 1817. The lightest of the alkali metals, lithium occurs naturally as a salt. The medical use of lithium can be traced back to ancient Greece, where Soranus of Ephesus recommended alkaline waters for the treatment of mania in the second century A.D. (Kline, 1973). Use of lithium for renal disorders and arthritic ailments began in the 1840s. The first published report did not appear until 1859, when Garrod described it as an effective treatment for gout. Several kinds of bottled water became available to the public in the late 1800s and were popularized for their high lithium content and curative powers for gout and other illnesses. Research suggested lithium as an effective sodium substitute. However, in the 1940s its use led to poisoning and deaths. The toxic hazards of lithium were not recognized before this, and these incidents led to extreme wariness of its use within the medical community.

Interest in the development of lithium for psychiatric use began in 1949. John Cade, an Australian physician, used lithium urate in guinea pigs to investigate connections between behavior and purine metabolism. He anecdotally noted lithium's calming effects on the animals and began experimenting with the drug as a sedative. European researchers such as Schou in Denmark began extensive research on the use of lithium as an antimanic agent in the 1950s and 1960s, and a number of controlled evaluative studies were reported. This effort gave rise to large-scale cooperative studies in the United States involving the Veterans Administration and the National Institute of Mental Health. Experimental and clinical evidence points to the effectiveness of lithium in the treatment of manic states (Prien, Caffey, & Klett, 1971). Research on the use of lithium for unipolar and other disorders is showing great promise as well.

Lithium was not authorized for use in the United States until 1970. The delay between discovery and introduction of this drug into clinical practice stemmed from several issues. First, the relative professional and geographic isolation of its discovery in Australia slowed interest in its acceptance. Additionally, psychiatrists of the 1950s were not strongly interested in pharmacological treatment of disorders, and manic patients made up a small diagnostic group that was not of major concern to mental health providers. Another reason for the delayed interest in the use of lithium was the risk associated with its toxic hazards. It is highly probable, however, that a major factor impeding the development and acceptance of lithium involved the low cost and ready availability that made it unprofitable for manufacture by private drug companies. As a result, marketing did not begin until the 1960s after pressure was applied to manufacturers by the psychiatric community.

PHARMACOLOGY AND METABOLISM

Lithium is a salt that is similar to sodium in its chemical properties but has a lower abundance in nature. In the body it exists as a small ion with a single positive charge. Unlike other ions that take part in psychopharmacological processes, lithium is not protein bound, is easily monitored by blood levels, and is distributed throughout the body. More than 50 formulations of lithium are available, including acetate, citrate, glutamate, orotate, and carbonate. Lithium carbonate is the predominate form and is generally available in 300-mg tablets or capsules. Also available are 450-mg controlled-release tablets and lithium citrate syrup.

After oral administration, the drug is rapidly absorbed into the bloodstream through the gastrointestinal tract. Peak blood levels are reached 2 to 4 hours after a single dosage. As an unbound ion, lithium is found in all body fluids and is actively transported across many cell membranes. It is distributed unevenly in the tissues of the body, however, with high concentrations in kidney tissue, moderate concentrations in the liver, bone, and muscles, and low concentrations in brain tissue. After approximately 1 week of administration, a steady state is established in the body.

Like sodium, lithium is almost completely excreted by the kidneys, with insignificant amounts excreted in sweat and feces. Lithium is fully filtered in the kidneys, and about 80% of it is reabsorbed in the proximal renal tubules and the loop of Henle. Lithium and sodium compete for absorption in the proximal renal tubules, and sodium is additionally absorbed in the distal tubules. The amount of lithium filtered and absorbed remains constant under normal body conditions. Excretion is thus proportional to plasma concentrations of the drug. Within 5 to 8 hours after administration of a single dose, 50% is excreted. The half-life is about 24 hours for those patients ingesting lithium on a maintenance basis.

The regulation of lithium levels is closely related to the sodium, potassium, and fluid balance of the body. The balance between sodium and lithium is the most important clinically, because sodium depletion increases lithium retention and the potential for toxicity. Decreased intake of fluids can also decrease the excretion of lithium. Excretion through body fluids after long-term use is generally rapid, but toxicity may persist because of lithium deposits in other tissues. Lithium leaves brain tissue quite slowly, and toxicity may persist for several days after the drug is discontinued (Bassuk, Hoover, & Schnoonover, 1977).

MECHANISM OF ACTION

The exact effective mechanism of lithium is unclear. Several ideas have been advanced to explain its therapeutic effectiveness in the treatment of mood disorders. Particular consideration has been given to the role of lithium in changing the electrolytic balance across cell membranes. It has been postulated that replacement of sodium with lithium may interrupt neuronal transmission. Although sodium is replaced by lithium during an action potential, once inside the cell lithium is not removed by the sodium pump. This results in diminished sodium-potassium exchange and intracellular replacement of potassium with lithium. The polarization required for an action potential is diminished, and electrical conduction drops off. There are indications, however, that at the clinically used concentrations the amount of lithium is insufficient to produce this effect (Baldessarini, 1985).

It has also been suggested that a less prominent interaction between lithium, sodium, potassium, and calcium exists. Lithium administration is believed to normalize the temporarily raised intracellular sodium levels associated with major affective disorders (Baldessarini, 1985).

A third type of mechanism considers the effect of lithium at receptor sites for neurotransmitters and hormones. This may explain some of its side effects as well as its primary therapeutic effects. Strong support exists for the blocking of hormonal stimulation of adenyl cyclase at receptor sites. This process could affect central nervous system changes involving prostaglandins and catecholamines as well as lead to the development of diabetes insipidus and interfere with thyroid-stimulating hormone (TSH) (Baldessarini, 1985).

Studies of the effects of lithium on monoamine transmitters support the notions that either serotonin underactivity or catecholamine neurotransmitter overactivity forms the basis for mania (Gershon & Shopsin, 1973). The introduction of norepinephrine has been reported to inhibit the release of norepinephrine and dopamine and to stimulate serotonin release (Baldessarini, 1985). This information, however, does not account for the ability of lithium to counteract the depressive states of recurrent affective disorders.

TREATMENT CONSIDERATIONS

Although lithium has been used primarily in the treatment of acute mania and bipolar disorders (also known as manic-depression), it has also been applied to various other disorders. Use in any of these disorders requires a number of treatment considerations, including phase, dosage, and monitoring requirements. In determining whether treatment with lithium is indicated, both psychological and physical evaluations should be performed.

First, a complete diagnostic assessment should be done. Delineation of the nature of the affective disorder is essential. Attempts to rule out schizophrenia are important, because lithium can result in marked worsening of psychotic symptoms or neurotoxicity in schizophrenic individuals. The clinical status of the patient is also a factor in deciding whether lithium will be used on a short-term basis, in combination with other drugs, or on a long-term maintenance schedule.

The second area of assessment concerns the physical status of the patient. It is crucial that a thorough physical examination be performed and that lithium levels be monitored. In addition, a complete medical history and laboratory tests are required. Medical evaluation should include blood cell count, blood sugar levels, renal and electrolyte analyses, and an electrocardiogram. Subsequent evaluation is usually recommended two to four times annually. Patients should be screened for thyroid disease, epilepsy, renal disease, cardiovascular disease, brain damage, and pregnancy, as these conditions necessitate cautious administration. Contraindications for lithium therapy include the first trimester of pregnancy, significant renal disease, cardiac disease, or brain damage. Both elderly individuals and children warrant special consideration before the application of lithium.

Acute Manic Episodes and Bipolar Affective Disorder

Lithium has been effective in controlling acute manic episodes. Although there is some debate over the relative effectiveness of lithium compared to antipsychotic drugs, it is felt that lithium has a greater antimanic specificity. Since there is a latent period of 5 to 14 days before the onset of its antimanic effect, however, lithium may be combined with an antipsychotic drug such as chlorpromazine or haloperidol in treating severe manic episodes. These neuroleptic agents provide behavioral control through sedation and by decreasing motor activity. Although these drugs appear to suppress the outward manifestations of mania, many patients nevertheless report a continued feeling of internal disorder.

The administration of either chlorpromazine or haloperidol together with lithium appears to be generally safe, but certain precautions should be followed. As always, lithium levels should be monitored for toxicity. Careful screening is necessary because of the increased risk of neurotoxicity in schizophrenic individuals. In general, dosages and duration of combined drug therapy should be minimized because administration of neuroleptics to manic patients may result in mood shifts toward depression. Sensitivity to the patient's subjective experience is also important in determining the duration of coadministration. Bassuk, Hoover, and Schnoonover (1977) suggest that neuroleptics be withdrawn only after (1) the patient has regained physical control, (2) clinical assessment indicates alteration of the manic symptoms, and (3) no less than 5 days of lithium treatment. Withdrawal of any drug used in combination with lithium alters electrolyte balance and should be done with care to avoid toxicity. Blood samples should be analyzed and dosage of the drug reduced slowly.

Lithium is initially administered in slowly increasing amounts because abrupt increases in blood levels often result in unwanted gastrointestinal side effects and because the margin between therapeutic and toxic blood lithium levels is narrow. The time lag to onset of effectiveness may be related to this, as it delays the time required for an adequate amount of the drug to cross the blood-brain barrier and neuronal cell membranes. Lithium treatment is generally initiated in divided dosages of 600 to 900 mg, which are increased over the next few days until concentrations of 1.0 to 1.25 mEq per liter of plasma or serum are reached. Levels of 2.0 mEq/liter or higher are considered toxic, thus illustrating the narrow safety margin for lithium. Exact dosages are related to the clinical and physical status of the patient as well as to serum blood levels. Manic patients may require three to four times more lithium than nonmanic patients to obtain desired blood levels. As the clinical condition of the patient improves, dosages may need to be decreased.

Daily dosages should always be divided because of the rapid excretion of the drug and possible side effects resulting from dramatic changes in blood levels. Blood level checks are initially done on a daily to biweekly basis, followed by weekly and then monthly checks; samples are always drawn 12 hours after the last dose of the day and before the morning dose to obtain consistent measurements. Typical inpatient dosages range from 1200 to 2400 mg, and outpatients generally have daily divided dosages of 600 to 1500 mg. These dosages result in a blood serum lithium level of 0.5 to 1.0 mEq/liter, with the effective level for each individual determined empirically. For further information about recommended dosage considerations, see Baldessarini (1985) and Bassuk, Hoover, and Schnoonover (1977).

The primary use of lithium is in the management of bipolar disorders, where it appears to exert a prophylactic effect on the occurrence of marked mood swings. Both clinicians and researchers now feel that lithium is more effective for this group than hospitalization, multiple courses of electroshock treatments, and various psychopharmacological treatments (Gershon & Shopsin, 1973). Nevertheless, 20% to 30% of patients with bipolar disorder do not respond well to lithium. Among those who do react favorably, there is great variation in response. Some individuals no longer experience manic episodes but continue to experience depressions, while others have no recurrence of either mania or depression.

The decision to continue lithium administration on an outpatient maintenance basis requires careful consideration of several factors, including the incidence and severity of manic episodes. Circumstances encouraging use would be an established history of manic episodes on an annual or biannual basis. Frequency is important, because occasional though severe episodes of mania or depression would probably not warrant chronic lithium therapy.

The ability and willingness of the patient to take the medication must also be considered. Patients must be reliable enough to maintain the medication schedule. Individuals who enjoy the feelings of euphoria associated with their manic state may be unwilling to take their medication regularly. Individuals may also be inclined to discontinue use after stabilization of mood swings and successful suppression of symptoms or because of annoying side effects. Those patients characterized as impulsive or at risk for suicide are unlikely candidates for outpatient maintenance regimens because of the risk of toxicity if even a slight overdose is attempted. A decision to use lithium on a long-term basis must also weigh the risks of side effects and complications of toxicity.

Depression

Recent investigations have looked at the effects of lithium in the treatment of depression. Lithium does appear to have an antidepressant effect in selected cases of acute depression, despite conflicting earlier reports (Cooper, 1979). A family history of lithium-responsive bipolar illness may have some predictive value in determining whether a patient with acute depression will respond to the drug.

Lithium may also be beneficial in the treatment of unipolar endogenous depression and for the prophylaxis of depression. The use of lithium in conjunction with antidepressants has shown some promise for those patients whose unipolar depressions did not respond to antidepressants alone (Schou, 1983). Patients with unipolar endogenous depression are more likely to respond to lithium if there is an early age of onset and a family history of bipolar disorder, mild hypomania, cyclothymia, or postpartum depression.

Numerous studies have examined the prophylactic use of lithium in depression. Baastrup and Schou (1983) and others have found lithium to be equally effective in the prophylaxis of unipolar and bipolar depression. Continued research in the application of lithium treatment to depression should enhance the understanding of its therapeutic implications.

Schizoaffective Disorders and Schizophrenia

Although lithium may be useful in the treatment of schizoaffective disorders, it is contraindicated in schizophrenia because of the possible exacerbations of psychotic symptoms and neurotoxicity. Symptoms include dyskinesias, memory impairment, confusion, disorientation, and facial grimacing. The differential diagnosis among manic-depression, schizoaffective disorder, and schizophrenia may be difficult but is important in making treatment recommendations. Lithium is indicated for manic states with psychotic symptoms and for "atypical" manic presentations that may be schizoaffective in nature. Lithium has not been useful in treating thought disorders, and its application in questionable cases warrants carefully monitored trials of the drug.

Other Applications

Beneficial effects have been achieved when lithium has been used in the treatment of affective disorders associated with certain physical conditions, including cerebrovascular accidents with subsequent injuries, brain stem injuries, hemodialysis, and closed head injuries (Rosenbaum & Barry, 1975). Patients with affective disorders combined with organic brain syndromes have also experienced some beneficial effects from lithium. According to Hale and Donaldson (1982), patients treated with lithium demonstrated improvements in affective instability as well as in cognitive functions such as memory and speech.

Lithium has been reported to result in positive effects in the treatment of anorexia nervosa. Jefferson, Griest, and Ackerman (1983) note that patients experienced weight gains of about 30% and sustained mood improvements for up to 4 years.

Treatment of other disorders has also included lithium when standard methods have been ineffective. Clinical administration of lithium has been included in the treatment of alcoholism with affective disorder, impulsive-aggressive behaviors, cyclothymic disorder, stimulant-induced euphoria, and premenstrual tension (Bassuk, Hoover, & Schnoonover, 1977; Baldessarini, 1985).

SIDE EFFECTS AND TOXICITY

Lithium rarely produces any adverse effects on emotional and intellectual functioning but may produce various physiological side effects. Most of those that occur at therapeutic blood levels can be annoying but are generally not serious and can be treated. They generally result from long-term lithium use and do not usually suggest discontinuation of treatment. Worsening of certain symptoms can be indicative of toxicity and of the need to stop drug administration. Side effects vary in intensity and duration and may affect a number of systems in the body.

Endocrinologic Effects

Lithium may induce hyperthyroidism, hypothyroidism, and the development of goiter. These may be related to previous thyroid deficits. The presence of underlying thyroid disease indicates the need for caution in administration but does not necessarily contraindicate lithium therapy. Enlargement of the goiter usually occurs after 5 months to 2 years of lithium treatment and is more frequent in women. After discontinuation of lithium, the condition returns to normal.

Polydipsia and polyuria are common side effects, especially in the elderly. These side effects are not dose dependent and usually occur early in treatment but may appear later as well. A diabetes insipidus–like syndrome may occur, in which patients are unable to concentrate their urine. Certain drugs such as chlorothiazide may ameliorate the diuresis associated with this condition, but ineffective treatment of this condition usually results in discontinuation of lithium because of the insatiable thirst and frequent urination. Lithium may also induce diabetes mellitus because of the impairment of insulin release. This condition indicates the need to terminate treatment with lithium. Lithium also elevates serum growth hormone levels, but the clinical significance of this is unclear. Serious problems may result with an increase in serum lithium level, which include anorexia, vomiting, nausea, diarrhea, and abdominal pains. Severe symptoms can be altered by changing the dosage and frequency of administration. Persistent diarrhea may result in significant electrolyte loss and lithium retention and should therefore be medically treated and given follow-up care.

Neuromuscular and Central Nervous System Effects

It is common to see some neuromuscular side effects with lithium treatment. A frequent early side effect is muscular weakness, which generally improves after the first few weeks of treatment. Another common side effect is a fine hand tremor, which may persist and vary in severity. Occasionally tremulousness may appear in the lower jaw or eyelid. These may develop into greater tremors of the upper extremities and face and can progress to facial spasms. Symptomatic progression such as this may indicate neurotoxicity and may be grounds for discontinuation of the drug.

Lithium can result in such uncommon side effects as dizziness, headaches, and a feeling of dullness. These may worsen as toxicity approaches. Apathy, memory impairment, disorientation, somnolence, fatigue, slurred speech, hyperreflexia, seizures, and incontinence may occur. The appearance of any central nervous system disorders should be addressed by lithium discontinuation and monitoring of patient status. Fairly rare reactions include grand mal seizures and clinical depression. Blurred vision and tinnitus have also been reported as side effects.

Miscellaneous Side Effects

Weight gain is a fairly common side effect of lithium therapy, but the basis for this is unclear. Other side effects include increased uric acid excretion, pretibial edema, and a metallic taste in the mouth.

Toxicity

The patient and significant others should be thoroughly educated about the toxic effects of lithium. Signs of toxicity should be called to the attention of the administering physician or psychiatrist.

The more adverse side effects are indicative of lithium toxicity; these include the neuromuscular side effects listed above. Symptoms usually begin with dysarthria and ataxia. Muscle twitching and slurred speech may also occur. Toxicity may result in marked neuromuscular irritability, seizures, loss of consciousness, irreversible neurological damage, coma, and death (Pary, Goolsby, & Rodriguez, 1985). Acute intoxication requires immediate discontinuation of lithium. The maintenance of vital functions, gastric lavage, and the specialized services of a toxicology unit are needed to provide appropriate management in most cases until the normal excretion process lowers lithium levels. Dialysis techniques have been effective for treatment of severe overdoses.

CONTRAINDICATIONS

Lithium treatment is not indicated for patients with organic brain damage, schizophrenia, or severe cardiac or renal disease. Patients with moderate medical conditions that may cause the retention of either sodium or fluid require careful assessment before lithium is prescribed. Use during pregnancy should be limited to extremely severe circumstances because of the tetatogenic effects of lithium; the first and final trimesters appear to be the peak risk periods. Elderly patients have a lowered tolerance for lithium and are at increased risk of cerebral intoxication, especially when the drug is used in combination with other drugs affecting the central nervous system or if dementia is present. With cautious administration, however, elderly patients can safely benefit from lithium.

DRUG INTERACTIONS

Drug interaction effects are mainly due to the decreased retention of sodium or increased retention of lithium, both of which can result in the increased blood levels of lithium associated with toxicity. Some drugs that adversely interact with lithium include certain neuroleptics such as chlorpromazine and thioridazine, the anti-inflammatory drugs indomethacin and ibuprophin, and antibiotics such as tetracycline and metronidazole. Certain diuretics such as the thiazides facilitate lithium loss, and caffeine increases its retention. The combination of lithium with drugs that depress the central nervous system, such as alcohol, sedatives, anti-hypertensives, neuroleptics, and antidepressants, may produce excessive sedation or confusion. The use of lithium in conjunction with haloperidol has been implicated in several cases of irreversible or fatal central nervous system intoxication, but the combination of the two has generally been considered safe and standard practice.

REFERENCES

Baastrup, P.C., & Schou, M. (1983). Lithium as a propylic agent: Its effect against recurrent depressions and manic-depressive psychosis. *American Journal of Psychiatry, 140,* 11–20.

Baldessarini, R.J. (1985). *Chemotherapy in psychiatry* (2nd rev. ed.). Cambridge, MA: Harvard Univ. Press.

Bassuk, E.L., Hoover, J., & Schnoonover, S.C. (1977). *The practitioner's guide to psychoactive drugs.* New York: Plenum.

Cooper, T.B. (Ed.). (1979). *Lithium: Controversies and unresolved issues.* Princeton: Excerpta Medica.

Gershon, S., & Shopsin, B. (Eds.). (1973). *Lithium: Its role in psychiatric research and treatment.* New York: Plenum.

Hale, M.S., & Donaldson, J.O. (1982). Lithium carbonate in the treatment of organic brain syndrome. *Journal of Nervous and Mental Disorders, 170,* 362–365.

Jefferson, J.W., Griest, J.H., & Ackerman, D.L. (1983). *Lithium encyclopedia for clinical practice.* Washington, DC: American Psychiatric Press.

Kline, N.S. (1973). A narrative account of lithium usage in psychiatry. In S. Gershon & B. Shopsin (Eds.), *Lithium: Its role in psychiatric research and treatment* (pp. 275–282). New York: Plenum.

Chapter 12

Antianxiety Medications

Jerry Williams and Gary W. Lawson

In a 1984 study conducted by the National Institute of Mental Health, it was found that during a 6-month period 29 million Americans, a full 19% of the total adult population, suffered from at least one psychiatric disorder. Of this population of 29 million, more than 13 million reported anxiety disorders (*Archives of General Psychiatry*, 1984). If these findings are valid, is it appropriate to conclude that more people are experiencing anxiety or simply that more people are reporting anxiety? Regardless of any solutions proposed to answer this seemingly unanswerable question, one conclusion can be made: anxiety is and will continue to be a major treatment issue for mental health professionals.

ANXIETY REVISITED

Conceptualization of Anxiety

Both within the ranks of mental health professionals and among the public at large, anxiety has come to be conceptualized in a number of ways. For the traditional psychodynamic therapist, anxiety is an ego state that arises out of the conflict, and resultant defensive functioning, between the id seeking gratification and the superego seeking to restrain the id. The Rogerian humanist views anxiety as resulting from a developing incongruence between the self as perceived and the real world as perceived. The behaviorist views anxiety either classically, as originating from the association between an object or situation and a fear-eliciting event, or operantly, at learning that as a particular response is made it will be followed by a particular stimulus event (in this case a perceived negative consequence).

In general, anxiety is understood to be an exaggerated or excessive response to either a verifiable or an unrecognized danger. Anxiety is also the name given when the response is incongruous or inappropriate in relation to the objective reality. Anxiety and fear also overlap when the danger is external and real.

Anxiety is best known by its physical manifestations or symptomatology. Descriptions of the external manifestations of anxiety states usually include at least some of the following: tenseness, nervousness, inability to relax, jitteriness, fatigue, restlessness, stomachache, cold hands, sweating, lump in the throat, pounding heart, hyperventilation, fearfulness, irritability, inability to sleep or concentrate, and lack of patience. The *Diagnostic and Statistical Manual of Mental Disorders* (Third Edition) (DSM-III; American Psychiatric Association, 1980) also specifies duration of the anxious state and differential diagnosis with other mental disorders.

Types of Anxiety States

Types of anxiety states have been proposed to aid treatment planning.

Anxieties Associated with Pre-existing Medical Conditions

There are many anxiety conditions that may present with clear-cut anxiety symptoms. In keeping with the philosophy that one can never know too much, the nonmedical mental health practitioner must be increasingly cognizant of medical issues. These general considerations should be helpful in determining whether a patient is in need of further differential diagnosis.

Refer for medical evaluation any patient who presents with pre-existing physical pain of any type, either localized (such as angina pectoris or cerebral headache) or general (such as severe pains in the limbs or spine); pre-existing pharmacological reactions such as drug toxicities (allergic responses and overdoses); pre-existing loss of neurological functioning (seizures, amnesias, aphasias, paralyses); history of heart dysfunction; history of thyroid dysfunction; premenstrual tension; history of diabetes; and symptoms of withdrawal from a central nervous system depressant (such as barbiturates).

Psychotic Terror

Psychotic terror is usually associated with psychosis and its accompanying paranoia and hallucinations. Drug-induced toxic psychosis also falls in this category.

Anxious Depression

This type of anxiety occurs in patients who demonstrate affectual manifestations of depression concurrently with agitated behavioral symptoms. These patients frequently complain of an inability to sleep.

Traumatic Anxiety

Except in the case of amnesia, this type of anxiety is readily traceable to a traumatic event.

Situational Anxiety

Situational anxiety is viewed as a reaction to a situationally specific stressful stimulus such as an examination or interview. This type of anxiety usually abates once the event is started or completed.

Phobic Anxiety

Phobic anxiety refers to a reaction in which the primary motivation of the patient is avoidance. Phobic reactions can occur in association with both objects and events.

Anticipatory Anxiety

Anticipatory anxiety refers to the eliciting of an anxious response through purely cognitive mechanisms. Differing from phobic reactions in which actual contact with the feared stimulus is necessary to elicit the anxious response, anticipatory anxiety occurs simply by thinking of either the feared stimulus or the personal response to that stimulus.

Free-Floating Anxiety

Free-floating anxiety is not readily traceable to either events or stimuli that elicit anxiety and is one of the more difficult types to treat. Panic attacks and fear of life-threatening physical illness are included in this type of anxiety.

Importance of a Precise Diagnosis

The need for precision in diagnosing anxiety cannot be understated. It is estimated that between 10% and 40% of those persons who present with anxiety suffer from a pre-existing physical disorder that is responsible for their symptoms. As previously mentioned, in most cases these symptoms can be attributed to endocrine, cardiovascular, pulmonary, infectious, and pharmacological reactions. Anxiety can also be attributed to pre-existing psychiatric or psychological disorders including schizophrenic, paranoid, and other personality disorders (*Internal Medicine for the Specialist*, 1985).

The importance of a precise diagnosis becomes even clearer when viewed in light of the fact that an estimated nine of ten prescriptions for antianxiety agents are issued by general practitioners (Spiegel & Aebi, 1984). Therefore, nonmedical mental health professionals are responsible not only for monitoring the effects of the prescribed medication but also, by virtue of their access to information that reveals itself progressively during the one-to-one therapeutic interplay, for determining whether the type of anxiety presented to the physician was accurately depicted by the patient. This is not to say that the patient would knowingly deceive the physician (although that is sometimes a possibility), but rather that the mental health professional needs to stay aware of and communicate to the physician, where necessary, any alterations of the original diagnosis. For example, if a patient was receiving diazepam (Valium) and as therapy progressed it was revealed that this individual had a cardiovascular dysfunction that was not communicated to the physician, then this new information, if not communicated to the physician, could result in a disastrous therapeutic and physical outcome. Other examples include individuals who originally seek pharmacological treatment for a traumatic anxiety that later shifts to an agitated depression. The list of examples is infinite.

PHARMACOLOGICAL TREATMENT OF ANXIETY

Any discourse on antianxiety agents presents a bit of a conceptual dilemma to the student of psychopharmacology. From a liberal point of view, almost every pharmacological agent has at one time or another been considered or actually used to treat anxiety. From traditional pharmacological and psychological therapies, the range of treatments for anxiety soon expands to include everything from alcohol ingestion to xylophone playing. In the interest of brevity, however, this section focuses on pharmacological treatments, their appropriateness for a particular anxiety type, limitations, contraindications, and possible side effects.

The Barbiturates

The barbiturates are commonly used in the treatment of anxiety, particularly with patients (Shader, 1977). Amobarbital, butabarbital, and phenobarbital are the long-acting barbiturates most often prescribed. Other than in research settings, the short-acting barbiturates have not been used. In comparison to the benzodiazepines, the barbiturates are more toxic and addicting and produce a higher incidence of severe central nervous system depression (Spiegel & Aebi, 1984). Overall, the barbiturates have no utility as antianxiety agents, regardless of the anxiety type, and thus should not be used.

Common side effects of barbiturates are central nervous system depression ranging from mild sedation to hypnosis, stupor, coma, and death. Depression of cardiac, skeletal, and smooth muscle has been noted. Severe neurogenic, chemical, and hypoxic respiratory depression occur. Barbiturates also have a central and peripheral depressant effect on the secretions and tone of the gastrointestinal tract. Overdoses are frequently lethal, with death resulting from respiratory failure. Barbiturates are rated high in the potential for both physical and psychological addiction, and tolerance does develop.

The Propanediols

Meprobamate, tybamate, and various carbamates are widely prescribed for anxiety states, although research has yielded that meprobamate is only equivocally better than placebo, no better than the barbiturates, and considerably less effective than the benzodiazepines in the treatment of acute anxiety states. Meprobamate is more effective in the treatment of chronic anxiety states than placebo and the barbiturates and is possibly as effective as the benzodiazepines. The carbamates are similar to the barbiturates, but because they are more toxic, addicting, and associated with a higher degree of morbidity and mortality their use is not recommended. Research on tybamate is at this time limited and inconclusive (Trimble, 1983). Overall, this class of drugs is not recommended in the treatment of anxiety.

The side effects of propanediols include impairment of motor function; potentiation (amplification) of the effects of ethanol; allergic responses in 2% of patients, resulting in rashes, bronchial spasms, blood disorders, and hypotension (especially in the elderly); and fetal abnormalities if ingested during pregnancy (Spiegel & Aebi, 1984). Their potential for both physical and psychological addiction is high, and tolerance does develop.

The Neuroleptics

The use of low dosages of antipsychotic agents such as Thorazine (chlorpromazine) as antianxiety agents is very controversial. Some authors regard any use of neuroleptics as entirely unethical (not to mention dangerous); others list specific criteria for their use. Some of the possible applications include anxious and agitated elderly patients showing signs of senile dementia, especially when aggressive behaviors are present; patients in whom anxiety is associated with a high degree of distractibility; patients with racing thoughts or thought blocking; obsessional patients with strong imagination; and patients who are unresponsive to other antianxiety treatments. Overall, because of the difficulty of differential diagnosis and the severity of side effects, the use of neuroleptics is contraindicated for all but psychotic terror anxiety states.

Side effects include drowsiness, ataxia, dry mouth, blurred vision, weakness, and feelings of unreality (Honigfeld & Howard, 1978). Extrapyramidal side effects and hypotension also occur at low dosages. The neuroleptics have a low potential for physical addiction and moderate potential for psychological addiction. Tolerance does develop.

The Antidepressants

The tricyclic antidepressants amitriptyline, imipramine, and doxepin and the monoamine oxidase inhibitors (MAOIs) phenelzine and tranylcypromine have been found to yield positive results with panic states (free-floating anxiety) and agitated depression. Because of problems with side effects and toxicity, MAOIs are generally considered inferior to the tricyclics (see Chapter 10 for a complete discussion). Contraindications for tricyclics include situations in which cholinergics (sleeping aids) or histaminergics (cold preparations) are to be ingested concurrently.

Side effects for MAOIs include convulsions brought on by overstimulation, orthostatic hypotension, hypertensive crisis, liver toxicity, and weight gain (Bassuk & Schoonover, 1978). Tricyclic side effects include sedation, jaundice, mild parkinsonian symptoms, hypotension, dryness of mouth, dizziness, tachycardia, palpitations, blurred vision, excessive sweating, and impotence (Honigfeld & Howard, 1978). Both types of antidepressant have a low potential for physical addiction and moderate potential for psychological addiction.

The Antihistamines

Diphenhydramine (a piperazine preparation), promethazine (a phenothiazine derivative), and hydroxyzine (an ethanolamine) are antihistamines that may be used if the benzodiazepines are not effective or are not tolerated by the anxious patient. The phenothiazines are also antipsychotics but can be effective antianxiety agents if used in lower dosages. Hydroxyzine is an effective antianxiety agent and has fewer and less serious side effects than the phenothiazines; it is considered to be a relatively safe preparation for the treatment of anxiety and follows, in order of choice, directly after the benzodiazepines. Diphenhydramine is also available over-the-counter in most cold preparations. The antihistamines can be used for all types of anxiety excluding psychotic terror, agitated depression, and that associated with medical conditions.

Side effects include hypotension, drowsiness, and (for hydroxyzine specifically) dry mouth and tremors. Temporary tinnitus (ringing in the ears) has also been noted when the antihistamines are used in combination with acetaminophen

(Bassuk & Schoonover, 1978). They have low potential for both physical and psychological addiction.

The β-Adrenergic Blocking Agents

Beta blockers such as L-(*d*)-propanolol (Inderal) are the most recently proposed antianxiety substances. Specific contraindications are the presence of asthma, bronchospasms, and certain cardiovascular diseases. The major advantage of β-blockers compared to traditional tranquilizers lies in the fact that wakefulness and alertness are unimpaired (*Internal Medicine for the Specialist*, 1985).

Inderal is currently being researched by the Food and Drug Administration. Its side effects and potential for addiction are currently being documented. This drug is not approved for use as an antianxiety agent in the United States.

The Benzodiazepines

Because they are less toxic and addicting than the other sedative hypnotics while remaining superior to placebo and the barbiturates, the benzodiazepines are the drugs of choice for the treatment of anxiety unaccompanied by depression or psychosis. Chlordiazepoxide, diazepam, oxazepam, and clorazepate are the benzodiazepines most commonly prescribed (Trimble, 1983).

Contraindications include the presence of depression, psychosis, and pregnancy. Side effects, although less severe and less frequent than those of other types of antianxiety agents, occur across a range of functions. Drowsiness and disinhibition are among the most frequently reported side effects. Respiratory depression occurs in some patients. Allergic skin reactions may occur, and blurred vision and hypoglycemia have been noted. Several drug interactions including the potentiation of alcohol, amphetamines, barbiturates, and hypnotic agents have also been noted. Concurrent use of tricyclic antidepressants impairs the metabolism of the benzodiazepines, thus potentiating their effect (Bassuk & Schoonover, 1978). There is high potential for both physical and psychological addiction, and tolerance does develop.

OVERVIEW

Whereas previously the responsibility for monitoring pharmacological therapy was strictly the domain of the psychiatrist, now, with general practitioners prescribing the bulk of antianxiety drugs, an increasing burden of responsibility is being placed on the nonmedical mental health professional to be able to distinguish between appropriate and inappropriate pharmacological therapy. In light of this development, it has become necessary for the mental health professional to gain a fundamental understanding of the various antianxiety drugs and their application.

REFERENCES

American Psychiatric Association. (1980). *Diagnostic and statistical manual of mental disorders* (3rd ed.). Washington, DC: Author.

Archives of General Psychiatry. (1984). *41*(Suppl. 10), 921–1012.

Bassuk, E., & Schoonover, S.C. (1987). *The practitioners guide to psychoactive drugs*, (2nd ed.). New York: Plenum.

Honigfeld, G., & Howard, A. (1978). *Psychiatric drugs: A desk reference*. New York: Academic Press.

Internal Medicine for the Specialist. (1985). Special supplement: Proceedings of a symposium, "Anxiolytic evolution in today's anxious world," held 21 May in Dallas, TX.

Shader, R. (1977). Manual of psychiatric therapeutics (5th ed.). Boston: Little, Brown & Co.

Spiegel, R., & Aebi, H.J. (1984). *Psychopharmacology: An introduction* (K. Kerr, Trans.). New York: Wiley.

Trimble, M. (1983). *Benzodiazepines divided: A multidisciplinary review*. New York: Wiley.

BIBLIOGRAPHY

Green, B. (1981). *Goodbye blues: Breaking the tranquilizer habit the natural way*. New York: McGraw-Hill.

Swonger, A., & Constantine, L.L. (1976). *Drugs and therapy: A psychotherapist's handbook of psychotropic drugs*. Boston: Little, Brown & Co.

Part III

The Major Psychoactive Medications

This section provides some of the basic information that the nonmedical psychotherapist needs to know about psychoactive medications. It should be noted, however, that there are constant changes in the field of psychopharmacology. For example, several years ago Valium, an antianxiety medication, was the most frequently prescribed drug in the United States; today the most frequently prescribed drug is Tagamet, an ulcer medication. For this reason, keeping up-to-date by reading journal articles and attending training courses on issues in psychopharmacology is most important for the nonmedical psychotherapist.

Chapter 13

Neurological Medications and Anticonvulsants

Gary R. Lewis and Gary W. Lawson

NEUROLOGICAL DISORDERS AND THEIR PHARMACOLOGICAL TREATMENT

The most common of the neurological medications are those that affect the central nervous system. It is with the side effects of these medications that the clinician will most likely be confronted. The most frequently occurring symptoms of neurological medications' side effects are extrapyramidal effects such as parkinsonian syndrome, dystonia, dyskinesia, and akathisia. Although drowsiness is also frequently present, it is a much less serious symptom.

Parkinsonian syndrome is especially frequent, particularly in the geriatric population (Chien, 1971); parkinsonian syndrome symptoms also occur as a side effect to antipsychotic medications as well as the major tranquilizers. (See Chapter 9.) The symptoms associated with parkinsonian syndrome include muscular rigidity, tremor, postural alterations, and akinesia or a decrease in spontaneous movements. When the latter symptom is present, the clinician must be careful not to diagnose the condition as a psychomotor retardation similar to that found in depressed clients. Other frequently occurring characteristics in this type of client are a fixed, masklike expression, a shuffling gait, drooling, and a loss of associated movement (such as the free swinging of arms while walking).

Dystonia refers to an increase in muscular rigidity that limits the client's ability to move the affected area. This condition usually affects certain muscle groups, resulting in asymmetric, distorted movements. Dystonia sometimes presents in a sudden onset and involves severe muscle cramping, which is referred to as acute dystonic reaction.

Dyskinesia is involuntary, repetitive movement that, when associated with the fine motor movements of the hand, appears as a type of "pill rolling" motion.

Akathisia manifests itself in involuntary motor restlessness, an inability to sit still, or constant fidgeting. Sometimes this condition is experienced completely subjectively as a feeling of strong inner tension, and the client may say "I feel as if I'm going to jump out of my skin." As such, this side effect may be hard to distinguish from the primary symptom of anxiety or agitation. Whether subjective symptoms of inner tension and restlessness are truly drug-induced side effects can be determined, as Van Putten (1975) suggests, by a trial of intramuscular antiparkinsonian medication such as biperiden (5 mg). If the symptoms constitute a side effect, there will be symptomatic relief for several hours.

Medications that are commonly utilized in attempts to overcome these extrapyramidal symptoms are biperiden (Akineton), trihexyphenidyl (Artane), benztropine mesylate (Cogentin), and procyclidine (Kemadrin). These medications appear to reduce the number of nerve impulses passing to peripheral effector cells by way of the postganglionic nerve fibers. They also appear to prevent neurotransmitter molecules from fulfilling their impulse-transmitting functions at tissues and organs innervated by postganglionic cholinergic nerve fibers (Dowd, 1986).

Neurological medications are, however, also associated with various side effects. These include dry mouth, blurred vision, skin dryness or rash, fever, palpitations (tachycardia), constipation, nausea and vomiting, urinary retention, drowsiness, mental confusion, headache, dizziness, excitement, weakness, and poor coordination.

CONVULSIVE DISORDERS AND ANTICONVULSANT MEDICATIONS

The next class of medications to be considered comprises those used to treat convulsive disorders or epilepsy. The term epilepsy is derived from a Greek word meaning to seize or fall upon and has long been applied to a group of "explosive" reactions that at one time was believed to constitute a disease entity of its own. There is now general agreement that epilepsy is not a disease entity but a symptom complex characterized by periodic, transient episodes of an alteration in the state of consciousness that may be associated with convulsive movements or disturbances in feeling or behavior (or both).

The kind of pharmacological intervention that is utilized for convulsive disorders is dependent on the type of seizure and the accompanying symptoms. The three major types of seizures are usually described as grand mal, petit mal, and psychomotor seizure or their equivalent. It is of great importance that the clinician be able to recognize psychomotor epilepsy, since it is characterized by trancelike attacks and confusional episodes that often lead to its misdiagnosis as schizophrenia. Included under this heading of psychomotor seizure are narcolepsy, a sudden irresistible desire to sleep, and cataplexy, a paralysis of voluntary movements and postural collapse of the whole body.

The primary aim of the pharmacological intervention is to administer a medication that will counteract the explosive tendency of the brain cells. This was accomplished for more than 60 years by the use of bromides, which were first introduced in 1857. These appear to have been largely replaced by several newer classes of medications that have become available (Stevens, 1966).

Barbiturates

Phenobarbital

Phenobarbital is a long-acting barbiturate and the most broadly used anticonvulsant. Its principal mode of action is in major motor, psychomotor, and focal seizures.

Drowsiness, which is usually transient, is the drug's most common adverse effect, although some children can become hyperactive. If the clinician observes these symptoms, underlying attentional disorders with or without hyperactivity should be suspected (Conners, 1971; Campbell, 1975); such a disorder could be the root cause of both the seizures and the response. Gastrointestinal upset is also noted occasionally and can include nausea, vomiting, and diarrhea.

Mephobarbital (Mebaral)

Mebaral is metabolized in the same manner as phenobarbital; thus it has similar properties and uses. Its major drawback is that larger dosages are necessary. Side effects are the same as those listed for phenobarbital.

Metharbital (Gemonil)

Gemonil has the same structural relation to barbital as mephobarbital has to phenobarbital. Its properties and uses are similar to those of phenobarbital, but this barbiturate requires even larger dosages than mephobarbital and is dependent on the patient's weight.

Primidone (Mysoline)

Mysoline is not a barbiturate by traditional classification but is considered with this group because of its close chemical relation. The primary use for Mysoline is in clients not responding adequately to a barbiturate-hydantoin regime (see below). Larger doses are needed than those for phenobarbital, however.

Sedation often diminishes with continuation of this medication over a period of time. When the dosage is increased gradually, incapacitating drowsiness can be avoided. Gastrointestinal upset and other minor adverse reactions are similar to those listed for phenobarbital.

Hydantoins

Diphenylhydantoin and diphenylhydantoin sodium (Dilantin and Dilantin Sodium)

Dilantin and Dilantin Sodium are the most frequently used drugs for major motor, psychomotor, and focal epilepsies. They often are used together with phenobarbital or primidone when a single drug is inadequate. Dilantin and Dilantin Sodium are the most common initial medications chosen, particularly in adults.

The medications have the advantage of producing little or no sedation in usual doses. Blurred vision and spots before the eyes may occasionally occur and can be treated by a reduction in the dosage of the medication. Gingival hyperplasia is commonly seen, particularly in children; this can be avoided by conscientious oral hygiene. Rare but serious side effects are hirsutism in the young, skin eruptions, hepatitis, bone-marrow depression, systemic lupus erythematosus, Stevens-Johnson syndrome, and lymphadenopathy.

Ethotoin (Peganone)

Peganone is only moderately effective in grand mal epilepsy and only slightly so in psychomotor epilepsy. It is seldom used alone for this reason. Its toxicity resembles that of Dilantin, but the incidence of reactions is generally lower. Thus this drug is less toxic but less effective than Dilantin.

Mephenytoin (Mesantoin)

Mesantoin is effective in major motor, psychomotor, and focal epilepsies but is more toxic than Dilantin. It is usually only used with those clients who do not respond to the drugs of choice. Mesantoin has a sedative effect that is usually absent with Dilantin; otherwise it lacks or has a lower incidence of some of the more minor adverse effects of Dilantin. Life-threatening and other serious reactions are considerably more common, however.

Succinimides

Within this classification are three major medications used to treat psychomotor or grand mal epilepsy: ethosuximide (Zarontin), methsuximide (Celontin), and phensuximide (Milontin). These are the drugs of choice for grand mal seizures. They are also effective for minor motor seizures in some clients but are generally effective for psychomotor or grand mal epilepsy or in clients with considerable organic brain damage.

The most common adverse reactions of the succinimides are gastrointestinal disturbances. Drowsiness, ataxia, headache, dizziness, euphoria, hiccups, rashes, and behavioral changes have also been reported. Major side effects occur considerably less frequently than with the oxazolidinediones (see below). Aplastic anemia, thrombocytopenia, leukopenia, pancytopenia, and eosinophilia are noted rarely.

Oxazolidinediones

The medications in this classification are principally effective in controlling petit mal seizures. They include trimethadione (Tridione) and paramethadione (Paradione). Although these drugs are among the most effective treatments for this condition, they should only be used in the most difficult clients because of their toxicity. Serious reactions, some of them fatal, include rashes that may progress to exfoliative dermatitis or erythema multiforme, nephropathy, hepatitis, and bone-marrow depression. Reversible visual disturbances, particularly hemeralopia, are quite common. Hiccups and hair loss may also be noted.

Other Anticonvulsants

Miscellaneous anticonvulsants are classified as primary and secondary. The primary medications include carbamazepine (Tegretol), diazepam (Valium), paraldehyde, and phenacemide (Phenurone). The secondary drugs are acetazolamide (Diamox) and lidocaine hydrochloride (Xylocaine hydrochloride).

REFERENCES

Campbell, M. (1975). Psychopharmacology in childhood psychosis. *International Journal of Mental Health, 4,* 238–254.

Chien, C.P. (1971). Psychiatric treatment for geriatric patients: "Pub" or drug? *American Journal of Psychiatry, 127,* 1070–1075.

Conners, C.K. (1971). Recent drug studies with hyperkinetic children. *Journal of Learning Disabilities, 4,* 476(a).

Dowd, A.L. (Ed.). (1986). *Physicians Desk Reference* (40th ed.). New Jersey: Medical Economics.

Stevens, J.R. (1966). Psychiatric implications of psychomotor epilepsy. *Archives of General Psychiatry, 14,* 461–471.

Van Putten, T. (1975). The many faces of akathisia. *Comprehensive Psychiatry, 16,* 43–47.

Chapter 14

Central Nervous System Stimulants

Thomas Young and Gary W. Lawson

Medically, central nervous system stimulants (amphetamines) have been primarily used to treat obesity. They are not often used for that purpose today. They are still used to treat some rare diseases such as narcolepsy and in the treatment of hyperactive children. However, their medical value is far outweighed by their potential for abuse.

The principal central nervous system stimulants or amphetamine compounds that are available in the United States include preparations of racemic amphetamine sulfate (Benzedrine), dextroamphetamine sulfate (Dexedrine, Ferndex), dextroamphetamine hydrochloride (Daro), dextroamphetamine tannate (Obotan), methamphetamine hydrochloride (Desoxyn, Methampex), amphetamine complex (Biphetamine), amphetamine combined (Obetrol, Delcobese), *d*-amphetamine plus amobarbital (Dexamyl), and *d*-amphetamine plus prochlorperazine (Eskatrol). In addition, there are a number of amphetamine-like psychostimulants, such as benzphetamine (Didrex), chlorphentermine (Pre-Sate), chlortermine (Voranil), diethylpropion (Tenuate), fenfluramine (Pondimin), methylphenidate (Ritalin), phendimetrazine (Plegine), phenmetrazine (Preludin), and phentermine (Ionamin). These drugs differ chemically from the amphetamine compounds but are similar in both their pharmacology and effect (Ellinwood & Petrie, 1977; Morgan, 1981; Young, Young, Klein, Klein, & Beyer, 1979).

Psychostimulants were once capriciously prescribed in the treatment of depression, epilepsy, Parkinsonian syndrome, narcolepsy, obesity, and hyperkinetic behavior in children (Ellinwood, 1973; Griffith, 1968). Today, their clinical use is primarily limited to the last three disorders, with approximately 80% to 85% of the prescriptions for amphetamines being utilized for their anorexiant effect (Morgan, 1981; Ray, 1972). Actually, these drugs have limited utility as anorexiants for two reasons: first, they lose their dietary effectiveness as tolerance increases; second, in most cases obesity is due to maladaptive behavior patterns that need to be changed (Schachter, 1971; Stunkart, 1968). The practice of prescribing Ritalin for hyperactivity has also been criticized by conflict sociologists and existential psychologists on the grounds that this "disorder" is as much the result of objective physiological reality (see, for example, Conrad, 1975, 1976, 1980; Schraf & Divoky, 1975; Zola, 1972).

At least three patterns of amphetamine abuse can be described, each manifesting somewhat different motives but all affecting consciousness in some manner (Tinklenberg, 1972). The first pattern features the use of low dosages for limited periods to overcome fatigue and to improve psychomotor functioning. Consequently, this type of abuse is seen in such situations as long-distance driving, military maneuvers, "cramming" for examinations, and athletic competition. In a survey of university students, for example, Rabins, Swanson, and Gallant (1974) found that 26% of the sample had used amphetamines as a study aid. In a survey of professional football players, Johnson (1973) discovered that 60% of the athletes regularly used amphetamines in game situations. Grinspoon and Hedblom (1975) estimated that more than 180 million amphetamine tablets were supplied to U.S. troops during World War II.

The second pattern of abuse involves the sustained consumption of oral doses in gradually increasing amounts. In these cases, the abuser is often trying to overcome obesity, fatigue, or depression through a process of self-medication. This can eventually lead to adverse behavior effects, however, since it not only can intensify pre-existing psychotic symptoms but also can induce a paranoid psychosis in nonschizophrenic individuals (Angrist and Gershon, 1970; Griffith, 1969; Segal and Janowsky, 1978).

The third pattern of abuse entails the intravenous injection of an amphetamine several times a day with a total dosage of between 1 and 2 g. This type of consumption typically leads to "runs" of 10 to 14 days of repeated amphetamine injections without food or sleep. Once the user "crashes," he or she may sleep for several days and may experience lethargy and depression upon awakening. During this period, the user may seek relief through alcohol and other sedatives, including heroin. Considering this clinical picture, it is not surprising that chronic intravenous amphetamine users are often marked by polydrug abuse, hepatitis, anorexia, malnutrition, physical deterioration, psychotic symptoms, and antisocial behavior (Morgan, 1981).

CLINICAL DIAGNOSIS AND TREATMENT OF AMPHETAMINE ABUSE OR DEPENDENCE

A diagnosis of amphetamine or similarly acting sympathomimetic abuse is made if there is a pattern of pathological use for at least 1 month with impairment in social or occupational functioning. If the essential clinical picture is either tolerance or withdrawal, a diagnosis of amphetamine or similarly acting sympathomimetic dependence is made.

The diagnostic criteria for amphetamine or similarly acting sympathomimetic intoxication are listed in the *Diagnostic and Statistical Manual of Mental Disorders* (Third Edition) (DSM-III; American Psychiatric Association, 1980) as follows.

1. Recent use of amphetamine or similarly acting sympathomimetic.
2. Within 1 hour of use, at least two of the following psychological symptoms:
   —psychomotor agitation
   —elation
   —gradiosity
   —loquacity
   —hypervigilance.
3. Within 1 hour of use, at least two of the following physical symptoms:
   —tachycardia
   —pupillary dilation
   —elevated blood pressure
   —perspiration or chills
   —nausea or vomiting.
4. Maladaptive behavioral effects (e.g., fighting, impaired judgment, interference with social or occupational functioning).
5. The symptoms are not due to any other physical or mental disorder. (p. 148)

Acute psychostimulant intoxication is generally handled by providing the client reassurance in a quiet environment. In cases of marked agitation, diazepam (Valium) can be given intramuscularly or orally in dosages of 10–20-mg every 2 hours. Severe intoxication is a medical emergency requiring such life-supportive measures as assisted ventilation, cardiac monitoring, and intravenous fluids and electrolytes (Steinhart, 1976).

A diagnosis of amphetamine or similarly acting sympathomimetic delirium is indicated if the essential clinical feature is a delirium within 24 hours of substance use. In most cases, however, the onset is within 1 hour and is also less commonly seen after intoxication. Associated features include tactile and olfactory hallucinations, labile affect, and violent behavior. Complications include syncope, seizures, and death from cardiac dysrhythmias and respiratory paralysis.

A diagnosis of amphetamine or similarly acting sympathomimetic delusional disorder is made when the essential feature is an organic delusional syndrome due to the recent consumption of a psychostimulant during a period of long-term use of moderate or high dosages. The diagnostic criteria for this disorder feature persecutory delusions and at least three of the following: (1) ideas of reference, (2) aggressiveness and hostility, (3) anxiety, or (4) psychomotor agitation. Although the delusional state can linger for more than a year, in most cases the course does not exceed more than 1 week. The length of this syndrome can be shortened by the use of antipsychotic medications such as chlorpromazine (Thorazine), which is given intramuscularly in dosages of 25 to 50 mg every 3 to 4 hours (Steinhart, 1976).

The clinical picture of amphetamine or similarly acting sympathomimetic withdrawal features depressed mood, fatigue, disturbed sleep, and increased dreaming. The onset of the syndrome occurs within 3 days of cessation of or reduction in substance abuse. Usually the symptoms peak in 2 to 4 days, but depression and irritability may last for several months. Since suicide is a complication associated with this syndrome, the patient should be closely observed by the clinician and significant others.

REFERENCES

American Psychiatric Association. (1980). *Diagnostic and statistical manual of mental disorders* (3rd ed.). Washington, DC: Author.

Angrist, B.M., & Gershon, S. (1970). The phenomenology of experimentally induced amphetamine psychosis. *Biological Psychiatry, 2*, 95.

Conrad, P. (1975). The discovery of hyperkinesis: Notes in the medicalization of deviant behavior. *Social Problems, 23*, 12–21.

Conrad, P. (1976). *Identifying hyperactive children: The medicalization of deviant behavior.* Lexington, MA: D.C. Heath.

Conrad, P. (1980). On the medicalization of deviance. In D. Ingleby (Ed.), *Critical psychiatry* (pp. 102–119). New York: Pantheon.

Ellinwood, E.H., Jr. (1973). Amphetamine and stimulant drugs. In *Drug use in America: Problems in perspective* (second report of the National Commission on Marijuana and Drug Abuse). Washington, DC: U.S. Government Printing Office.

Ellinwood, E.H., Jr., & Petrie, W.M. (1977). Dependence on amphetamine, cocaine, and other stimulants. In S.N. Pradhan & S.N. Dutta (Eds.), *Drug abuse: Clinical and basic aspects.* St. Louis, MO: C.V. Mosby.

Griffith, J.D. (1968). Psychiatric implications of amphetamine abuse. In J.R. Russo (Ed.), *Amphetamine abuse.* Springfield, IL: Charles C Thomas.

Griffith, J.D. (1969). Schizophreniform psychosis inducted by large administration of amphetamine. *Journal of Psychiatric Drugs, 2*, 42.

Grinspoon, L., & Hedblom, P. (1975). *The speed culture: Amphetamine use and abuse in America.* Cambridge, MA: Harvard Univ. Press.

Johnson, L.A. (1973). Amphetamine Abuse in Professional Football (Doctoral dissertation, Ann Arbor, MI, *73-11*, 437).

Morgan, J.P. (1981). Amphetamines. In J.H. Lowinson & P. Ruiz (Eds.), *Substance abuse: Clinical problems and perspectives* (pp. 167–184). Baltimore, MD: Williams & Wilkins.

Rabins, P., Swanson, W.C., & Gallant, D.M. (1974). A comparison of two methods of determining drug use among university students. *Journal of the Louisiana State Medical Society, 126*, 1.

Ray, O.S. (1972). *Drugs, society, and human behavior.* St. Louis, MO: C.V. Mosby.

Schachter, S. (1971). Some extraordinary facts about obese humans and rats. *American Psychologist, 26*, 129–144.

Schraf, P., & Divoky, D. (1975). *The myth of the hyperactive child.* New York: Pantheon.

Segal, D.S., & Janowsky, D.S. (1978). Psychostimulant-induced behavioral effects: Possible models of schizophrenia. In M.A. Lipton, A. Dimascio, & K.F. Killam (Eds.), *Psychopharmacology: A generation of progress.* New York: Raven.

Steinhart, M. (1976). Drug abuse. In C. Ekert (Ed.), *Emergency room care* (pp. 437–459). Boston: Little, Brown & Co.

Stunkart, A.J. (1968). Environment and obesity: Recent advances in our understanding of regulation of food intake in man. *Federation Proceedings, 27*, 1367–1373.

Tinklenberg, J.R. (1972). A current view of the amphetamines. In P.H. Blachly (Ed.), *Progress in drug abuse.* Springfield, IL: Charles C Thomas.

Young, L.A., Young, L.G., Klein, M.M., Klein, D.M., & Beyer, D. (1979). *Recreational drugs.* New York: Berkley Books.

Zola, I.K. (1972). Medicine as an institution of social control. *Sociological Review, 20*, 487–504.

Part IV

Special Populations

There are two populations that do not respond to drugs in the ways that the average adult population might respond. These groups are children and the elderly, and both have their own special issues. Many therapists have made the mistake of treating children as if they were small adults. They are not. Their thinking, their values, and their issues in life are different from those of adults. The same can be said of the elderly; for developmental reasons they see the world differently than younger people. For these reasons, the two chapters in this section have been added to provide the nonmedical psychotherapist with the special insights needed to work with these two populations.

Chapter 15

Geriatric Populations and Drugs

Ann W. Lawson

The geriatric population is often overlooked and sometimes hidden in our society. Yet it is a rapidly growing population with increasing needs. Of the estimated 250 million people in the United States, 20 million are older than 65. It is predicted that 35 million people will be in this age bracket by 1990. Offer (1974) predicts that by the year 2000, one half of the population will be older than 50 and one third will be older than 65. Brotman (1980) reports that life expectancy is 70 for males and 77 for females. With advances in technology and medical care these estimates may rise even higher, and the life expectancy could increase. Even though the elderly population is increasing, its problems continue to be overlooked or misdiagnosed.

Although it may seem that the elderly have more physical problems than other populations, they are rarely thought of as drug abusers. Yet the elderly are at high risk for misuse and at considerable risk for abuse of legal drugs, and there is a small group of elderly opiate addicts (Glantz, 1983). These misuses and abuses include alcohol, prescription drugs, and over-the-counter drugs. These problems are often complicated by mental disorders or confused with the symptoms of aging. Furthermore, the elderly use three times as many prescription drugs as all other groups combined (Hanan, 1978). This puts them at risk for drug interactions that often go undiagnosed because of the similarity between drug interaction symptoms and the symptoms of old age (forgetfulness, weakness, confusion, tremor, anorexia, and anxiety).

The aging process creates new physical and psychological stresses that increase the risk of drug abuse and misuse for the elderly. The physical changes alter the way in which a drug is absorbed and distributed through the body, metabolized, and then excreted. The elderly experience decreased tolerance for drugs, and drugs stay in the body longer and have prolonged biologic activity. They have more clinical and toxic effects, and they tend to accumulate in fatty tissues (Shader, 1975). Psychologically, the elderly face a number of late-life stresses including bereavement from the loss of family and friends, loss of occupation because of retirement, loneliness, boredom, and impaired health and physical abilities. They are often victims of self-neglect, falls, and aggressive and violent behavior, sometimes at the hands of their relatives.

Considering the difficulties of aging, it becomes more understandable how the elderly could be at risk for drug abuse. It is interesting to compare this aging population with adolescents, an age group that is more easily recognizable as drug abusing. The similarities include uncertain and changing roles and self-concepts, low social status, disadvantages in employment and income, shifting and uncertain social supports, and limited resources for coping. Both groups also find drugs readily available. One difference is that adolescents use illicit drugs more often, whereas the elderly use licit drugs (Mandolini, 1981). This difference is understandable for people who grew up in the Prohibition era, which colored their views of alcohol consumption and the use of illegal substances. This same group spent a lifetime learning to trust physicians and to use medications when they were sick. Often their physicians are important social contacts who give them drugs to relieve symptoms and stresses.

Drugs most often prescribed for elderly patients are cardiovascular medication (22%), tranquilizers (10%), diuretics (9%), and sedative-hypnotics (9%) (Mandolini, 1981). These drugs are prescribed for heart disease, hypertension, arthritis and rheumatism, and mental and nervous conditions. It is common for the elderly to combine their prescription drugs with over-the-counter drugs, increasing the potential for harmful interactions.

In addition to prescription drug misuse, the elderly have alcohol problems, psychiatric disorders, and reduced resources. These difficulties are hard to diagnose, and they overlap. The elderly may not seek psychological care or drug and alcohol rehabilitation, and they may have lost many of the social contacts who could intervene and get help for them: The threat of job loss is no longer there, and they may be living alone with little contact with family and friends. To complicate the picture further, the elderly may be experiencing new physical limitations. Busse (1983) points out that two of five males aged 65 and older have restricted activity, and one of four is unable to carry on some major activity. Those more than 75 years of age are even more limited.

This chapter focuses specifically on mental disorders of late life, drug misuse and abuse, alcohol problems, and the best methods of helping the geriatric client. There is limited literature on the problems of the elderly and the kinds of therapy most beneficial to them. As Glantz (1983) notes, "Research in this area is really just beginning and the relevant literature is limited, often inconclusive and sometimes contradictory" (p. 1). It is important, however, for therapists to be aware of potential problems and symptoms of these problems in their elderly clients.

MENTAL DISORDERS OF LATE LIFE

The most common mental disorders of the elderly are senile and presenile dementia, depression, suicide, and hypochondriasis. Although studies of organic brain disorders differ in their criteria and definitions, it is estimated that the prevalence of moderate and severe dementia varies from 5% to 7.1% (Busse, 1983). About 50% of the residents of nursing homes in the United States are there because of organic brain impairment. Presenile dementia is often called Alzheimer's disease and appears to be similar to senile dementia. The *Diagnostic and Statistical Manual of Mental Disorders (Third Edition)* (DSM-III; American Psychiatric Association, 1980) differentiates between these two disorders by the age of onset: presenile dementia occurs in younger people and often in those who have a familial history of Down's syndrome.

With aging comes increased frequency and depth of depressive episodes in the elderly. Often these episodes are linked to the loss of the functions or objects that created self-esteem earlier in life, such as a job, a family, friends, and a sense of life direction and worthiness. This form of environmentally induced depression should be distinguished from major depressive illness, which requires medication and possible hospitalization. According to DSM-III, major depression lasts at least 2 weeks, and there are four to eight symptoms that are persistent and significant, including appetite and weight changes, sleep changes, loss of energy, psychomotor agitation or retardation, loss of interest in pleasurable activities, decrease in sex drive, feelings of self-reproach or inappropriate guilt, decreased ability to think, indecisiveness, and suicide ideation. The elderly may not have the same symptoms of depression found in young people. They may show an increased sensitivity to pain and refuse to get out of bed when they do not require bed rest. They may exhibit poor concentration, a narrowing of coping styles, and increased physical complaints. Depression can often be confused with dementia in the elderly and thus not given proper treatment.

As a result of the same problems that increase depression in the elderly, there is also an increase in suicides. Of all suicides, 25% to 30% occur in people older than 65. This rate is five times that of the general population and jumps to eight times higher in the group older than 75. Women tend to have a peak in suicide rate between ages 45 and 64, whereas the rate for men increases after age 64; this may be due to retirement and loss of purpose. Women, however, tend to be more depressed after age 65 than men (Busse, 1983).

Hypochondriasis is prevalent among women late in life. It is often associated with depression and is complicated by actual chronic disabilities. Although it is difficult to know which complaints are real and which are imagined, Busse (1983) suggests that outpatient treatment reduces the risk of reinforcing the hypo-chrondriasis while hospitalization convinces the patient that an organic explanation does exist but was missed in the examination. These complaints should not be disregarded because, as Salzman, Vander Kolk, and Shader (1975) state, "Depressed elderly patients, especially white males, may be high suicide risks; the only warning may be hypochondriasis of recent origin" (p. 179).

SOMATIC TREATMENT OF MENTAL ILLNESSES IN THE ELDERLY

Most of the mental illnesses that require somatic treatment fall into four categories: behavioral disturbances, disorders of affect (depression and anxiety), impaired cognitive functioning, and problems with sleep (Shader, 1975).

Behavioral problems may be the result of psychotic, organic, or affective disorders. Many elderly patients with schizophrenia or other psychoses developed these conditions earlier in life. Those who develop psychosis after age 65 usually experience paranoia, which is characterized by agitation, paranoid delusions, emotional distress, grandiosity, thought disorder, and auditory hallucinations (Shader, 1975). Involutional psychotic reactions are characterized by depression, florid paranoid ideation, and agitated behavior; depression can also be associated with agitation. Organic problems may be associated with agitation, assaultiveness, inappropriate inquisitiveness, and wandering. These symptoms may become worse at night and are referred to as sundowner's syndrome (Shader, 1975). Neuroleptic agents are usually the treatment. There are many side effects of these agents (see Chapter 9), and the elderly are at risk of overmedication since they do not need the same dosages as younger patients.

Tricyclic antidepressants have been used successfully to treat mild to moderately severe depression. Shader (1975) points out that they may activate psychotic or manic symptoms in the elderly if there is underlying schizophrenia, schizoaffective disorder, or manic-depressive illness.

The losses suffered in late life may trigger old neurotic symptoms including anxiety, depression, and obsessive-compulsive behaviors. These symptoms are also common to the onset of organic brain syndrome. Antianxiety agents are used to treat these symptoms, but they may cause drowsiness, especially if they have a long half-life. The best treatments are psychotherapy, family therapy, and social intervention.

As mentioned above, probably 50% of the elderly in nursing homes and mental hospitals have organic brain syndrome, which is a mental disorder caused by or associated with diffuse impairment of brain tissue functioning. Up to 30% of those who are not institutionalized have some form of organic brain syndrome (Shader, 1975). Acute organic brain syndrome is reversible and characterized by sudden restlessness, confusion, disorientation, disordered behavior, incontinence, and hallucinations. It is important to diagnose and treat underlying causes. Symptoms can be controlled with phenothiazines. Chronic organic brain syndrome is characterized by impaired recent and remote memory, deficit in immediate recall, disorientation, lack of attention and concentration, fluctuation of state of consciousness, and impaired judgment and social functioning. This condition may accompany other existing illnesses. The patient's response to organic brain syndrome is influenced by his or her premorbid personality and current circumstances; these responses may include anxiety, agitation, depression, apathy, withdrawal, paranoid ideation, delusions, and hallucinations. Although some drug therapies, such as cerebral vasodilators and dihydrogenated ergot alkaloids, have had modest success, individual, group, and family therapy with mental and physical stimulation are recommended. Depression may occur simultaneously with this disorder and increase its symptoms; this should be cleared up with therapy and possibly antidepressants.

Sleep disorders are also found in the elderly. These are defined as difficulty falling asleep or early-morning waking and may involve daytime napping, anxiety, or physical distress. Chloral hydrate given at bedtime may relieve these problems, and antianxiety drugs are also occasionally used. Depression should be considered when the patient experiences persistent early-morning waking. This bedtime sedation may lead to the problems of night confusion and potential for falls if the patient gets up at night.

There are difficulties with drug therapies for the elderly. Psychotropic drugs have a certain degree of toxicity, and the elderly are susceptible to these side effects because of a decreased ability to withstand stress, an impaired organ system, and modified pharmacological responses to drugs (Shader, 1975). Side effects to be aware of are cardiovascular difficulties, neurologic disorders, and symptoms such as dryness of the mouth, constipation, vertigo, sweating, urinary retention, parkinsonian effects, and tardive dyskinesia. These symptoms can be further complicated if elderly patients are also using over-the-counter drugs, other prescription drugs, or alcohol. Complete drug histories should be obtained, and unnecessary medications or interacting drugs should be deleted. Drug-free holidays may be needed to reduce toxicity.

ABUSE AND MISUSE OF LICIT AND PRESCRIBED DRUGS

In addition to the problems the elderly may have with psychotropic medications, they are at risk for overmedication by their physicians, drug interactions, erratic drug use, and misuse of over-the-counter drugs (Whittington, 1983b). Their unique life situations and the presence of chronic illnesses contribute to the misuse. The aging who are most at risk are alcoholics, the chronically painfully ill, and those who are troubled with chronic anxiety states, somatization disorders, and insomnia (Kofoed, 1985).

How common is substance abuse in late life? Use of illegal drugs such as marijuana, LSD, and opiates is usually found only in aging criminals. Older opiate users often switch to more readily available drugs such as hydromorphone (Dilaudid) and reduce their intake, or they use barbiturates or alcohol as substitutes on occasion. The abuse of cocaine and amphetamines is rare mainly because of the decreased effect of these drugs with aging and changing neurochemistry (Kofoed, 1985). Although this is a small problem with the elderly now, as the younger population currently abusing illicit drugs grows older it will probably increase.

More frequently, the elderly abuse prescription drugs. They comprise 10% of the population, yet they use 25% of all prescribed drugs (Basen, 1977), which are more available to the elderly than illicit drugs and are often prescribed for pain or insomnia. Sedatives and narcotics are the most common drugs of abuse, followed by narcotic analgesics (Kofoed, 1985). Women, twice as often as men, abuse analgesics (including opioids), antianxiety agents, and sedative hypnotics (Atkinson, 1984). Twenty-five percent of drugs prescribed for the elderly are psychoactive, and Stephens, Haney, and Underwood (1982) discovered that 18% of the elderly receive them. However, two-thirds were taking them as prescribed; those who were not were underusing them. The major problem with prescription use among elderly is omission (Schwartz, Wang, Zeitz, & Gross, 1962).

It is important to distinguish between drug abuse and misuse with the elderly; this distinction helps to locate the area in which intervention is needed. There are two major differences between abuse and misuse. First, abuse is intended, or the inappropriateness of use is known, whereas misuse is inadvertent. Second, abuse has some psychoactive or psychosocial consequence and may involve licit or illicit drugs, including alcohol (Glantz, 1983), whereas misuse does not.

To elucidate further, drug abuse is the nontherapeutic use of drugs, including alcohol, which adversely impacts on the user's life. The drug may be obtained from legal or illegal sources and used occasionally or habitually. As Glantz (1983) outlines, abuse entails some or all of the following.

1. using an illegal drug
2. using an illegally obtained drug (i.e., by falsified prescription)
3. using multiple prescriptions of the same or a similar drug
4. using a drug prescribed for another person
5. hoarding drugs and taking them all at one time
6. knowingly using a drug for purposes other than those for which it was prescribed
7. violating prescription directions, deviation in quantity or frequency, or consumption with other contraindicated drugs
8. excessively using alcohol
9. excessively consuming caffeinated beverages
10. smoking more than is considered safe

11. taking more of an over-the-counter drug than recommended by directions
12. combining over-the-counter drugs with alcohol or a prescribed drug (or both)

Drug misuse is the inappropriate use of drugs that were meant to be used therapeutically. Glantz describes misuse as the inappropriate prescription of drugs due to

1. physician's lack of knowledge
2. errors in physician's judgment
3. lack of supervision of a physician or lack of instructions
4. excessive use of over-the-counter drugs

Misuse of drugs usually takes four forms: overuse, underuse, erratic use, and contraindicated use (Peterson, Whittington, & Beer, 1979). The most common misuse of drugs among the elderly is underuse. This occurs most frequently when prescribed drugs are expensive, are used mainly to control symptoms, and are likely to produce side effects (Hemminki and Heikkla, 1975). Most often, misuse of drugs among the elderly is due to errors by the physician and in the prescription process. According to Whittington (1983), problems include

1. selecting an inappropriate medication
2. prescribing too high or too low a dosage
3. prescribing too many different drugs at a time
4. failing to check the potential for side effects or interaction
5. failing to check the patient's drug history, including over-the-counter drugs, current prescriptions, and alcohol intake
6. prescribing over the phone
7. providing inadequate oral or written instructions for taking the medications or inadequate information about possible reactions
8. allowing too many automatic renewals

Physicians may hold stereotypes of the elderly. They may feel that aging is synonymous with disease and that there is little that can be done to help the elderly. This may cause physicians to rely on medical (drug) solutions to nonmedical problems. This process is further complicated by the following problems of the elderly (Whittington, 1983).

1. They may have several simultaneous problems and medications.
2. They experience a slower rate of drug absorption, distribution, metabolism, and excretion.
3. They are at greater risk for side effects.

4. They often have cognitive deficits and may view the physician as a powerful authority whom they will not question.

Given this dilemma, it is difficult to know where to intervene. Do physicians need to be educated about the unique pharmacological and psychological needs of the elderly, or do the elderly need to be self-advocates? The answer, probably, is both, but therapists who work with elderly patients can also be teachers and advocates once they understand the risks that are inherent when such a patient seeks medical help.

Several investigators have studied the misuse of prescription drugs among the elderly to determine the reasons for the problem. Doyle and Hamm (1976) studied 405 people in Florida who were 60 years of age or older. When questioned about the process of receiving prescription drugs, 72% said they did not usually inform physicians if they were using drugs, only 13% saw the physician in person, and the rest received the prescription over the phone. Furthermore, 75% did not question the pharmacist about the drug's action, possible side effects, or cost. The Michigan Office of Services to the Aging and the Michigan Office of Substance Abuse Services (1979) surveyed 371 persons aged 60 or older to discover why they stopped taking or varied their prescription drugs. The responses indicated that 43% felt better when they stopped or varied their prescription drugs, 18% reported side effects as the reason, and 10% forgot to take the medication. Stephens, Haney, and Underwood (1981) found that their subjects stopped their medication or varied it for several reasons: 48% "did not like it" (or possibly did not like the physician), 23% used medication only when they needed it, 6.8% said that they got better results their way, 4.1% experienced bad side effects, 9.4% felt that the drug was too expensive, and 2.7% forgot. Although it is reported that the elderly hold physicians in high esteem, they often appear to make medical decisions themselves that are against the physician's advice.

Another area of prescription drug misuse is institutions. Often there is overuse of psychoactive medication, particularly sedatives and tranquilizers, because of the staff's desire to control agitated, unruly, or demanding patients (Learoyd, 1972; Gubrium, 1975). Misuse can include errors in administration of drugs in nursing homes (too much, too late, or with the wrong liquid); this is due to lack of staff training, poor controls, overloaded staff, and use of unlicensed nursing aides to distribute medications (Gubrium, 1975).

The main reason that abuse and misuse of prescription drugs by the elderly and those attending them is dangerous is the biological changes that cause the elderly to react differently than younger adults. With aging comes a decline of protein and an increase in fat. Moreover, metabolic rate declines 16% between 30 and 70 years of age and caloric requirements decrease by one third. Also, the loss of brain cells may make the elderly more sensitive to drugs, and brain enzymes and neurotransmitters are altered. The activity of monoamine oxidase increases, and dopamine, norepinephrine, serotonin, tyrosine hydroxylase, and cholinesterase activities decline. Furthermore, absorption of drugs is slow and erratic because of the low acid level in the stomach. Fat-soluble drugs (phenobarbital, diazepam, and chlorpromazine) tend to be stored for longer periods in the elderly. For these reasons there is a decrease in the intensity of the drug but a prolonged duration, which ultimately produces a toxic effect. Circulatory changes also alter drug absorption; drugs may accumulate in the brain and heart because these organs are the first to be supplied by a decreased cardiac output. The liver's capacity to metabolize drugs decreases with aging; this may be due to a reduced protein intake, which reduces available metabolizing enzymes and may cause prolonged effects of some drugs. Other drugs that must be metabolized for full effect are reduced in their effectiveness (Hanan, 1978). The kidneys also lose their functioning: there is a 30% glomerular filtration rate in individuals older than 65, so that drugs are excreted less efficiently.

Because of the potential for misuse of prescription drugs by the elderly, the therapist working with this population should be alert to signs of psychological reactions and behavior changes that could be due to toxicity or drug interaction. Antipsychotic drugs may cause oversedation, restlessness, withdrawal, and depression. Antidepressants may elicit confusional states and exacerbate schizophrenic and manic symptoms. Antianxiety drugs may lead to oversedation and occasionally disinhibition or uncontrolled rages. Antimanic drugs such as lithium can cause confusional states that can mimic organic brain syndrome if the drug level becomes toxic; this distinction is particularly crucial.

ABUSE AND MISUSE OF OVER-THE-COUNTER DRUGS

One of the most dangerous practices among the elderly is self-diagnosing and self-medicating with over-the-counter drugs. Kofoed (1984) reports that 69% of people 60 years of age and older use such drugs, and 40% use them daily. This is due partly to economics and possibly to bad experiences with health professionals. Over-the-counter medications can cause the elderly many problems, so that it is important to screen routinely for them when working with these clients.

In large doses, analgesics such as aspirin and acetaminophen can cause acute metabolic disturbances and organic mental disorders. Aspirin can cause stomach bleeding, and acetaminophen-elevated serum alkaline phosphatase levels and overdoses can cause liver damage (Stewart, Hale, & Marks, 1982). Laxatives are used by 10% of the elderly and can cause diarrhea and malabsorption syndromes. Antihistamines and anticholinergics, which include cold and allergy medications and sleeping aids, interact with alcohol and other drugs to enhance sedative effects. It is possible to develop toxic psychosis or delirium from anticholinergics. Antihistamines may be used by the elderly as sedatives and can produce acute toxic delirium resembling atropine psychosis (Shader, 1975). Sympatomimetics or decongestants can have a stimulant effect and produce psychoses similar to those induced by amphetamines, although this is rare in older persons. Alcohol-containing drugs, such as night cold medicines, are often used for the alcohol effect, but some elderly people consider them medicine and deny that they have alcohol-related problems. Antacids and bromides have been known to cause psychiatric symptoms; bromide toxicity can resemble schizophrenia.

Although caffeine and nicotine may not seem dangerous because they are in common, daily use, they can be problematic for the elderly. Caffeine overuse can contribute to anxiety and panic disorders, cardiac dysrhythmias, gastric disease, and osteoporosis. Caffeine is often found in over-the-counter medications as well as in beverages. Nicotine contributes to oral and lung cancer, osteoporosis, weight loss, decreased muscle strength, and decline in pulmonary functions. Heavy cigarette use in older men may indicate high alcohol consumption and should be investigated (Schuckit & Miller, 1976).

ALCOHOL ABUSE AND ALCOHOLISM

Research has indicated that alcohol abuse and alcoholism do exist among the elderly. An estimated 2% to 10% of the elderly suffer from alcoholism (Glantz, 1983). There is a higher than average incidence in widows, nursing home residents, patients on medical wards, and psychiatric patients (Zimberg, 1979; Schuckit & Miller, 1976).

Three factors contribute to the low rate of alcoholism among the elderly: (1) early mortality of alcoholics; (2) "spontaneous recovery" attributable to substitute dependencies (67%), medical problems induced by alcohol (48%), membership in Alcoholics Anonymous (38%), or a new love relationship (38%); and (3) underdiagnosis and underreporting (Vaillant & Milofsky, 1982). Alcoholism among the elderly is often hidden by family members or through isolation, or it is sometimes confused with normal aging because trembling, confusion, and mental lapses can be symptoms of alcohol abuse and dependency or aging.

Elderly alcoholics differ from younger alcoholics in several ways. They do not drink as much on each occasion, but they are likely to drink more frequently. They rarely reach the point of needing detoxification and rarely have withdrawal symptoms (National Institute on Alcohol Abuse and Alcoholism, 1978). They may be more psychologically dependent than physically dependent on alcohol.

Investigators have distinguished two types of elderly alcoholics: early onset and late onset (Zimberg, 1974). Approximately two thirds of the elderly alcoholics are early onset, and one third are late onset. The early-onset alcoholics are those who began to have drinking problems early in life and have survived into old age. They may or may not have developed physical problems as a result of their drinking, and they may have personality characteristics similar to those of younger alcoholics. Late-onset alcoholics have recently begun to experience alcohol problems, usually in response to stress in their lives. They do not have the personality characteristics of younger alcoholics, but they do experience the stresses and problems of aging: depression, bereavement, loneliness, retirement, marital stress, and physical difficulties (Rosin & Glatt, 1971). Most late-onset alcoholics begin drinking in an attempt to alleviate life stresses; the behavior is therefore seen as reactive. Because the alcohol enhances the feelings of isolation and boredom that led to the drinking in the first place, a destructive cycle of more isolation and more alcohol to relieve them becomes established. Late-onset alcoholics are generally responsive to treatment and have a good prognosis, but, they often go unnoticed and untreated. In a study conducted in Baltimore, Rathbone-McCuan, Lohn, Levenson, and Hsu (1976) found that 85% of those who could be diagnosed as alcoholic were not receiving treatment for their alcohol problems.

Although many of the alcohol problems of the elderly are stress related or hidden, older people who drink experience problems similar to those of younger alcoholics, including hangovers, blackouts, memory loss, shakes, psychological dependence, health problems and accidents due to existing health problems being exacerbated by alcohol use, financial problems, family and marriage problems, problems with friends and neighbors, job-related problems (if they are still employed), attitude problems, and legal problems (Carruth, 1973).

In a study of lifetime drinking patterns aimed at elucidating the drinking patterns of the elderly, Dunham (1981) interviewed 310 persons 60 years of age or older living in low-income housing in Dade County, Florida. Only 100 of those interviewed reported any drinking in their lifetime. Subjects were placed in five drinking categories: heavy drinkers, moderate drinkers, light drinkers, infrequent drinkers, or abstainers. Six life patterns were discovered: rise and fall (25%), rise and sustained (28%), light drinking throughout life (21%), light drinking with late rise (7%), late starter (11%), and highly variable (8%).

In the rise and fall pattern, the subjects' alcohol consumption began at age 21, increased at age 24, was heavy for 17 years, decreased at age 61, and terminated (complete abstention) at age 68. These subjects were usually women with low levels of education and an alcohol-related illness. In the rise and sustained pattern, the subjects' alcohol consumption began at age 17, increased at age 25, and was heavy for 36 years. The subjects were usually White or Black men with average education, and they were the least likely to have alcohol-related illnesses. Those who drank lightly throughout their lives began at age 30 and usually returned to abstinence at about age 72. These subjects were most often Latin women with less than high school education; they had a moderate chance of alcohol-related illnesses. Subjects who reported light drinking with a late rise in alcohol consumption began at age 31 and started drinking heavily at age 74; these were usually Latin men with low incidence of alcohol-related illness. In the late starter pattern, subjects began drinking at age 54 and continued for 17 years or began at age 49 and continued for 3 years and stopped. These subjects were mostly Black or White (not Latin) men; those who stopped early were mostly women. The alcohol-related illnesses were moderate. Those characterized as variable drinkers began at age 22, increased their drinking at age 30, crossed the light-moderate boundary three times, reached the first peak after 9.6 years, and decreased at ages 56 and 65. The subjects were usually Black men with alcohol-related illnesses.

Dunham (1981) points out that at least four of these drinking patterns can be problematic for the elderly: rise and sustained, light drinking with late rise, late starter, and variable patterns. Findings also indicated that women are likely to return to abstinence, whereas men often continue heavy drinking. Blacks often follow variable patterns and have many alcohol-related illnesses, and Whites most often follow the rise and sustained pattern. People following these two patterns are most likely to become early-onset alcoholics, while those who follow the light drinking with late rise or the late starter patterns are apt to become late-onset drinkers. This information may be useful to the therapist when obtaining drinking and drug use histories from patients; it helps identify those who are in high-risk groups and indicates treatment strategies.

There are additional risk factors for elderly alcoholics. Family and genetic factors play a part: there is an inverse relation between reported family alcoholism and the age of onset of alcoholism (Atkinson, 1984). Older alcoholics in treatment have a lower rate of family alcoholism than younger patients (Jones, 1972; Penick, Read, Crowley, & Powell, 1978). This is probably due to a complication of environmental factors in alcoholic families that produces early alcohol abuse among children of alcoholics. Late-onset alcoholics (after age 40) report familial alcoholism 41% of the time, and early-onset alcoholics report a family influence in 86% of the cases (Atkinson, 1984). This underscores the role of late-life stresses and adjustments as a risk factor for late-onset alcoholism. Not all stressed elderly people become alcohol abusers late in life, however, and stress may not be a factor in early-onset alcoholism.

One of the most dangerous problems for elderly people who drink is the interaction of alcohol and other drugs. As discussed earlier, the elderly use many prescription and over-the-counter drugs that can cause problems when combined with alcohol. States of confusion or sedation out of expected proportions can occur: "Unexpected response to prescribed medication may be the clinician's first clue to undisclosed substance abuse" (Atkinson, 1984, p. 12).

Because environmental stresses and psychological reactions to aging play an important part in the etiology of substance abuse in the elderly, they respond well to treatment that considers alleviating some of the environmental problems. Therapies that have been helpful with the elderly substance abuser are socialization, group therapy, case work, and cognitive therapy. Zimberg (1974b) recommends psychosocial interventions with the elderly. Antidepressant medications are sometimes necessary, but often cognitive therapy is more effective. Elderly alcoholics view their alcoholism differently than younger alcoholics; they feel that they do not need detoxification and are reluctant to undergo inpatient treatment. They may also feel out of place if they are referred to a program with younger alcoholics. Feelings of stigma are greater among the elderly, probably because they grew up before and during the Prohibition era, when little was known, mentioned, or done about drinking problems. These same people were conditioned to feel guilty and ashamed when they drank. As a result they use a strong denial system to hide their drinking (Buys and Saltman, 1984).

TREATMENT OF THE ELDERLY

The elderly are underrepresented in treatment populations. They do not seek assistance at traditional treatment sites and are often embarrassed to ask for help. Elderly persons may not consider therapy because they think that they are not able to make major changes in their lives or they lack hope for their future. Elderly alcoholics present special treatment difficulties. Inpatient alcohol wards may be reluctant to treat the elderly because of other physical problems that put them at high risk for injury with some treatment methods. For example, cardiovascular impairments in the elderly make it risky to use Antabuse. Aversive therapies, such as shock or nausea-producing medications, are also not recommended. Lack of hospitalization insurance keeps some elderly patients out of treatment centers, and some detoxification centers reject older people because they fear medical dangers. Yet when the elderly get help, they respond well.

The elderly need to be treated in places that they are already frequenting. Senior citizen centers in neighborhoods with a high population of older people are good places to work with the elderly. Alcoholics Anonymous groups in these centers are helpful. Efforts can be made to combine the expertise of therapists who specialize in geriatric populations and those who specialize in substance abuse. Many elderly citizens may need help in their homes.

Therapists who want to work with the elderly need more than just a liking of old people. They must have a genuine respect and a deep sense of caring for the elderly; a history of positive experiences with the elderly; an ability and desire to learn from them; a conviction that the last years of life can be challenging and fruitful; knowledge of the biological, psychological, and social needs of the elderly; a healthy attitude regarding their own eventual old age; an understanding of the developmental tasks of each period of life; an ability to deal with extreme feelings of depression, hopelessness, grief, hostility, and despair; personal characteristics such as humor, patience, enthusiasm, courage, endurance, hopefulness, tolerance, nondefensiveness, freedom from limiting prejudices, and a willingness to learn; and the ability to be both supportive and challenging and the sensitivity to know when each is needed (Corey & Corey, 1982).

In working with the elderly it is essential to obtain a complete history and to perform a comprehensive assessment. The history should include information about the client's social history, financial status, emotional well-being, medical condition, and self-care status. In doing the assessment, therapists should look for the client's strengths and remember that the elderly are survivors. When creating treatment plans, therapists should use all possible social networks. Family, social services agencies, senior citizen centers, special senior programs, transportation programs, medical help, public health nurses, and recreation and education programs are just a few possibilities. The therapy environment and materials need to be customized for the elderly. The room should be well lighted and in a safe place, and there may be a need for vocal amplification and large print. The pace of the therapy itself should be slow.

Goals for working with the elderly should be realistic and small. Therapists need to see small changes as important and not expect quick, radical changes. Therapists may have to take an active role and meet survival needs of food and shelter before proceeding to address other needs. Therapists' attitudes are also important: the elderly should be viewed as having dignity, intelligence, and something to contribute. They should not be talked to as if they were children or treated oversolicitously.

An important resource for the elderly is the elderly themselves. Peer support and help are valuable assets that provide help for others and improve the self-esteem of the one who is helping (Lawson & Hughes, 1980). An example of peer help can be seen in group work. Shere (1964) found in a group of people 85 years of age or older who met 47 times that feelings of loneliness and depression lessened, self-respect was regained, old pleasures were revived, social drives were reactivated, intellectual interests were reawakened, and community life was resumed.

Group therapy for seniors with the goal of making life more meaningful is especially beneficial. The groups need to take a positive approach and have clear goals; task-oriented groups work best. The sessions should go at a slow pace, and all members should be supportive. It is not advisable to mix regressed clients with those who are at a high level of functioning. Group themes can include loneliness; social isolation; loss; poverty; feelings of rejection; the struggle to find meaning in life; dependency; feelings of uselessness, hopelessness, and despair; fears of death and dying; grief over others' deaths; sadness over physical and mental deterioration; depression; and regrets over past events (Corey & Corey, 1982). Life review is healthy and often helpful to group members.

Marriage and family therapy should not be overlooked in working with the elderly. The elderly may need help in negotiating their new retirement status and the increase of time spent with marital partners, which may put a strain on the marriage if old marital problems were not resolved and surface after retirement or when the children have left home. Couples may have to renegotiate old contracts of relating and role behavior. Multigenerational family therapy may be useful in making changes in family systems that reinforce, hide, or protect substance abuse in the elderly. Because alcoholism is a multigenerational illness, it is likely that others in the family may have similar problems, especially early-onset alcoholics.

Although clinicians are just beginning to learn about the needs, problems, and life tasks of the elderly, it can be a rewarding experience to work with this population. Therapists need to look at their own issues with aging, because they too are aging and will someday join an even larger group of senior citizens. The therapist who learns to help the elderly will undoubtedly assure himself or herself of a job for life.

REFERENCES

American Psychiatric Association. (1980). *Diagnostic and statistical manual of mental disorders* (3rd ed.). Washington, DC: Author.

Atkinson, R.M. (Ed.). (1984). *Alcohol and drugs: Abuse in old age.* Washington, DC: American Psychiatric Press.

Basen, A.B. (1977). The elderly and drugs: Problem, overview and program strategy. *Public Health Report, 92*, 43–48.

Brotman, H.B. (1980). *Every ninth American, development in aging.* (Rev. ed.). Report to the Special Committee on Aging, United States Senate.

Busse, E.W. (1983). Geriatric psychiatry: Recent developments. In B.B. Wolman (Ed.), *International encyclopedia of psychiatry, psychoanalysis and neurology, progress volume* (pp. 182–186). New York: Van Nostrand–Reinhold.

Buys, D., & Saltman, J. (1984). *The unseen alcoholics—The elderly.* Public Affairs Committee, Inc.

Carruth B. (1973). Toward a definition of problem drinking among older persons: Conceptual and methodological considerations. In E.P. Williams (Ed.), *Alcohol and problem drinking among older persons.* Springfield, VA: National Technical Information Service.

Corey, G., & Corey, M.S. (1982). *Groups: Process and practice* (2nd ed.). Monterey, CA: Brooks/Cole.

Doyle, J.P., & Hamm, B.M. (1976). *Medication use and misuse study among older persons.* Jacksonville, FL: The Cathedral Foundation of Jacksonville.

Dunham, R.G. (1981). Aging and changing patterns of alcohol use. *Journal of Psychoactive Drugs, 13*(2), 143–151.

Glantz, M.D. (1983). Drugs and the elderly adult: An overview. In M.D. Glantz, D.M. Peterson, & F.J. Whittington (Eds.), *Drugs and the elderly: Research issues 32* (pp. 1–3). Rockville, MD: National Institute of Drug Abuse.

Gubrium, J. (1975). *Living and dying at Murray Manor.* New York: St. Martin's Press.

Hanan, Z.I. (1978). Geriatric medications: How the aged are hurt by drugs meant to help. *RN*, Jan., 57–59.

Hemminki, E., & Heikkela, J. (1975). Elderly people's compliance with prescriptions and quantity of medication. *Scandinavian Journal of Social Medicine, 3*, 87–92.

Jones, R.W. (1972). Alcoholism among relatives of alcoholic patients. *Quarterly Journal of Studies on Alcohol, 33*, 810.

Kofoed, L.L. (1984). Abuse and misuse of over the counter drugs by the elderly. In R.M. Atkinson (Ed.), *Alcohol and drug abuse in old age* (pp. 50–59). Washington, DC: American Psychiatric Press.

Kofoed, L.L. (1985). Substance abuse in the older patient. *Medical Aspects of Human Sexuality, 19*(2), 22–27.

Lawson, G., & Hughes, B. (1980). Some considerations for the training of counselors who work with the elderly. *Counseling and Values, 24*(3), 2045–2208.

Learoyd, B.M. (1972). Psychotropic drugs and the elderly patient. *The Medical Journal of Australia, 1,* 1131–1133.

Mandolini, A. (1981). The social contexts of aging and drug use: Theoretical and methodological insights. *Journal of Psychoactive Drugs, 13*(2), 135–142.

Michigan Office of Services to the Aging and Michigan Office of Substance Abuse Services. (1979). *Substance abuse among Michigan's senior citizens: Patterns of use and provider perspectives.* Lansing, MI: The Offices.

National Institute on Alcohol Abuse and Alcoholism. (1978). *Alcohol topics in brief: Alcohol and the elderly.* Rockville, MD: National Clearinghouse for Alcohol Information.

Offer, C. (1974). *At sixty-five work becomes a four letter word. Psychology Today, 7*(10), 40.

Penick, E.C., Read, M.R., Crowley, P.A., & Powell, B.J. (1978). Differentiation of alcoholics by family history. *Journal of Studies on Alcohol, 39,* 1944-1948.

Peterson, D.M., Whittington, F.J., & Beer, E.T. (1979). Drug use and misuse among the elderly. *Journal of Drug Issues, 9*(1), 5–26.

Rathbone-McCuan, E., Lohn, H., Levenson, J., & Hsu, J. (1976). *Community survey of aged alcoholics and problem drinkers.* Washington, DC: National Institute on Alcohol Abuse and Alcoholism.

Rosin, A.J., & Glatt, M.M. (1971). Alcohol excess in the elderly. *Quarterly Journal of Studies on Alcohol, 32,* 53–59.

Salzman, C., Vander Kolk, B., & Shader, R. (1975). Psychopharmacology and the geriatric patient. In R. Shader (Ed.), *Manual of psychiatric therapeutics* (pp. 171–184). Boston: Little, Brown & Co.

Schwartz, D., Wang, M., Zeitz, L., & Gross, M.E.W. (1962). Medical errors made by elderly chronically ill patients. *American Journal of Public Health, 52*(12), 2018–2029.

Shader, R. (Ed.). (1975). *Manual of psychiatric therapeutics.* Boston: Little, Brown & Co.

Shere, E. (1964). Group work with the very old. In R. Kastenbaum (Ed.), *New thought on old age.* New York: Springer.

Schuckit, M.A., & Miller, P.L. (1976). Alcoholism in elderly men: A survey of a general medical ward. *Annals of the New York Academy of Sciences, 273,* 558–571.

Stephens, R.C., Haney, C.A., & Underwood, S. (1981). Psychoactive drug use and potential misuse among persons aged 55 years and older. *Journal of Psychoactive Drugs, 13*(2), 185–193.

Stephens, R.C., Haney, C.A., & Underwood, S. (1982). *Drug taking among the elderly: National Institute on Drug Abuse Treatment Research Report* (DHHS Publication ADM83-1229). Washington, DC: U.S. Government Printing Office.

Stewart, R.B., Hale, W.W., & Marks, M.G. (1982). Analgesic drug use in ambulatory elderly populations. *Drugs, Intelligence, and Clinical Pharmacology, 16,* 1833–1836.

Vaillant, G.E. & Milofsky, E.S. (1982). Natural history of male alcoholism, Part IV: Paths to recovery. *Archives of General Psychiatry, 39,* 127–133.

Whittington, F.J. (1983). Consequences of drug use, misuse and abuse. In M.D. Glantz, D.M. Peterson, & F.J. Whittington (Eds.), *Drugs and the elderly adult: Research issues 32* (pp. 203–206). Rockville, MD: National Institute on Drug Abuse.

Whittington, F.J. (1983b). Misuse of legal drugs and compliance with prescription directions. In M.D. Glantz, D.M. Peterson, & F.J. Whittington (Eds.), *Drugs and the elderly adult: Research Issues 32* (pp. 63–69). Rockville, MD: National Institute on Drug Abuse.

Zimberg, S. (1974). The elderly alcoholic. *The Gerentologist, 14*(3), 221–224.

Zimberg, S. (1974b). Two types of problem drinkers: Both can be managed. *Geriatrics, 29,* 135–139.

Zimberg, S. (1979). Alcohol and the elderly. In D.M. Peterson, F.J. Whittington, & B.P. Payne (Eds.), *Drugs and the elderly: Social and pharmacological issues* (pp. 28–40). Springfield, IL: Charles C Thomas.

Chapter 16

Adolescents and Children

Robert Cohen and Gary W. Lawson

Attention deficit disorder with hyperactivity is a behavioral syndrome marked by hyperactivity, distractability, impulsivity, excitability, and a short attention span. Other symptoms may include perceptual deficits, conceptual deficits, aggression, learning disorders, speech difficulties, poor self-concept, and depression. The syndrome is more common in boys than in girls, with estimates as high as a 9:1 ratio of boys to girls (Campbell, 1976).

The most popular treatment approach, although not without controversy, is the use of stimulant medication. Children with attention deficit disorders taking stimulant medication display significant and dramatic improvement in impulse control and attention. Approximately 70% of hyperactive children respond positively to stimulant medication (Satterfield, Cantwell, & Satterfield, 1974).

Stimulant medication has been used to reduce hyperactivity in children since the condition was first described by Bradley in the late 1930s. He introduced the use of Benzedrine in children who had behavioral problems and reported a decrease in levels of high activity. Since Bradley's work, numerous studies have reported the value of such psychostimulants as methylphenidate (Ritalin), dextroamphetamine (Dexedrine), and pemoline (Cylert). Other stimulants such as caffeine have also been used (Schnackenberg, 1973).

Other medications that have been used with these children are the tricyclic antidepressants. Not long after the tricyclics began to be used for the treatment of enuresis, reports appeared on the use of these drugs with aggressive or hyperactive children. The reports indicated that the therapeutic effects achieved with these drugs were similar to those of the stimulants (Rapoport, 1965); other studies confirmed those early reports. These results demonstrated the beneficial effects of tricyclics for restless and antisocial behaviors (Kupietz & Balka, 1976; Rapoport, Quinn, Bradbard, Riddle, & Brooks, 1974). Rapoport (1984) states ''the responses are immediate and in some cases dramatic'' (p. 397). Ritalin, however, has been shown to be superior to the tricyclics. Rapoport (1984) states that the results of long-term treatment of children are "unsatisfactory" and need further study.

Gittelman-Klein, Klein, Katz, Saraf, and Pollack (1976) suggest that neuroleptics can be used along with psychostimulants; they report on the administration of Thorazine and Haldol (haloperidol) to children who have attention deficit disorder with hyperactivity. They also report a decrease in activity and impulsive behaviors. General beneficial effects of the phenothiazines on attention and learning have not been noted, however (Rapoport, 1984). Further, the growing recognition that tardive dyskinesia can and does occur in children has prompted clinicians to use stimulant medications, which are generally regarded as more effective and safe.

Despite the efficacy of the psychostimulants in treating attention deficit disorder with hyperactivity, there are several concerns. The most predominant side effect reported is the possible growth-reducing effects of the stimulants, although studies have provided conflicting results. Some (Satterfield et al., 1974) report that the psychostimulants have no effect on growth, and others report significant decrements in height over time (Safer, Allen, & Barr, 1972). Mattes and Gittelman (1983) treated children with Ritalin over a 4-year period and found a significant decrement in height percentiles over time. Because of this concern, the height of treated children should be monitored and drug holidays instituted if growth seems to be effected. Gittelman (1984) reports that drug withdrawal has induced significant gains in height.

Another concern is that periods of sustained use of psychostimulants may encourage the development of a drug-taking habit. This belief persists despite a lack of clinical data or evidence to support it (Grunspoon & Singer, 1973). A third concern is whether state-dependent learning occurs during treatment. It has been suggested that special teaching efforts could be compromised by drug treatment. Like the concern with height, however, the literature provides conflicting data. Some studies report that the use of psychostimulants affects learning, while others find little evidence to suggest less state-dependent learning during psychostimulant drug use (Swanson & Kinsbourne, 1976; Aman & Sprague, 1974).

Ayllon, Layman, and Kandel (1975) report their concern that psychostimulants control behavior but note that they do not have an effect on increasing academic performance. Behavior modification and cognitive training have been employed in the study of attention deficit disorder with hyperactivity. Although stimulant medication has been found to be effective in controlling behavior, behavior modification procedures have been effective in improving academic performance. Gittelman (1984) reports that when the psychostimulants are combined with behavior therapy excellent results are obtained. Therefore, since the two combined techniques produce beneficial results, it appears that when these two treatment approaches are used together, children with attention deficit disorder with hyperactivity will be able to maximize their performance in the classroom and at home.

CHEMICAL MANAGEMENT OF SCHIZOPHRENIC DISORDERS AND INFANTILE AUTISM IN CHILDREN AND ADOLESCENTS

Clinical experience has demonstrated that the prognosis for schizophrenic and autistic disorders in children and adolescents is guarded at best. Although many treatment interventions are utilized in treating these disorders, chemical management has been a beneficial component in treatment. Sprague (1972) maintains that a combination of behavioral therapy and pharmacotherapy is more advantageous then either treatment alone. Research has shown that, while behavior therapy can reduce maladaptive behavior and can also stimulate adaptive complex behaviors, the use of neuroleptics is effective in diminishing psychomotor excitement (Lovaas & Newsome, 1976).

Chemical management is only one of the components in the treatment plans of these children and adolescents. Other treatment modalities include "special education services; individual, group, and family therapy; behavior therapy; environmental therapy; and hospitalization" (Campbell, 1985, p. 115). The treatment plan depends on various factors, such as the severity of symptoms, environmental supports, and other handicaps of the individual. For technical reviews of the chemical management of schizophrenic and autistic children and adolescents, see Weiner (1985).

Campbell (1985) reports that psychoactive drugs are administered to schizophrenic children and adolescents regardless of measurable therapeutic results and that recommendations for such chemical treatment are based solely on general clinical experience. Green and colleagues (1984) indicate that these children respond to neuroleptics to a lesser degree than their adult counterparts and typically become sedated at low dosages. It has also been shown that haloperidol has less sedative properties than chlorpromazine or thioridazine at therapeutic dosages. Campbell (1985) further reports that most research on the "short- and long-term efficacy and safety of psychoactive drugs in the treatment of infantile autism is based on studies of haloperidol and trifluoperazine" (p. 155). Research has shown that autistic children with low I.Q. who are hyperactive, disruptive, or have temper tantrums respond well to haloperidol. Further, those autistic children who are exclusively anergic and hypoactive do not respond well to this drug.

Thompson and Schuster (1968) indicate that all psychoactive drugs can have unpleasant and adverse side effects. These reactions vary depending on the type of drug, the dosage, the duration of drug use, the patient's age, the presence or absence of brain damage or disease, and the conditions under which the drug is administered. Behavioral toxicity has been defined by DiMascio and Shader (1970) as the actions of a drug that produce changes in cognitive and perceptual functioning, mood, psychomotor performance, interpersonal relationships, motivation, or intrapsychic processes. Behavioral toxicity also refers to the physical hazards that occur within the dosage range that has been found to have clinical utility. Campbell (1985) reports that there have not been any reported studies of the adverse side affects of neuroleptics in schizophrenic children or adolescents. Campbell notes, however, that in her work with autistic children there were no adverse side effects on cognition at dosages that were effective in reducing behavioral symptoms.

It has frequently been observed that there is a deterioration of pre-existing behavioral symptoms or the emergence of new behavioral symptoms in schizophrenic or autistic children before any other unfavorable or adverse side effects, including irritability, temper tantrums, hyperactivity or hypoactivity, apathy, and decreased verbal productivity, are observed. Like adults undergoing treatment with phenothiazines, children and adolescents treated with neuroleptics can display extrapyramidal side effects. "These include acute dystonic reactions, dyskinesias, parkinsonian reactions, akathisia, and rabbit syndrome" (Campbell, 1985, p. 137). Other adverse side effects on the central nervous system include sedation, dizziness, confusion, headache, insomnia, ataxia, depersonalization, and seizures. Campbell reports that excessive sedation is the most common of the side effects associated with the use of neuroleptics in children. Autistic children reportedly have a relatively high incidence of seizures even without the use of neuroleptics (Campbell, Green, Anderson, & Deutsch, 1985). Tarjan, Loery, and Wright (1957) report that chlorpromazine will either increase the frequency of seizures or decrease the threshold for seizures in these children or adolescents.

Campbell, Green, and Bennett (1983) report that 8% to 51% of children and adolescents who are given neuroleptics will either develop tardive or withdrawal dyskinesias. In addition, these abnormal movements may develop during drug administration, after the dosage has been reduced, or during drug withdrawal. The earliest time at which tardive or withdrawal dyskinesias are observed is after 3 months of cumulative drug administration. For additional information about neuroleptic-induced tardive or withdrawal dyskinesias in children and adolescents, see Campbell and colleagues (1983).

Behavioral and withdrawal effects refer to the emergence of symptoms that develop after ending the use of a psychoactive drug. Manifestations include the deterioration of pre-existing symptoms, anxiety, restlessness, agitation, insomnia, irritability, anorexia, weight loss, stomach cramps, vomiting, diarrhea, chills, and cold sweats (Klein, Gittelman, Quitakin, & Rifinkin, 1980).

Other rare side effects that may occur in children involve the autonomic nervous system. These effects include dry mouth, constipation, and diarrhea. Campbell

(1985) reports that there has not been any systematic research conducted on the effect of neuroleptics on height and weight in schizophrenic or autistic children and adolescents. She states that there is a need for accurate measurements, along with the utilization of growth charts and appropriate and controlled study designs. For further information about the use of neuroleptics in children, see Winsberg and Yepes (1978).

CHEMICAL MANAGEMENT OF AFFECTIVE DISORDERS IN CHILDREN AND ADOLESCENTS

Antich, Ryan, and Rabinovich (1985) report that, partly because of progress in the assessment of affective disorders in juveniles, there have been four recent developments: (1) the demise of the concept of masked depression; (2) the verification of endogenous and psychotic forms of affective disorders (Strober, Green, & Carlson, 1982); (3) the initial validation of the diagnosis of the dysthymic disorder (Kovacs, Feinberg, Crouse, Paulaskas, & Finkelstein, 1984); and (4) the acknowledgment of the psychosocial and relationship deficits that accompany major depression in children.

Chambers and Puig-Antich (1982) found that developmental differences in the presentation of affective disorders are present in children and adolescents. These investigators, as well as Strober and co-workers (1982), indicate that a proportion of children and adolescents display depressive hallucinations and delusions and that this has implications for classification. It has been found that depressive delusions in prepubescent children are rare and that only juveniles who are psychotically depressed present with hallucinations alone. In adolescents, however, depressive delusions are typically frequent and hallucinations occur as well; in contrast, psychotically depressed adults predominantly exhibit delusions only. Antich and colleagues (1985) suggest that the young child's cognitive immaturity makes the development of a depressive delusional system improbable. Glassman, Kantor, and Shostak (1975) report that in adults psychotic depressions are less likely to respond to tricyclic antidepressant medications; recent psychopharmacological studies have not addressed psychotic subtypes in children.

The prognostic importance of dysthmic disorders in children and adolescents is equivalent to that in adults; Kovacs et al. (1984) describe and validate this type of prolonged disorder in children and adolescents. Because of its association with major depression, it has the potential to produce long-term psychosocial disability. Weissmann, Klerman, Paykel, Prusoff, and Hanson (1974) state that psychosocial deficits along with impairments in interpersonal relationships that are associated with major depression in prepubescence, as well as their lack of full resolution in spite of chemical management, resemble findings concerning the social functioning and recovery of depressive adults.

Evidence suggests that the justification for pharmacological treatment lies in the risk-benefit ratio compared to the risks inherent in the natural history of affective disorders. Antich and colleagues (1985) further suggest that the rates of recovery in childhood, adolescence, and adulthood from major depression and the risk of relapse are similar.

Rane and Wilson (1983) state that, in addition to age-related changes in affective disorders, the age of the patient must be considered in assessing drug effects. Despite the absence of differences in the rates of drug absorption, there are significant age-related differences related to body composition, the ratio of liver mass to body mass, metabolic pace, and renal excretion; these all influence drug distribution, metabolism, and elimination. Rane and Wilson maintain that because of these differences separate drug-efficacy studies in children are needed. For example, it is known that certain drugs, including the tricyclic antidepressant imipramine, react differently in children than in adults. Further, Weinberg Rutman, and Sullivan (1973); Saraf, Klein, and Gittelman-Klein (1974), state that children are more susceptible to cardotoxic effects of tricyclic antidepressants than adults. Usually school-aged children require somewhat higher weight-corrected dosages than adults. Further, it is possible that developmental variations in pharmacodynamics also affect treatment responses in juveniles and adolescents (Antich et al., 1985). For a more technical review of antidepressant medication that discusses clinical studies, see Weiner (1985).

Antich and co-workers report that data concerning the use of lithium in treating childhood affective disorders are limited. The results of controlled adult studies suggest that lithium may be used for treating mania and depression in children and adolescents (Goodwin, Murphy, Dunner, & Bunney, 1969; Baron, Gershon, Rudy, Jonas, & Buschbaum, 1975). Although there have been few controlled studies of children, it seems likely that the side effects experienced by children and adolescents are similar to those experienced by adults. For a review of the literature concerning the clinical studies of the use of lithium in children and adolescents, see Youngerman and Canino (1978).

Antich and colleagues (1985) maintain that a course of lithium is desirable for the treatment of mania in children and adolescents, despite a lack of controlled studies indicting its usage. In addition, these investigators suggest that neuroleptics may also be added for short-term control of mania. They conclude that the potential side effects of lithium (renal, thyroid, and bone effects) must be weighed against the long-term use of the drug. Lithium is indicated for longer-term preventative maintenance only after recurrent episodes of childhood bipolar illness. Because of the noted side effects, conservative approaches are usually taken in medicating the child who has experienced a single manic episode and who responds in a favorable manner to short-term use of lithium. This drug should be discontinued after 3 to 6 months, and it is essential that the treating physician and family members monitor the child for signs of an emergence of the manic symptoms.

In children who do not respond to standard forms of chemical management of affective disorders, the medicating physician usually uses pharmacological approaches that have been advantageous with adults who manifest similar symptomatology. As in the treatment of any disorder, the risks must be balanced against the risks of withholding medication. Antich and co-workers (1985) have found that adolescents with psychotic depression often respond to a combination of tricyclic antidepressants and neuroleptics. Despite this, these same investigators emphasize that there is a strong need for more clinical research in the chemical management of affective disorders in children and adolescents.

CHEMICAL MANAGEMENT OF ANXIETY DISORDERS

Two classes of medication, the antihistamines and the benzodiazepines, are used to treat mild to moderate anxiety states. These medications should be used only when feelings of anxiety are intense and overwhelming. Both these medications have been studied in clinical trials with children who were hospitalized with severe psychopathology.

Kandel (1983) defines anxiety as a "normal inborn response either to a threat to one's person, attitudes, or self-esteem or to the absence of people or objects that assure safety" (p. 1278). Anxiety is a human emotion that most people experience in mild and brief forms as part of their daily experiences. In more extreme forms, it becomes the central feature of child and adolescent psychiatric disorders. According to Jaffe and Magnuson (1985), mild to moderate anxiety is also experienced as a normal part of the developmental process. They maintain that these "developmental" anxieties are a prominent component of the clinical evaluation and assessment of anxiety in children and adolescents.

Anxiety can be classified in terms of objective and subjective features. Klein (1964) asserts that the subjective features of anxiety are indistinguishable from the experience of fear under authentic conditions. Subjective features range from a heightened sense of awareness and apprehension to a profound fear of impending disaster and tragedy. Objective features consist of signs of motor tension; autonomic hyperactivity; verbalized concerns, worries, and anticipated fears; and a heightened sense of responsiveness along with signs of distractibility and irritability.

Anxiety has been classified by Kandel (1983) into two types: (1) actual or automatic anxiety, which comprises in-born responses to either external or internal danger, and (2) acquired anxiety, which is subdivided into panic attacks, anticipatory anxiety, and chronic anxiety. Panic attacks involve spontaneous episodes of terror associated with sympathetic crisis. Jaffe and Magnuson (1985) note that this type of anxiety responds well to tricyclic antidepressants. Anticipatory anxiety refers to brief periods of anxiety that are associated with real or imagined signals. This form of anxiety responds to the benzodiazepines. The benzodiazepines are also used in treating chronic anxiety, which is a persistent feeling of apprehension not related to external dangers or fears.

Jaffe and Magnuson (1985) state that there are no controlled studies of medication in the treatment of children with the diagnoses of avoidant or overanxious disorders. They add that only separation anxiety disorder has been studied. As recently as 1980, Gittelman noted that there were no controlled studies examining the efficacy of antianxiety medication in treating children who exhibited symptoms of anxiety. Jaffe and Magnuson (1985) state that the lack of controlled studies is partly due to the recent diagnostic categories outlined in the *Diagnostic and Statistical Manual of Mental Disorders* (Third Edition) (DSM-III; American Psychiatric Association, 1980). Therefore, making diagnostic distinctions has led some investigators to compare separation anxiety in children to agoraphobia in adults.

Gittelman-Klein and Klein (1971, 1973) studied the use of imipramine in school-phobic children. This drug in dosages of 1.0 to 5.0 mg/kg/day is recommended in conjunction with other forms of psychotherapeutic measures. Although there are no controlled studies of the efficacy of antihistamines, benzodiazepines, and low dosages of major tranquilizers, Jaffe and Magnuson (1985) report that these medications are used clinically for treating children who are diagnosed with overanxious disorder. These investigators report that obsessive-compulsive disorder is quite rare in children. It has been found that in children who have the disorder the clinical presentation of symptoms resembles that of those in adults. Multimodal psychotherapy is somewhat effective in treating children, but complete recovery is uncommon. Jaffe and Magnuson report that new evidence suggests that clomipramine is helpful in treating some children who manifest the disorder. In addition, they suggest that "anxiolytic tranquilizers may be used selectively to provide relief from the anxiety which accompanies the disorder" (Jaffe & Magnuson, 1985, p. 207).

Jaffe and Magnuson (1985) strongly maintain that it is essential that the treating clinician identify pathological anxiety states that are "overwhelming, persistent, and disruptive" (p. 208), even if not yet formed into a distinct DSM-III clinical disorder. They contend that, although the antihistamines and benzodiazepines may be useful as adjunctives to treating anxiety, anxiety states also respond to other treatment techniques as well. They state that feelings of anxiety related to normal development respond to the following additional treatment measures: empathic understanding and support, individual psychodynamic psychotherapy, family therapy, behavior modification, and cognitively oriented treatment approaches. As for any medication, the risk-benefit ratio must be taken into consideration.

CHEMICAL MANAGEMENT OF CONDUCT DISORDERS

Conduct disorders are the most common reason why children and adolescents are referred for psychiatric evaluation and treatment. Two thirds to three quarters of children diagnosed with a conduct disorder are boys. Further, boys present with a higher percentage of the aggressive conduct disorders (O'Donnell, 1985). O'Donnell asserts that the traditional treatment methods for conduct disorders have tended to be ineffective. Despite the lack of data supporting the efficacy of pharmacological agents in treating conduct disorders, they are widely used. O'Donnell states that, regardless of the type of agent used for chemical management, it should be only a part of the total treatment plan. O'Donnell suggests using the following management strategies in addition to medication: "social skills training, parenting skills training, individual and/or group therapy, identification and proper treatment of parental psychiatric illness, decreasing parental and marital stress, control of parental alcoholism, direct behavioral management of aggressive behavior, and proper management of learning disabilities" (p. 260).

It seems apparent that many children and adolescents who are diagnosed with conduct disorders also experience undiagnosed psychiatric or neurological disorders that subsequently influence the development, perpetuation, or maintenance of the conduct disorder. Pharmacological agents should be used only when there is ample evidence that there will be beneficial effects, regardless of sociological and psychological explanations for the behavior. Medications that are used include: neuroleptics, lithium carbonate, anticonvulsants, stimulants, and tricyclic antidepressants (O'Donnell, 1985).

OTHER DISORDERS

Some other areas of consideration for the application of psychopharmacology in treating children and adolescents include Tourette's syndrome, tic disorders, eating disorders, enuresis, and sleep disorders. For further information about these particular disorders, see Weiner (1985).

REFERENCES

Aman, M., & Sprague, R. (1974). The state-dependent effects of methylphenidate and dextroamphetamine. *Journal of Nervous and Mental Disease, 158*, 268–279.

American Psychiatric Association. (1980). *Diagnostic and statistical manual of mental disorders* (3rd ed.). Washington, DC: Author.

Antich, J.P., Ryan, N., & Rabinovich, H. (1985). Affective disorders in childhood and adolescence. In J. Weiner (Ed.), *Diagnosis and psychopharmacology of childhood and adolescent disorders* (pp. 152–178). New York: Wiley.

Ayllon, T., Layman, D., & Kandel, H. (1975). A behavioral educational alternative to drug control of hyperactive children. *Journal of Applied Behavior Analysis, 8,* 137–185.

Baron, M., Gershon, E., Rudy, V., Jonas, W., & Buschbaum, M. (1975). Lithium carbonate response in depression. *Archives of General Psychiatry, 32,* 1107–1111.

Bradley, C. (1937). The behavior of children receiving Benzedrine. *American Journal of Psychiatry, 94,* 577–585.

Campbell, M. (1985). Schizophrenic disorders and pervasive developmental disorders/infantile autism. In J. Weiner (Ed.), *Diagnosis and psychopharmacology of childhood and adolescent disorders* (pp. 114–150). New York: Wiley.

Campbell, M., Green, W.H., Anderson, L.T., & Deutsch, S.I. (1985). *Childhood pharmacology.* Beverly Hills: Sage Publications.

Campbell, M., Green, W.H., & Bennett, W.G. (1983). Neuroleptic-induced dyskinesias in children. *Clinical Neuropharmacology, 6,* 207–222.

Campbell, S.B. (1976). Hyperactivity: Course and treatment. In A. David (Ed.), *Child personality and psychopathology: Current Topics* Vol. 3. (pp. 221–278). New York: Wiley.

Chambers, W.J., & Puig-Antich, J. (1982). Psychotic symptoms in prepubertal major depressive disorder. *Archives of General Psychiatry, 39,* 921–927.

DiMascio, H., & Shader, R.I. (1970). Behavioral toxicity. Part I: Definition and Part II: Psychomotor functions. In R.I. Shader & H. DiMascio (Eds.), *Psychotropic drug side effects* (pp. 124–131). Baltimore: Williams & Wilkins.

Gittelman, R. (1980). Diagnosis and drug treatment of childhood disorders. In D.F. Klein, R. Gittelman, F. Quitkin, & A. Rifkin (Eds.), *Diagnosis and drug treatment of psychiatric disorders: Adults and children* (2nd ed.) (pp. 590–776). Baltimore: Williams & Wilkins.

Gittelman, R. (1984). Hyperkinetic syndrome: Treatment issues and principles. In M. Reutter (Ed.), *Developmental neuropsychiatry* (pp. 437–449). London: Plenum.

Gittelman-Klein, R., & Klein, D.F. (1971). Controlled imipramine treatment of school phobia. *Archives of General Psychiatry, 25,* 204–207.

Gittelman-Klein, R., & Klein, D.F. (1973). School phobia: Diagnostic considerations in the light of imipramine effects. *Journal of Nervous and Mental Diseases, 156,* 199–215.

Gittelman-Klein, R., Klein, D.F., Katz, S., Saraf, K., & Pollack, E. (1976). Comparative effects of methylphenidate and Thorazine in hyperactive children. *Archives of General Psychiatry, 33,* 1217–1231.

Glassman, A.H., Kantor, S.J., & Shostak, M. (1975). Depression, delusions, and drug response. *American Journal of Psychiatry, 132,* 716–719.

Goodwin, F.K., Murphy, D.L., Dunner, D., & Bunney, W.E. (1969). Lithium carbonate treatment in depression and mania. *Archives of General Psychiatry, 21,* 486–496.

Green, W.H., Campbell, M., Wolsky, B.B., Deutsch, S.I., Golden, R.R., & Cicero, S.D. (1984). *Effects of short and long term haloperidol administration on growth in young autistic children.* Paper presented at the 31st Annual Meeting of the American Academy of Child Psychiatry, Toronto, Canada, October 1984.

Grunspoon, L., & Singer, S.B. (1973). Amphetamines in the treatment of hyperactive children. *Harvard Educational Review, 45*, 515–555.

Jaffe, S.L., & Magnuson, J.V. (1985). Anxiety disorders. In J. Weiner (Ed.), *Diagnosis and psychopharmacology of childhood and adolescent disorders* (pp. 200–214). New York: Wiley.

Kandel, E.R. (1983). From metapsychology to molecular biology: Explorations into the nature of anxiety. *American Journal of Psychiatry, 140*(10), 1277–1293.

Klein, D.F. (1964). Delineation of two drug-responsive anxiety syndromes. *Psychopharmacologia, 5*, 397–408.

Klein, D.F., Gittelman, R., Quitakin, F., & Rifinkin, A. (1980). *Diagnosis and drug treatment of psychiatric disorders: Adults and children*. Baltimore: Williams & Wilkins.

Kovacs, M., Feinberg, T.L., Crouse, M.A., Paulaskas, S., & Finkelstein, R. (1984). Depressive disorders in childhood. *Archives of General Psychiatry, 41*, 229–237.

Kupietz, S., & Balka, E. (1976). Alterations in vigilance performance of children receiving amitriptyline and methylphenidate pharmacotherapy. *Psychopharmacology, 50*, 24–33.

Lovaas, O.I., & Newsome, C.D. (1976). Behavior modification with psychotic children. In H. Leitenberg (Ed.), *Handbook of behavior modification and behavior therapy* (pp. 303–360). Englewood Cliffs, NJ: Prentice-Hall.

Mattes, J., & Gittelman, R. (1983). Growth of hyperactive children on maintenance regimen of methylphenidate. *Archives of General Psychiatry, 40*, 317–321.

O'Donnell, D. (1985). Conduct disorders. In J. Weiner (Ed.), *Diagnosis and psychopharmacology of childhood and adolescent disorders* (pp. 250–287). New York: Wiley.

Rane, A., & Wilson, J.T. (1983). Clinical pharmacokinetics in infants and children. In M. Gibaldi & L. Prescott (Eds.), *Handbook of clinical pharmacokinetics* (pp. 142–168). New York: Adis Health Sciences Press.

Rapoport, J. (1965). Childhood behavior and learning problems treated with imipramine. *International Journal of Neuropsychiatry, 1*, 635–642.

Rapoport, J. (1984). The use of drugs: Trends in research. In M. Reutter (Ed.), *Developmental neuropsychiatry* (pp. 385–403). London: Plenum.

Rapoport, J., Quinn, P., Bradbard, G., Riddle, K., & Brooks, E. (1974). Imipramine and methylphenidate treatment of hyperactive boys. *Archives of General Psychiatry, 30*, 789–794.

Safer, D., Allen, R., & Barr, E. (1972). Depression of growth in hyperactive children in stimulant drugs. *New England Journal of Medicine, 287*, 217–220.

Saraf, K.R., Klein, D.F., Gittelman-Klein, R. (1974). Imipramine side effects in children. *Psychopharmacologia, 37*, 265–274.

Satterfield, J.H., Cantwell, D.P., & Satterfield, B.T. (1974). Pathophysiology of the hyperactive child syndrome. *Archives of General Psychiatry, 31*, 839–844.

Schnackenberg, R. (1973). Caffeine as a substitute for schedule-II stimulants in hyperkinetic children. *American Journal of Psychiatry, 130*, 796–798.

Sprague, R.L. (1972). Psychopharmacology and learning disabilities. *Journal of Operational Psychiatry, 3*, 56–67.

Strober, M., Green, J., & Carlson, G. (1982). Phenomenology and subtypes of major depressive disorders in adolescents. *Journal of Affective Disease, 3*, 281–290.

Swanson, G., & Kinsbourne, M. (1976). Stimulant-related state-dependent learning in hyperactive children. *Science, 192*, 1354–1356.

Tarjan, G., Loery, V.E., & Wright, S.W. (1957). Use of chlorpromazine in two hundred seventy-eight mentally deficient patients. *Journal of Diseases of Children, 94*, 294–300.

Thompson, T., & Schuster, C.R. (1968). *Behavioral pharmacology*. Englewood Cliffs, NJ: Prentice-Hall.

Weinberg, W.A., Rutman, J., & Sullivan, L. (1973). Depression in children referred to an educational diagnostic center: Diagnosis and treatment. *Journal of Pediatrics, 83*, 1065–1072.

Weiner, J. (1985). *Diagnosis and psychopharmacology of childhood and adolescent disorders*. New York: Wiley.

Weissmann, M.M., Klerman, G.L., Paykel, E.S., Prusoff, B., & Hanson, B. (1974). Treatment effects of the social adjustment of depressed patients. *Archives of General Psychiatry, 30*, 771–778.

Winsberg, B.G., & Yepes, L.E. (1978). Antipsychotics. In J.S. Werry (Ed.), *Pediatric Psychopharmacology* (pp. 234–273). New York: Brunner/Mazel.

Youngerman, J., & Canino, I.A. (1978). Lithium carbonate use in children and adolescents: A survey of the literature. *Archives of General Psychiatry, 35*, 216–224.

Part V

Major Drugs of Abuse

In 1978, a study of medical schools in the United States revealed that, on average, the medical student received only 1 day per year of training on both drug and alcohol abuse. Since that time training in this area for medical doctors has improved, but not to the point that it may be assumed that the medical professional is well trained in substance abuse. Even today, many nonmedical psychotherapists receive little or no training in substance abuse. Many who are trained receive only a brief lecture or a visit from a member of Alcoholics Anonymous during a course in psychopathology. This section provides the nonmedical psychotherapist with valuable information regarding treatment, diagnosis, and intervention processes with various drugs that are abused; of special interest may be the detailed chapter on cocaine.

Chapter 17

Alcohol

Gary W. Lawson

Alcohol presents people with more personal and social problems than any other drug. Alcohol is the drug that is not thought of as a drug. Most people do not consider alcohol in the same category as heroin, barbiturates, and cocaine, yet from a pharmacological standpoint there are some strong similarities. There are many facets to alcohol, but for the purposes of this chapter alcohol is the drug that represents the source of more of the problems of those who seek counseling from nonmedical (and medical) psychotherapists than any other drug, and perhaps more than all other drugs combined. A therapist could be working with patients with alcohol-related problems without even being aware of it. Some therapists have their own issues associated with alcohol. Children who grow up with one or more alcoholic parents often have problems later in life that are directly related to their early family life and their parents' use of alcohol. Yet for many families alcohol has offered nothing but good times and pleasure, and still other families are never in direct contact with alcohol.

An excellent illustration of the diverse ways in which alcohol can be seen is the following address to the legislature by a Mississippi senator in 1958.

> You have asked me about whisky. All right, here is just how I stand on this question:
>
> If, when you say whisky, you mean the devil's brew, the poison scourge, the bloody monster that defiles innocence, yea, literally takes the bread from the mouths of little children; if you mean the evil drink that topples the Christian man and woman from the pinacles of righteous, gracious living into the bottomless pit of degradation and despair, shame and helplessness and hopelessness, then certainly I am against it with all of my power.
>
> But if, when you say whisky, you mean the oil of conversation, the philosophic wine, the stuff that is consumed when good fellows get

together, that puts a song in their hearts and laughter on their lips and the warm glow of contentment in their eyes; if you mean Christmas cheer; if you mean the stimulating drink that puts the spring in the old gentleman's step on a frosty morning; if you mean the drink that enables a man to magnify his joy, and his happiness, and to forget, if only for a little while, life's great tragedies and heartbreaks and sorrows, if you mean that drink, the sale of which pours into our treasuries untold millions of dollars, which are used to provide tender care for our little crippled children, our blind, our deaf, our dumb, our pitiful aged and infirm, to build highways, hospitals and schools, then certainly I am in favor of it.

This is my stand. I will not retreat from it; I will not compromise. (Goodwin, 1981, p. 4)

It appears that alcohol use is an emotional as well as a political issue. Each therapist has his or her personal views related to alcohol, as do patients and clients. There is an extensive and ever-growing body of literature related to alcohol, alcohol-related problems, and alcoholism. It is suggested that anyone who will be seeing patients for psychotherapy be well versed in the issues and problems related to alcohol and its abuse.

This chapter presents a comprehensive yet brief review of alcohol and alcohol-related problems. Alcohol is considered from pharmacological, biological, sociological, and psychological perspectives. Treatment and prevention of alcohol-related problems are also briefly considered.

PSYCHOPHARMACOLOGICAL AND BIOLOGICAL EFFECTS OF ALCOHOL

Ethyl alcohol is a central nervous system depressant similar in most aspects to sedative-hypnotic compounds such as barbiturates. Nevertheless, alcohol is sometimes thought of as a stimulant because of the initial feelings of increased energy many people experience after the first drink or two. This is due to an increase in the blood sugar level and the release of inhibition that accompanies alcohol use (it is postulated that inhibitory synapses are depressed slightly earlier than excitatory ones). This initial effect may also lead intoxicated people to believe that they can perform certain tasks, such as driving or dancing, better than they really can. Carefully controlled experiments have shown, however, that in general alcohol increases neither physical nor mental abilities.

The brain is extremely sensitive to the depressant effects of alcohol. The highest centers—speech, cognition, restraint, and judgment—are depressed first, followed by lower brain function, respiration, and spinal cord reflexes as the quantity of alcohol in the blood rises. When alcohol is consumed in large quantities over a short period of time it can depress the respiratory reflex center, and death may occur. This happens most often when alcohol is mixed with other central nervous system depressants, usually in pill form. There is a dangerous synergistic effect when alcohol and other drugs such as barbiturates are mixed. Death also may occur when novice drinkers have contests to see who can drink the most or get the drunkest.

Fermentation forms the chemical basis for most alcoholic products. This takes place when yeast acts on sugar in the presence of water. Chemically, $C_6H_{12}O_6$ (glucose) and H_2O (water) are transformed into C_2H_6O (ethyl alcohol) and CO_2 (carbon dioxide). In natural fermentation, such as occurs in wine making, the yeast dies of acute alcohol intoxication when the alcohol content reaches 12% to 13%. Most drinkers are not aware that they are drinking the dessication of yeast.

Alcohol is rapidly absorbed into the body from the stomach, small intestine, and colon. Vaporized alcohol can be absorbed through the lungs. Many factors modify the rate of absorption of alcohol from the stomach, such as the volume, character, and dilution of the alcoholic beverage. The presence of food in the stomach, the length of time during which the drink is consumed, and individual physiological peculiarities are major factors as well.

Once the alcohol is absorbed it is distributed rapidly, since its molecules diffuse readily across capillary walls. Recent research suggests that women may become more intoxicated than men from the same amount of alcohol, even when body weights are the same. One explanation for this finding is that a woman generally has less body fluid and more body fat than a man of the same weight. Since alcohol does not diffuse as rapidly into body fat, its concentration in a woman's blood will be higher even if she drinks the same amount as a man.

Alcohol is metabolized in the liver as follows:

Ethyl alcohol ⟶ acetaldehyde ⟶ acetate ⟶ heat-energy (calories)

Although alcohol is metabolized as a carbohydrate, it exhibits none of the properties expected of a food. It does not remain in the stomach, nor can it be stored. Research has demonstrated that the rate of alcohol metabolism, like that of absorption, can be influenced by several factors. One study showed that both alcoholic and nonalcoholic subjects maintained on good diets can moderately increase their rate of alcohol metabolism if they consume substantial amounts of alcohol over a long period of time. In general, it appears that the rate of alcohol metabolism may have a small influence on behavioral tolerance of alcohol, but no significant differences in ability to metabolize alcohol differentiate the alcoholic from the nonalcoholic (Mendelson & LaDou, 1964). At the Karolinska Institute in Stockholm, it has been reported that normal drinkers can metabolize approximately 7 g of pure alcohol per hour, 8 g in the form of whiskey, 9 g in the form of dessert wines, 12 g in the form of table wines, and 9 to 11 g in the form of beer (Goldberg, 1963).

Because of variations among individuals, it is not possible to determine the exact alcohol concentrations at which certain behavioral changes occur. For most people, however, it is usually accepted that blood alcohol levels up to 0.05% will induce some sedation or tranquility; 0.05% to 0.15% may produce lack of coordination; 0.15% to 0.20% induces obvious intoxication; 0.30% to 0.40% may produce unconsciousness; and 0.50% or more is usually fatal (Blum, 1984).

Physical effects of alcohol with both long- and short-term use vary from individual to individual. Nevertheless, alcohol is known to cause damage to the heart and circulatory system, the gastrointestinal and genitourinary systems, the liver, and every other major system and organ in the body (Blum, 1984). On the other hand, there have been reports that the moderate use of alcohol can reduce heart ailments and increase longevity. Then again, heavy or in some cases even moderate alcohol use by women during pregnancy can result in a characteristic pattern of severe mental and physical defects in neonates termed fetal alcohol syndrome (Liska, 1986).

One further note on the physiological aspects of alcohol is that for an unknown biological reason some individuals are more prone or at risk to become alcoholic than others. Many studies have indicated this, but thus far there is no conclusive evidence that any one physical factor can be identified as the major one in the transmission of alcoholism. Nonetheless, it is apparent that alcoholism does run in families and that there are some genetic factors involved. The nonmedical psychotherapist must not underestimate the effects of alcohol and the harm this drug can cause. Alcohol can only be considered good or bad in each individual's context; not to consider it at all is a mistake the nonmedical psychotherapist cannot afford to make.

SOCIOLOGICAL ASPECTS OF ALCOHOL USE AND ABUSE

As indicated by Lawson, Peterson, and Lawson (1983), the three areas that must be considered in relation to the use of alcohol are the physical, the psychological, and the sociological aspects. Of these three the one most likely not to be considered by the therapist is the sociological aspect. Tarter and Schneider (1976) identify 13 variables that affect an individual's decision to start, continue, or stop drinking. These are (1) childhood exposure to alcohol and drinking models, (2) the quantity of alcohol that is considered appropriate or excessive, (3) drinking customs, (4) the type of alcoholic beverage used, (5) levels of inhibition that are considered safe, (6) the symbolic meaning of alcohol, (7) attitudes toward public intoxication, (8) the social group associated with drinking, (9) activities associated with drinking, (10) the amount of pressure exerted on the individual to drink or continue drinking, (11) the use of alcohol in social or private contexts, (12) the individual's mobility in changing drinking reference groups, and (13) the social rewards or punishment for drinking.

There are numerous studies of how cultures differ in their views of alcohol and how individuals with different cultural or religious backgrounds respond under the influence of alcohol. MacAndrew and Edgerton (1969) surveyed evidence from many diverse societies provided by anthropologists, historians, missionaries, explorers, and other observers and found that in many parts of the world drinking is followed by either no change in behavior or by a wide variety of changes. The drunken "misconduct" that does take place occurs within socially defined limits. Their conclusion was that drunken behavior cannot be explained simply as a result of alcohol's effect on the brain. Instead, these changes in behavior can be explained on the basis of social definitions of drunkenness as a state of reduced responsibility or of "time out." Armyr, Elmer, and Herz (1982) present a comprehensive review of drinking practices in 23 countries. The differences are striking. What citizens of one country consider normal drinking could be considered alcoholism by those of another. This becomes a problem in the United States because of the diverse cultural and ethnic backgrounds of its citizens.

Also complicating the differences between individual attitudes toward alcoholism is the unique dynamic structure of individual families. For the nonmedical psychotherapist to have a complete understanding of patients or clients and their relationship to alcohol, family dynamics must be taken into account. This becomes especially important if the therapist is working to change a patient's behavior, feelings, or thinking regarding alcohol.

One reason why social variables have largely been discounted by many people in the field of alcoholism rehabilitation is the incompatibility of sociological theories with the predominantly accepted "disease model" of alcoholism (discussed later).

PSYCHOLOGICAL ASPECTS OF ALCOHOL USE AND ABUSE

Lawson, Peterson, and Lawson (1983) and Lawson, Ellis, and Rivers (1984) discuss two major factors to be considered in relation to the psychological risk for alcoholism: the psychological effect of the use or abuse of alcohol on the individual, and the psychological profile of an individual with regard to the probability of use or abuse of alcohol by that individual. In other words, how does alcohol affect personality, what type of personality exhibits what type of alcohol use pattern, and is there an alcoholic personality? As explained by Lawson and colleagues (1983), there are personality types that are at risk for alcoholism, but physical and social factors must be considered in the formulation of any theory. Personality is only one aspect of the overall picture. There are also vast differences in the ways in which individuals respond to the use of alcohol, but again the physiological makeup of the individual and the social customs regarding alcohol use are equally important in evaluating why a person behaves in a certain way under the influence of alcohol.

A review of the literature on personality traits associated with alcoholism suggests that chronic alcoholics may indeed have a distinct personality type. Characteristics such as dependency, denial, depression, superficial sociability, emotional instability, suspiciousness, low tolerance for frustration, impulsiveness, self-devaluation, and chronic anxiety occur with high frequency among alcoholics. Gross and Carpenter (1971) report that 266 male alcoholics tested on the 16 Personality Factors (16PF) personality inventory showed traits that differentiated them from the general population, with significant differences on 12 of the 16 personality traits on the inventory.

There seems to be an important relation between the self-image of the individual and the likelihood that he or she will drink alcohol to excess. Those with a low self-image and who experience self-doubt as to their ability to get along in the world are likely to use alcohol to excess and, as a result, to become alcoholic. As they take this course, the use of alcohol may dull their feelings of low self-worth but also decrease the probability that they will be successful in everyday living; this will increase their feelings of low self-worth, thus increasing the need to drink more alcohol. What this means for the therapist working with an alcoholic is that treatment should include every means possible to enhance the patient's self-esteem, confidence, and ability to negotiate the everyday problems of living.

TREATMENT AND PREVENTION OF ALCOHOL ABUSE AND ALCOHOLISM

As with the treatment of dependence on any central nervous system depressant, the first consideration for the nonmedical psychotherapist in the treatment of alcoholism is detoxification. This is best left to the medical professionals who have the equipment, medication, and training for such a task. The job of the nonmedical therapist at this time is to be sure that the patient is aware that the detoxification process is sometimes life threatening and therefore is best done under medical supervision.

Not all people with alcohol problems, or even all alcoholics, are physically addicted to alcohol. The amount of alcohol the patient consumes and length of time he or she has been drinking determine physical addiction and the likelihood of withdrawal symptoms. Most people with alcohol problems will not need medical detoxification, but if there is a doubt a physician should make the decision.

Early in the withdrawal process is an excellent time for the nonmedical therapist to begin therapeutic intervention with patients because their motivation to seek help for their drinking problems is often high at this point. It is also an excellent time to obtain a commitment from patients to alter their drinking habits. From then on the choice for a course of treatment varies depending on the needs of the patient.

There are many valuable resources on the treatment of alcoholism (Davis, 1987; Edwards & Grant, 1980; Heather & Robertson, 1981; Lawson et al., 1983, 1984; Pattison & Kaufman, 1982). These resources will assist the nonmedical psychotherapist in acquiring a working knowledge of various treatment approaches to alcoholism, even if he or she does not specialize in working with alcoholics. The choice of a referral source is often critical to the success of the patient in treatment, and the well-educated therapist will make the best decisions for his or her patients.

For most alcoholic patients, "traditional wisdom" in the alcohol treatment field indicates a course of treatment that includes a stay in a 1-month hospital-based inpatient treatment program, where patients are advised as to the probable course of their "disease" if they do not stop drinking (death, of course). They also receive training in the 12 steps of Alcoholics Anonymous and are encouraged to attend meetings both during and after treatment. This inpatient treatment is followed by an aftercare program, consisting of group therapy through the agency providing the inpatient treatment. These groups are often led by volunteer ex-alcoholic patients who have received about 1 day of training in group therapy. These groups meet one night a week. Patients are also encouraged to attend meetings at other times depending on how much support the individuals need to "stay sober."

The ideal course of treatment for the alcoholic or problem drinker is entirely based on the needs of each individual. For some, inpatient treatment is a must. On the other hand, far fewer people need inpatient treatment than are placed in such programs. Many inpatients could be equally well or perhaps better served on an outpatient basis. In most cases, family therapy is the best course of treatment (Lawson et al., 1983). For the nonmedical psychotherapist the choice is between following the dictates of "traditional wisdom," which are not based on research or the needs of individual patients, and following a course of treatment based solely on the needs of the patient. There is a price for going against traditional wisdom in the field of alcohol rehabilitation, as pointed out by Peele (1986) and Shaffer (1987), but the need to do so was called for long ago (Cain, 1964). The basis of the controversy is: Should alcohol abuse be called a disease when other abuse behaviors, such as smoking and overeating, are considered merely bad habits? The important considerations of the issue are the pros and cons of the "disease" approach to alcohol abuse and the alternatives to such an approach. One obvious motive for the decriminalization of alcoholic behavior is that it increases the likelihood that the alcoholic will seek help, but there are those who believe that decriminalization is an ineffective way of addressing the problem (e.g., Vogler & Bartz, 1982). Possibly the most unfortunate consequence of the disease model is that total abstinence is offered as the only cure. There are those who recommend treatment approaches that are not within these limits (Miller, 1982; Heather & Robertson, 1981), and the scientific data seem to support their recommendations. At the other extreme, there are also those who advocate diagnosing everyone connected with the alcoholic as having a disease, including the alcoholic's children, grandchildren, and spouse (see Miller, 1987).

The nonmedical psychotherapist must be well informed and well read on the issues and must keep in mind that the use or abuse of alcohol (or any drug for that matter) is a compulsive behavior. Many who have supported the disease model of alcoholism are beginning to recognize the learned nature of drinking habits. Dr. Alfred Smith, a psychiatrist who spent 15 years seeking a biological cause for alcoholism, remarked before the National Safety Congress in Chicago, "It is a terrible disappointment to me to finally face up to the fact that alcoholism is a behavior disorder" (Vogler & Bartz, 1982, p. 17). There are social costs (such as the loss of friends or jobs) for those who admit to not drinking sensibly. To encourage the problem drinker to seek help early these social costs must be reduced, and perhaps there should be social gains involved in learning early to drink responsibly if an individual chooses to drink.

Lawson and colleagues (1983) suggest the family as the appropriate place to learn drinking behavior. By the legal drinking age of 21, however, most children are no longer under the direct influence of the family. They must learn well ahead of the time that they actually start drinking what is expected of them if they choose to drink. This cannot be done if they have as models parents who themselves abuse alcohol. The key to prevention is therefore to involve the whole family in the treatment of the alcoholic and to treat the family as well by helping to reduce the risk of the generational transmission of alcoholism.

The prevention of alcoholism and problem drinking must also involve a change in public attitude about what is acceptable behavior with regard to drinking in American society. Other societies and cultures for hundreds of years have not accepted drunkenness as acceptable behavior; the result is an extremely low rate of alcoholism and problem drinking in those societies. Problem drinking is not likely to decrease in this country. It is more likely to increase. Nevertheless, as this condition becomes better understood, the nonmedical psychotherapist can provide help for those who suffer as a result of the inappropriate use of alcohol.

REFERENCES

Armyr, G., Elmer, A., and Herz, U. (1982). *Alcohol in the world of the 80's.* Stockholm: Sober Forlags AB.

Blum, K. (1984). *Handbook of abusable drugs.* New York: Gardner Press.

Cain, A. (1964). *The cured alcoholic.* New York: John Day.

Davis, D. (1987). *Alcoholism treatment.* New York: Gardner Press.

Edwards, G., & Grant, M. (Eds.). (1980). *Alcoholism treatment in transition.* Baltimore: University Park Press.

Goldberg, L.A. (1963). The metabolism of alcohol. In S.P. Lucia (Ed.), *Alcohol and civilization* (pp. 237–295). New York: McGraw-Hill.

Goodwin, D. (1981). *Alcoholism: The facts* (pp. 4–5). New York: Oxford Press.

Gross, W.F., & Carpenter, L. (1971). Alcoholic personality: Reality or fiction. *Psychological Reports, 28,* 375–378.

Heather, N., & Robertson, I. (1981). *Controlled drinking.* London: Methuen.

Lawson, G., Ellis, D., & Rivers, C. (1984). *Essentials of chemical dependency counseling.* Rockville, MD: Aspen Publishers.

Lawson, G., Peterson, J., & Lawson, A. (1983). *Alcoholism and the family: A guide to treatment and prevention.* Rockville, MD: Aspen Publishers.

Liska, K. (1986). *Drugs and the human body.* New York: Macmillan.

MacAndrew, C., & Edgerton, R.B. (1969). *Drunken comportment: A social explanation.* Chicago: Aldins Publishing Co.

Mendelson, J., & LaDou, J. (1964). Experimentally induced chronic intoxication and withdrawal in alcoholics: Part 2. Psychophysiological findings. *Quarterly Journal of Studies of Alcohol,* 2(suppl.), 14.

Miller, W. (1982). Treating problem drinkers: What works? *The Behavior Therapist, 5,* 15–17.

Miller, W. (1987). Adult cousins of alcoholics. *Psychology of Addictive Behaviors, 1,* 74–76.

Pattison, E.M., & Kaufman, E. (Eds.). 1982. *Encyclopedic handbook of alcoholism.* New York: Gardner Press.

Peele, S. (1986). Denial of reality and freedom in addiction research and treatment. *Bulletin of the Society of Psychologists in Addictive Behaviors, 5,* 149–166.

Shaffer, H. (1987). Academic freedom and the development of science. *Psychology of Addictive Behaviors, 1,* 62–69.

Tarter, R.E., & Schneider, D.V. (1976). Models and theories of alcoholism. In R.E. Tarter & A.A. Sugleman (Eds.), *Alcoholism: Interdisciplinary approaches to an enduring problem* (pp. 603–636). Reading, MA: Addison-Wesley Publishing Co.

Vogler, R., & Bartz, W. (1982). *The better way to drink.* Oakland, CA: New Harbinger Press.

Chapter 18

Phencyclidine: A Clinical Review*

Thomas Young, Gary W. Lawson, and Carl B. Gacono

Phencyclidine (PCP) is a Schedule II controlled substance. According to Section 201, Criteria of the Controlled Substance Act, a Schedule II controlled substance has a high potential for abuse, an accepted medical use in treatment in the United States, or a currently accepted use with severe restrictions, and may lead to severe psychological or physical dependence. Many factors such as the availability of phencyclidine, the ease of its production, the large profits involved in its sale, the unpredictable behavior of its users, and the health hazards posed by PCP labs have caused some states, such as California, to view PCP as "the single greatest drug problem to law enforcement" (McAdams, Linder, Lerner, & Burns, 1980). PCP abuse is a drug problem that warrants special training for professionals in the mental health, law enforcement, and medical professions.

Not the least of PCP-related problems has been the appropriate classification of the drug itself (Cohen, 1981). PCP has been referred to both as an "upper" and as a "downer" and has stimulant- or depressant-like properties. Some investigators include PCP with drugs of the hallucinogenic category (Julien, 1981). PCP, however, is not an upper, a downer, or strictly a hallucinogen but what McAdams and colleagues (1980) refer to as an "insider-outer" drug.

PCP represents a new class of drugs containing some 30 analogs, of which the anesthetic ketamine is also well known (see Figure 18-1). Unlike any other street drug, its psychological effects are often nearly indistinguishable from the symptoms of schizophrenia (Linder, Lerner, & Burns, 1981). The unique properties of PCP, coupled with the characteristic personality pattern of the chronic user, have led Cohen (1981) and others to focus much attention on the specific management issues involved in the treatment of PCP abuse.

---

*From "Clinical Aspects of Phencyclidine" by Thomas Young, Gary W. Lawson, and Carl B. Gacono, 1987, *International Journal of the Addictions*, 22(1), pp. 1-15. Copyright 1987 by Marcel Dekker, Inc. Adapted by permission.

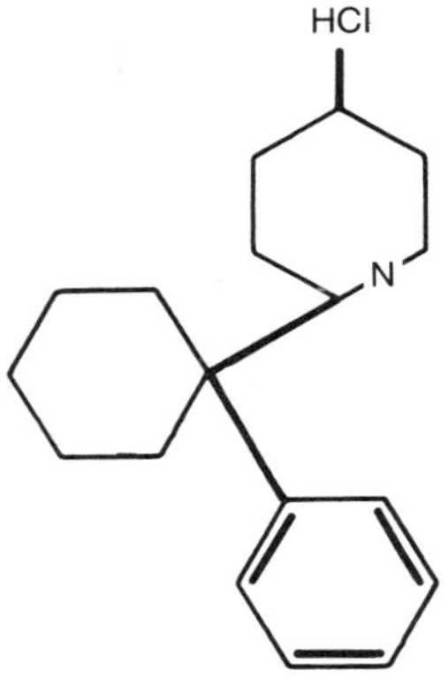

HCl

N

Figure 18-1 Chemical Structure of Phencyclidine [1-(1-phenylcyclohexyl)piperidine hydrochloride].

HISTORY

PCP [1-(1-phencyclohexyl)piperidine hydrochloride] was first synthesized by Parke-Davis Laboratories in 1956. It was found to produce a state of serenity in laboratory monkeys; hence its trade name, Sernyl. Early research on phencyclidine was directed into three areas: as a surgical anesthetic for humans, as an experimental drug in producing model psychoses, and as a veterinary tranquilizer. Postoperative psychotic reactions and acute agitations, especially among young and middle-aged patients, ended the potential use of phencyclidine as a general surgical anesthetic (Griefenstein et al., 1958; Johnstone, 1960; Julien, 1981). As an experimental drug, PCP produces two types of psychotic effects: a schizophrenic syndrome lasting several hours in normal volunteers, and an extreme exacerbation of schizophrenia lasting up to 6 weeks in chronic schizophrenic patients (Bakker & Amini, 1961; Davies & Beach, 1960; Luby et al., 1959; Rosenbaum et al., 1959). In 1965 Parke-Davis withdrew PCP from experimental use in humans (Reed & Kane, 1972). As an animal tranquilizer, PCP was marketed under the name Sernylan but was outlawed in 1978 and replaced by the structural analog ketamine (Luisada, 1981).

As an illicit street drug, PCP was first reported in Los Angeles in 1965 (McAdams et al., 1980). In 1967 it surfaced in San Francisco under the name "PeaCe Pill." Because of bad press surrounding the high incidence of "bummer" experiences, the drug disappeared from the Haight-Ashbury area. PCP later (1968) reappeared on the East Coast as "hog." During the next 12 years the incidence of its use increased geographically to include 44 of the 50 states (McAdams et al., 1980). Today the drug is illegally sold under various street names, such as amoeba, angel dust, CJ, cadillac, crystal, crystal joints, cyclones,

DOA, embalming fluid, horse tranquilizer, Mr. Lovely, pig tranquilizer, rocket fuel, scuffle, supergrass, soma surfer, THC, whack, whacky weed, and window pane (Perry, 1975; Siegel, 1978a; Young et al., 1977). Luisada (1981) has pointed out that this ever-expanding list of street names "has generated a rule of thumb among those treating PCP abuses: a new drug with a bizarre name that is smoked or snorted can be assumed to be PCP unless proven otherwise" (p.211).

PCP appears as a crystalline powder and as tablets and capsules in various colors, shapes, and sizes. PCP is one of the most widely misrepresented street drugs. It is often used to adulterate, or is sold as, such drugs as LSD, MDA (methylenedioxyamphetamine), STP (dimethoxymethylamphetamine), psilocybin, mescaline, synthetic cocaine, and most commonly as THC (tetrahydrocannabinol). PCP is taken for its euphoric effects, pseudo-hallucinogenic potential, ability to decrease inhibitions, and ability to instill feelings of power and to eliminate pain. Easily manufactured by "lay chemists," it is inexpensive to produce. McAdams and colleagues (1980) report that an initial investment of $625 can yield up to $200,000 worth of PCP. These factors make PCP very attractive as an illicit drug.

PCP is now believed to be one of the most widely used and most widely available psychoactive drugs in the United States. In fact, some investigators have suggested that it may be approaching marijuana as the drug of preference among substance abusers (Graeven, 1977, 1978; Khajawall et al., 1982; Micik, 1980; Petersen & Stillman, 1978; Showalter & Thorton, 1977; Snyder, 1980). According to national surveys, approximately 8 million people have used PCP. In 1979 almost 13% of graduating high school seniors reported that they had used PCP (Nicholi, 1984). In a survey of students in New York, 22% in grades 11 through 12 and 7.5% in grades 7 through 8 indicated that they had tried PCP (Sharp & Korman, 1981).

In all likelihood, however, this information is extremely conservative and does not represent the true scope of PCP use. At least six reasons may account for this problem. First, that PCP is known by a wide variety of street and regional names may result in an inability to recognize the nomenclature used in drug surveys. Second, since PCP is often used as an adulterant, many users may be totally ignorant of its presence. Third, PCP is often misrepresented as THC or as some other kind of psychoactive drug. Fourth, PCP can cause amnesia and an inability to recall drug use (Cohen, 1981; McAdams et al., 1980). Fifth, the role of PCP may be overlooked and misdiagnosed in cases marked by schizophrenic reactions and affective disorders (Fauman & Fauman, 1977). Sixth, it is also believed that the role of PCP is overlooked in hundreds of cases of accidental deaths and suicides (Nicholi, 1984).

Regardless, there is no question that PCP has gained access into the "gray market" of the middle class. One group of typical PCP users can be distinguished from other drug users by the fact that they are more likely to be white, to live in the suburbs, to have a higher socioeconomic status, and to have a higher level of education (Luisada, 1981; Schuckit & Morrissey, 1978). The heaviest incidence of PCP use is generally found in males in their late teens and early 20s. Several studies of PCP use among adolescents have found that the average age of first use is 14 years. In most cases the adolescent is introduced to PCP through a friend (Lerner & Burns, 1978, Luisada, 1981; Siegel, 1978a).

The widespread use of PCP is marked by particularly dangerous consequences. Chronic PCP users are characterized by various clinical problems that are attributed to direct effects of the drug on both physical and psychological functioning as well as the adjunct effects caused by poor personal care and the exacerbation of areas of poor premorbid personality adjustment. These clinical problems include anorexia, insomnia, constipation, urinary hesitancy, organic memory impairment, speech problems, rhabdomyolysis, teratogenic effects, severe affective disorders, personality changes, and psychotic episodes (Allen & Young, 1978; Rosen, 1979; Strauss et al., 1981). In addition, the tendency for explosive rage to develop during the course of PCP intoxication has been cited as a contributory factor in the rise of violent acts and antisocial behavior (Cohen, 1977; Fauman & Fauman, 1979; Sandler, 1979; Sidoff, 1979; Siegel, 1978b; Wright, 1980).

That PCP use is a serious clinical problem is also illustrated by reports that some psychiatric emergency units in large urban hospitals have indicated that ''in up to 70% of their admissions, the urine has been positive for phencyclidine'' (Nicholi, 1984, p. 197). One study of a metropolitan hospital revealed that PCP psychoses exceeded both schizophrenia and alcoholism as the cause of psychiatric admission (Luisada & Brown, 1976). Another study conducted in Detroit disclosed that PCP was the most commonly used substance in 1,000 cases of drug intoxication (Horwitz et al., 1976). Since PCP has become an increasingly encountered clinical problem, professionals in the field of psychiatric care should be familiar with its effects, diagnosis, and treatment.

CLINICAL EFFECTS

Pollack (1976) has noted that PCP intoxication is ''a clinical condition that is defined by clinical signs and symptoms ranging from mild, moderate, to severe, with coma and eventual death'' (p. 258). As a clinical condition, PCP intoxication is influenced by a number of important variables related to the drug itself, such as preparation, purity, dosage, and route of administration. Intoxication is also affected by characteristics of the user such as age, medical history, drug history, behavioral history, and personality (Siegel, 1978b). This multivariate perspective helps to explain that PCP intoxication ''may produce either depression or stimulation of the central nervous system, depending on the dose and route of administration''; it also helps to explain how PCP can produce a mental state that ''ranges from euphoria to acute psychosis'' (Tong et al., 1975, p. 512).

In most cases, the effects of PCP begin within 1 hour if the drug is orally ingested or within 5 minutes if the drug is smoked, insufflated, or injected. PCP is also taken rectally or in eye drops. The most popular method is smoking PCP sprinkled on mint, parsley, or other kinds of leaves. The typical high from PCP lasts 4 to 6 hours and is followed by a ''come down'' that lasts 6 to 24 hours. Depending on the chronicity of use, it may take up to 4 weeks for the person to feel normal once again (Linder et al., 1981; McAdams et al., 1980). The specific effects of the drug are clearly related (see Table 18-1). A dosage of 1 to 5 mg of phencyclidine normally produces feelings of euphoria and numbness. The user can be best described as being in a giddy, drunken state that resembles ethyl alcohol intoxication. Disinhibition and emotional lability are also regularly observed at low dosages. A moderate dosage of 5 to 10 mg often results in an excited, confused intoxication marked by ataxia and dysarthria. Other clinical manifestations include depersonalization, repetitive motor movements, myoclonus, vomiting, flushing, diaphoresis, fever, decreased peripheral sensations, and horizontal and vertical nystagmus. Psychotic reactions in the form of stu-

---

Table 18-1 Dosage-Related Effects of Phencyclidine

Low to moderate dose (5 mg)
  Blank stare
  Horizontal and vertical nystagmus
  Ataxia and dysarthria
  Assaultive, agitated behavior
  Increased blood pressure
  Increased deep tendon reflexes

Moderate to high dose (20 mg or greater)
  Coma
  Unresponsive stare; eyes fixed open
  Spontaneous nystagmus
  Muscle rigidity
  EEG: diffuse, theta and delta slowing
  Increased blood pressure
  Increased deep tendon reflexes

High to extremely high dose (up to 500 mg)
  Prolonged coma
  Extensor posturing
  Seizures
  Hypoventilation or apnea
  Sustained increased blood pressure
  EEG: diffuse, slowing, and periodic; slow-wave complexes

porous catatonia, excited catatonia, or paranoid schizophrenia may emerge with both moderate and high dosages. With pharmacological overdose, the primary cause of death is respiratory depression caused by seizure activity and, in rare cases, extreme hypertension or uncontrollable increase in body temperature. Prolonged coma, convulsions, and death may result from 20 mg of PCP or more (American Psychiatric Association, 1980; Cohen, 1977; Linden et al., 1975; Ungerleider & DeAngelis, 1981).

In general, PCP is more likely to result in impaired thought, anxiety, psychosis, and other negative effects than either LSD or mescaline (Showalter & Thorton, 1977). It has been estimated, for example, that somewhere "between 70 to 80 percent of PCP users have experienced at least one 'bad trip' " (Luisada, 1981, p. 212). In addition, Fauman and Fauman (1978) discovered that 48% of their sample of PCP users had experienced multiple "bad trips." Of note in one study is that one fourth of patients originally treated for PCP psychosis returned within 1 year with a schizophrenic psychosis in the absence of the drug (McAdams et al., 1980). This is indicative that one of the specific characteristics of chronic PCP users is their poor premorbid functioning (that is, they are vulnerable to decompensation). The most frequently described dysphoric symptoms are "numbness and loss of motor control, or paralysis, confusion, sensory distortions and loss of consciousness" (Fauman & Fauman, 1978, p. 192). Other adverse reactions include cramps, nausea, emesis, hallucinations, and violent psychotic behavior. Despite the adverse effects, 72% of subjects in Fauman and Fauman's study continued to use PCP because of its potent psychological effects, availability, and relatively low cost. Although there is evidence of personality disorganization in cases of PCP use, evidence of tolerance development or of a withdrawal syndrome is incomplete (Cohen, 1981).

Smith and colleagues (1978) have noted that the PCP abuse syndrome is marked by four behavioral phases: acute PCP toxicity, PCP toxic psychosis, PCP-precipitated psychotic episodes, and PCP-induced depression. Acute PCP toxicity is characterized by the "four C's": combativeness and catatonia at lower dosages and convulsions and coma at higher dosages. Some individuals develop a toxic psychosis after the acute PCP toxicity phase. The symptomatology of PCP toxic psychosis includes impaired judgment, agitation, paranoid delusions, auditory and visual hallucinations, and flattened affect. The duration of this behavior phase is normally around 24 hours to 7 days. Apparently, PCP toxic psychosis is most commonly seen among chronic abusers. Patients can also move from a PCP toxic psychosis into a PCP-precipitated psychotic episode that can last 7 to 30 days or more. According to Smith and co-workers (1978), "The characteristics of the episode are of the schizoaffective type with paranoid features and a waxing and waning thought disorder" (p. 235). It is generally believed that most patients in this phase have psychotic or prepsychotic personalities. Nevertheless, individuals with no history of pre-existing psychosis have experienced a PCP-precipitated episode after a single administration of the drug. Finally there is the clinical problem of PCP-induced depression, which can follow any of the preceding stages and can last anywhere from 1 day to several months. During this phase, the patient is at high risk for suicide and may attempt to self-medicate the depression. Consequently, follow-ups are a clinical imperative in providing professional psychiatric care for the PCP user.

DIAGNOSIS

In medical and mental health facilities the PCP-intoxicated patient is often misdiagnosed and consequently treated inappropriately. In one study, trained emergency room physicians correctly identified PCP intoxication in only 8 of 61 cases in which the drug was later confirmed (Fauman & Fauman, 1977).

Nystagmus is induced by PCP at low dosages and offers the best single indication of PCP intoxication. A blank stare and muscle rigidity are also characteristic of PCP intoxication. Presence of nystagmus or ataxia rules out central nervous system stimulants or LSD with the acutely excited and confused patient. Hypertension and hyperreflexia differentiates PCP intoxication from an overdose of a sedative-hypnotic. Of diagnostic significance is the presence of diffuse theta activity with periodic, slow-wave complexes on electroencephalography (McAdams et al, 1980). Toxicological screening and electroencephalography are recommended in verification of the final diagnosis.

The *Diagnostic and Statistical Manual of Mental Disorders* (Third Edition) (DSM-III; American Psychiatric Association, 1980) provides the following diagnostic criteria for PCP intoxication (pp. 151–152).

1. Recent use of phencyclidine.
2. Within 1 hour (less when smoked, insufflated, or used intravenously) at least two of the following physiological symptoms:
   —vertical or horizontal nystagmus,
   —increased blood pressure and heart rate,
   —numbness or diminished responsiveness to pain,
   —ataxia, or
   —dysarthria.
3. Within 1 hour, at least two of the following psychological symptoms:
   —euphoria,
   —psychomotor agitation,
   —marked anxiety,
   —emotional lability,
   —grandiosity,

—sensation of slowed time, or
—synesthesis.
4. Maladaptive behavioral effects (e.g., belligerence, impulsiveness, unpredictability, impaired judgment, assaultiveness).
5. Not due to any other physical or mental disorder or to delirium.

Obtaining an accurate drug history from the patient is often difficult or impossible. This is particularly true if the patient is mute, amnesic, or unaware of the nature of the consumed substance. Consequently, the use of laboratory tests, such as gas chromatography, is extremely helpful in determining whether the patient has recently used PCP. Some clinicians consider the absence of dilation of the pupils and the presence of gross ataxia with vertical and horizontal nystagmus sufficient clinical evidence for a working diagnosis of PCP intoxication (Nicholi, 1984).

If a moderate dosage of PCP results in stupor, the clinician may find it difficult to differentiate this clinical state from an overdose of a sedative-hypnotic. As a general rule, PCP intoxication is induced from the presence of hypertension and hyperreflexia and the absence of significant respiratory depression. In the case of coma, the presence of opisthotonic posturing, status epilepticus, hypertension without prominent respiratory depression, and a prolonged recovery phase indicate PCP overdose (Nicholi, 1984; Senay et al., 1977).

TREATMENT

Medical

The effects of PCP on the user are unpredictable. During a period of excitation, the user can be extremely dangerous. McAdams and colleagues (1980) recommend a backup of at least five large people when dealing with one average-sized patient. Use of body weight, rather than physical strength, tends to be the only effective method of control.

In uncomplicated cases of PCP intoxication, the immediate clinical task is to prevent the patient from injuring himself or herself or others. This primarily involves reducing sensory stimulation by isolating the patient in a quiet room with reduced lighting. If possible, the patient's behavior and vital signs should be closely monitored through unobstrusive medical means (e.g., video cameras and physiological monitoring equipment) in place of direct personal interaction. If acutely agitated, the patient "should not be approached unless there are adequate staff available" (Luisada, 1981, p. 214). As Petersen and Stillman (1978) have noted, "patients are often so unmanageable that restraints are necessary, and the help of four or five (not one) burly aides will often be needed to prevent injury to staff and patients'' (p. 12). The acutely agitated patient can also be managed by administering 10 to 20 mg of diazepam intramuscularly or orally (Luisada, 1981; Smith et al., 1978; Tong et al., 1975). Since the use of PCP causes environmental sensitivity, "talk down" techniques commonly used in cases marked by "bad trips" from hallucinogens are contraindicated (Linden et al., 1975; Showalter & Thorton, 1977; Stein, 1973).

Treatment of PCP overdose requires intensive medical management of the most acute physical effects of PCP, such as hyperactive crisis, convulsions, and coma. Consequently, "treatment of this phase frequently requires the full life support capabilities of a good intensive care unit" (Petersen & Stillman, 1978, p. 11). In addition to supportive measures, treatment of PCP overdose includes "the removal of phencyclidine enriched gastric secretions from the patient's stomach and the enhancement of urinary excretion of phencyclidine" (Luisada, 1981, p. 216). The former is accomplished by continuous gastric suction and the latter by first reducing the urinary pH to 5 or lower through the use of ammonium chloride in conjunction with ascorbic acid and then by promoting diuresis with 20 to 40 mg of furosemide (Lasix) intravenously (Aronow et al., 1981). Other treatment is symptomatic since there is no specific antagonist for PCP. Nasopharyngeal suctioning, for example, may be needed since PCP can induce hypersecretion in the pharynx (Kline & Lindenmayer, 1981; Smith et al., 1978). Patients should also be observed for myoclonic movements, which typically precede the onset of seizures (Nicholi, 1984). Seizures are treated with diazepam intravenously in 2- or 3-mg increments, up to 5 mg/minute (Kline & Lindenmayer, 1981). Blood pressure should also be closely monitored for hypertension. Severe hypertension can be reduced with diazoxide (Hyperstat) or hydralazine (Apresoline) (Eastman & Cohen, 1975; Luisada, 1981; Smith et al., 1978). Respiratory depression can develop in cases in which PCP was taken in high dosages or in combination with alcohol, sedative-hypnotics, or opiates. In this situation, respiratory assistance with the use of a respirator is necessary (Smith et al., 1978). In most cases, however, pure PCP rarely results in significant or prominent respiratory depression (Senay et al., 1977; Smith et al., 1978).

Nonphenothiazine tranquilizers such as haloperidol (Haldol) are commonly used in the treatment of PCP toxic psychosis, although some clinicians prefer to use sedative-hypnotic medication. In general, the drugs are primarily used because they render the patient more manageable in a ward, but they do not appear to shorten the length of the psychosis (Smith et al., 1978). In PCP-precipitated psychosis, however, Luisada and Brown (1976) recommend the administration of chlorpromazine (Thorazine), starting with 400 mg/day in divided dosages and increasing as necessary by 200 mg/day to an average dosage of 1600 mg/day. The need for long-term antipsychotic drug maintenance in cases of PCP-precipitated psychosis makes it clinically important to differentiate these patients from those with PCP-induced toxic psychosis (Luisada, 1981; Smith et al., 1978).

PCP-induced depression has been successfully treated through the daily administration of the tricyclic antidepressant amitriptyline (Elavil) and imipramine (Tofranil). On an outpatient basis, antidepressant medication should be dispensed in a limited quantity, and the patient should be warned about the "possible interaction of tricyclic antidepressants with PCP, alcohol, and other drugs" (Smith et al., 1978, p. 238). The patient should also be told to discontinue medication if the use of PCP is resumed.

Psychotherapeutic

Psychotherapy is necessary once the patient no longer represents a medical emergency. DeAngelis and Goldstein (1978) have noted that drug users frequently present their substance abuse as the therapeutic focus in order to prevent the therapist from dealing with underlying conflicts and issues. Consequently the psychotherapeutic process should focus on internal and external conflicts as well as on the presenting problem. In some cases PCP use may reflect a problem within the family and the need for family therapy (see, for example, Haley, 1980). Other cases may be marked by pre-existing affective and personality disorders. As the DSM-III points out, "Frequently individuals who develop substance abuse disorders also have pre-existing personality disorders and affective disorders with concomitant impairment in social and occupational functioning" (p. 164).

As a group, chronic PCP drug abusers are often more disturbed than abusers of other drugs. They tend to show greater signs of pathology on the Minnesota Multiphasic Personality Inventory and on psychotic indexes or projectives such as the Rorschach Test (Linder et al., 1981). Other addicts are often put off by the poor coping skills and schizoidlike style of PCP abusers, viewing them as "low-class" abusers (McAdams et al., 1980). As a group, chronic PCP abusers lack social skills, are prone to periods of primary process thinking, have difficulty in modulating emotions (with a tendency toward lability), and are more likely to act out predictably than are normal subjects or heroin addicts. Chronic users tend to have a history of premorbid adjustment, often with personality organizations at the lower continuum of development (that is, schizoid, borderline, schizophrenic disorders).

Treatment-such as Synanon-style therapy, which is often used with heroin addicts, may be inappropriate for the chronic PCP abuser (McAdams et al., 1980). Treatment of PCP abuse requires a supportive, comprehensive program, including various therapy modalities, vocational and educational counseling, and case-management functions as well as medical consultation (see, for example, Gacono, 1985). At least for one group of chronic PCP abusers, treatment is similar to that for schizophrenics, whose symptomatology the PCP patient often mirrors.

PCP use is a complex multivariate problem that requires multiple therapeutic approaches. In other words, there are multiple patterns of dysfunctional PCP use that occur "in different types of personalities, with multiple combinations of adverse treatment interventions" (Lawson, 1984, p. 35). Thus therapeutic decisions should always be based on a professional evaluation of the patient's biological, psychological, and sociological profile (see, for example, Lawson, Peterson, & Lawson, 1983).

CONCLUSION

PCP use is not only a clinical problem but a sociological dilemma, especially among adolescents and young adults. Very little attention has been directed at the question of why some individuals use this substance. In general, however, it can be speculated that PCP is used as an alloplastic and as an autoplastic mode of adaptation to intra- and extrapsychic problems. That some people choose PCP in place of other modes of adaptation may be due to the interaction of biological, psychological, and sociological variables that are not yet fully understood (Halleck, 1967).

From a social-psychiatric perspective, PCP use is both an alloplastic and an autoplastic response to alienation, particularly feelings of helplessness (see, for example, Freud, 1959) and powerlessness (see, for example, Marx, 1939; Mills, 1957; Weber, 1946). This is especially true for adolescents, since they are characterized by social, political, and economic marginality (Goodman, 1960; Greenberg, 1978; Keniston, 1960; Kvaraceus, 1972; Vexler, 1972). Consequently it is not surprising that many adolescents use PCP because they enjoy the feeling of omnipotence that the substance can induce (Lerner & Burns, 1978). As an autoplastic adaptation, PCP use may allow an individual to change the external environment through violence, psychotic behavior, and other actions that indicate suffering (Halleck, 1967).

Lawson (1984) and Lawson and colleagues (1983) outline approaches for the assessment of the substance-abusing client, and Gacono (1985) discusses treatment strategies. McAdams and colleagues (1980) recommend strategies for the prevention and treatment of PCP abuse. Nevertheless, it has not been determined with certainty which strategies are the most predictable, usable, and successful. Further research is needed to determine the most effective combination of approaches for preventing and treating PCP abuse.

REFERENCES

Allen, R.M., & Young, S.J. (1978). Phencyclidine-induced psychosis. *American Journal of Psychiatry, 135*, 1081–1084.

American Psychiatric Association. (1980). *Diagnostic and statistical manual of mental disorders* (3rd ed.). Washington, DC: Author.

Aronow, R., et al. (1981). Clinical observations during phencyclidine intoxication and treatment based on ion-trapping. In R.C. Petersen & R.C. Stillman (Eds.), *Phencyclidine (PCP) abuse: An appraisal*. Rockville, MD: National Institute on Drug Abuse.

Bakker, C.B., & Amini, F.B. (1961). Observations on the psychotomimetic effects of Serynl. *Comparative Psychiatry*, *2*, 269–280.

Cohen, S. (1977). Angel dust. *Journal of the American Medical Association*, *238*, 515–516.

Cohen, S. (1981). *The substance abuse problem*. New York: Haworth Press.

Davies, B.M., & Beach, H.R. (1960). The effect of 1-arlycyclonexylamine (Sernyl) on twelve normal volunteers. *Journal of Mental Science*, *106*, 912–924.

DeAngelis, G.G., & Goldstein, E. (1978). Long-term treatment of adolescent PCP abusers. In R.C. Petersen & R.C. Stillman (Eds.), *Phencyclidine (PCP) abuse: An appraisal*. Rockville, MD: National Institute on Drug Abuse.

Eastman, J.M., & Cohen, S.N. (1975). Hypertensive crisis and death associated with phencyclidine poisoning. *Journal of the American Medical Association*, *232*, 1270–1271.

Fauman, M.A., & Fauman, B.J. (1977). The differential diagnosis of organic-based psychiatric disturbance in the emergency department. *Journal of the American College of Emergency Physicians*, *6*(7), 315–323.

Fauman, M.A., & Fauman, B.J. (1978). The psychiatric aspects of chronic phencyclidine (PCP) abuse: A study of phencyclidine users. In R.C. Petersen & R.C. Stillman (Eds.), *Phencyclidine (PCP) abuse: An appraisal*. Rockville, MD: National Institute on Drug Abuse.

Fauman, M.A., & Fauman, B.J. (1979). Violence associated with phencyclidine abuse. *American Journal of Psychiatry*, *136*, 1584–1586.

Freud, S. (1959). Inhibitions, symptoms and anxiety. In J. Strachey (Ed.), *Standard Edition of the Complete Psychological Works of Sigmund Freud* (vol. 20). London: Hogarth Press.

Gacono, C. (1985). Mental health work in a county jail: A heuristic model. *Journal of Offender Counseling*, 5(1), 16–22.

Goodman, P. (1960). *Growing up absurd*. New York: Random House.

Graeven, D.B. (1977). Phencyclidine (PCP): A local and national perspective. *Addictive Diseases*, *3*, 243–252.

Graeven, D.B. (1978). Patterns of phencyclidine use. In R.C. Petersen & R.C. Stillman (Eds.), *Phencyclidine (PCP) abuse: An appraisal*. Rockville, MD: National Institute on Drug Abuse.

Greenberg, D.P. (1978). Delinquency and the age structure of society. In P. Wierkman & P. Whitten (Eds.), *Readings in criminology*. Lexington, MA: D. C. Heath.

Griefenstein, F.E., et al. (1958). A study of 1-arlcyclohexylamine for anesthesia. *Anesthesia and Analgesia*, *47*, 283–294.

Haley, J. (1980). *Leaving home: The therapy of disturbed young people*. New York: McGraw-Hill.

Halleck, S.L. (1967). *Psychiatry and the dilemmas of crime*. New York: Harper & Row.

Horwitz, J.E., et al. (1976). Adjunct hospital emergency toxicology service. *Journal of the American Medical Association*, *235*, 1708–1712.

Johnstone, M. (1960). The use of Sernyl in clinical anesthesia. *Anaesthesist*, *9*, 114.

Julien, R. (1981). *A primer of drug action*. New York: W.H. Freeman.

Keniston, K. (1960). *The uncommitted*. New York: Dell.

Khajawall, A.M., et al. (1982). Chronic phencyclidine abuse and physical assault. *American Journal of Psychiatry, 139,* 1604–1606.

Kline, N.S., & Lindenmayer, J.P. (1981). *Psychotropic drugs: Manual for emergency management of overdoses.* Oradell, NJ: Medical Economics Co.

Kvaraceus, W.C. (1972). Alienation as a phenomenon of youth. In W.C. Bier (Ed.), *Alienation: Plight of modern man.* New York: Fordham Univ. Press.

Lawson, G., et al. (1983). *Alcoholism and the family.* Rockville, MD: Aspen Publishers.

Lawson, G. (1984). Characterizing clients and assessing their needs. In G. Lawson, D. Ellis, & P.C. Rivers (Eds.), *Essentials of chemical dependency counseling.* Rockville, MD: Aspen Publishers.

Lerner, S.E., & Burns, R.S. (1978). Phencyclidine use among youth: History, epidemiology, and acute and chronic intoxication. In R.C. Petersen & R.C. Stillman (Eds.), *Phencyclidine (PCP) abuse: An appraisal.* Rockville, MD: National Institute on Drug Abuse.

Linden, C.B., et al. (1975). Phencyclidine: Nine cases of poisoning. *Journal of the American Medical Association, 234,* 513–516.

Linder, R., Lerner, S., & Burns, R. (1981). *PCP: The devil's dust.* Belmont, CA: Wadsworth.

Luby, E.D., et al. (1959). Study of a new schizophrenic omimetic drug—Sernyl. *Archives of Neurological Psychiatry, 81,* 363-369.

Luisada, P.V. (1981). Phencyclidine. In J.H. Lowinson & P. Ruiz (Eds.), *Substance abuse: Clinical problems and perspectives.* Baltimore, MD: Williams & Wilkins.

Luisada, P.V., & Brown, B.I. (1976). Clinical management of the phencyclidine psychosis. *Clinical Toxicology, 9,* 539–545.

Marx, K. (1939). *The German Ideology.* New York: International Publishers.

McAdams, M., Linder, R., Lerner, S., & Burns, R. (1980). *Phencyclidine abuse manual.* Los Angeles: University of California Extension.

Micik, S. (1980). PCP update. *Western Journal of Medicine, 132,* 62–63.

Mills, C.W. (1957). *White collar.* New York: Oxford Univ. Press.

Nicholi, A.M., Jr. (1984). Phencyclidine hydrochloride (PCP) use among college students: Subjective and clinical effects, toxicity, diagnosis and treatments. *Journal of the American College of Health, 32,* 197–200.

Perry, D.C. (1975). PCP revisited. *PharmChem Newsletter, 4,* 1–6.

Petersen, R.C., & Stillman, R.C. (1978). Phencyclidine: An overview. In R.C. Petersen & R.C. Stillman (Eds.), *Phencyclidine (PCP) abuse: An appraisal.* Rockville, MD: National Institute on Drug Abuse.

Pollack, S. (1976). *Forensic psychiatry in the defense of diminished capacity.* Los Angeles: University of Southern California.

Reed, A., & Kane, A.W. (1972). Phencyclidine (PCP): Another illicit psychedelic drug. *Journal of Psychedelic Drugs, 5,* 8–12.

Rosen, A. (1979). Case report: Symptomatic mania and phencyclidine abuse. *American Journal of Psychiatry, 136,* 118–119.

Rosenbaum, G., et al. (1959). Comparison of Sernyl with other drugs. *Archives of General Psychiatry, 1,* 651–656.

Sandler, J.N. (1979). *Psychopharmacology of aggression.* New York: Raven.

Schuckit, M.A., & Morrissey, E.R. (1978). Propoxyphene and phencyclidine (PCP) use in adolescents. *Journal of Clinical Psychiatry, 39,* 7–13.

Senay, E.C., et al. (1977). *Emergency treatment for the drug abusing patient.* Rockville, MD: National Institute on Drug Abuse.

Sharp, C.W., & Korman, M. (1981). Volatile substances. In J.H. Lowinson & P. Ruiz (Eds.), *Substance abuse: Clinical problems and perspectives.* Baltimore: Williams & Wilkins.

Showalter, C.V., & Thorton, W.E. (1977). Clinical pharmacology of phencyclidine toxicity. *American Journal of Psychiatry, 134,* 1234–1238.

Sidoff, M.L. (1979). Phencyclidine: Syndromes of abuse and modes of treatment. *Topics in Emergency Medicine, 1,* 111–119.

Siegel, R.K. (1978a). Phencyclidine and ketamine intoxication: A study of four populations of recreational users. In R.C. Petersen & R.C. Stillman (Eds.), *Phencyclidine (PCP) abuse: An appraisal.* Rockville MD: National Institute on Drug Abuse.

Siegel, R.K. (1978b). Phencyclidine, criminal behavior, and the defense of diminished capacity. In R.C. Petersen & R.C. Stillman (Eds.), *Phencyclidine (PCP) abuse: An appraisal.* Rockville, MD: National Institute on Drug Abuse.

Smith, D.E., et al. (1978). The diagnosis and treatment of the PCP abuse syndrome. In R.C. Petersen & R.C. Stillman (Eds.), *Phencyclidine (PCP) abuse: An appraisal.* Rockville, MD: National Institute on Drug Abuse.

Snyder, A. (1980). Phencyclidine. *Nature (London), 285,* 355–356.

Stein, J.N. (1973). Phencyclidine-induced psychosis: The need to avoid unnecessary sensory influence. *Military Medical Journal, 138,* 590–591.

Strauss, A.A., et al. (1981). Neonatal manifestations of maternal phencyclidine (PCP) abuse. *Pediatrics, 68,* 550–552.

Tong, T.G., et al. (1975). Phencyclidine poisoning. *Journal of the American Medical Association, 234,* 512–513.

Ungerleider, J.T., & DeAngelis, G.G. (1981). Hallucinogens. In J.H. Lowinson & P. Ruiz (Eds.), *Substance abuse: Clinical problems and perspectives.* Baltimore: Williams & Wilkins.

Vexler, S. (1972). General alienation of youth. In W.C. Bier (Ed.), *Alienation: Plight of modern man.* New York: Fordham Univ. Press.

Weber, M. (1946). *Essays in sociology.* New York: Oxford Univ. Press.

Wright, H.H. (1980). Violence and PCP abuse [Letter to the editor]. *American Journal of Psychiatry, 137,* 752–753.

Young, L.A., et al. (1977). *Recreational drugs.* New York: Berkeley Books.

Chapter 19

Cocaine

Gene Ondrusek

Cocaine is a bitter, white crystalline alkaloid prepared from the leaves of the coca plant. There are some 250 varieties of coca plants in the genus *Erythroxylon*, the most noteworthy being *Erythroxylon coca*, known for its high concentration of cocaine alkaloids. The coca plant flourishes in the continuously moist forest conditions in the *montañas* of South America; it is not known to grow anywhere else in the world because these climatic and environmental conditions are not matched by any other geographic area. Most of the coca that is grown, either legally or illegally, comes from Peru and Bolivia, although there is still extensive illegal cultivation and use in Columbia, Argentina, Brazil, and Ecuador.

The use of coca by natives of South America is quite extensive and has a long history. In Bolivia alone, it is estimated that more than half the native population (approximately three million people) uses coca, consuming some 10,000 metric tons per year (Carroll, 1977). Eradication of coca production is therefore probably not a realistic possibility, as it is a mainstay of the South American economy; such an attempt would be akin to having American farmers cease production of tobacco and barley, hops, potatoes, and other raw ingredients for alcoholic beverages.

Current coca use by the natives of South America extends from the *mestizo* farmers to truck drivers, fishermen, stevedores, and miners. It is consumed by intellectuals and artists and is used by medicine men in healing and for religious rituals. The differential use by age, sex, social class, and so forth varies not only from one country to another, but within regions of the same country. Essentially, coca leaves are used for the following reasons: (1) for stimulation and to ward off fatigue, (2) as an adjunct to work, and (3) to combat hunger, cold, and "psychic distress." Very few reviewers, historical or contemporary, have found adverse reactions to health resulting from chronic coca use, as most users titrate or adjust their intake to avoid any undesirable effects (Siegel, 1984a). It is noteworthy, however, that as common abusive practices involving more concentrated forms of cocaine (snorted as a crystalline powder or smoked as a dried paste or base) have been introduced by foreign smugglers and dealers, the native South American population has in recent times begun to experience severe abuse problems. This has now become a problem of major and epidemic proportions in South America as well as in the United States. It is also important to note that, as the revenue from illegally exported cocaine rises, cocaine has become more involved in political and economic corruption.

CURRENT EPIDEMIOLOGY OF COCAINE USE

In the late 1960s and early 1970s, cocaine appeared in the United States as a drug of choice. Prevalence of use began to rise starting in the early 1970s. As shown in Figure 19-1 (Abelson & Miller, 1985), two major trends have emerged. First, for young adults (18 to 25 years of age), use of cocaine increased over the decade from 1972 to 1982; use in this group remains the highest of all age groups. Second, although the prevalence rates for youth and older adult groups are less than for younger adults, the two former groups show a pattern of increased use. The conclusion is that, as age cohorts pass into higher age groups, these numbers will increase; therefore, even if there is no increase in use in the young population (and there probably will be), the total number of persons who have used or are using cocaine can be expected to increase in coming years. This means that of all persons in the U.S. household population (which does not include transients and people in college dormitories, military bases, and the like) 22 million have used cocaine at some time during their lives. If it is assumed that only 10% of these Americans are ''at risk'' for continuing use or progression to abuse, and that only one half of those will have significant problems requiring treatment, this nevertheless yields a conservative underestimate of 550,000 problem users.

Other indicators point to increasing utilization of cocaine in this country. For instance, in 1968, drug enforcement efforts netted only 50 pounds of cocaine. This sort of effort today hardly receives notice. Recent evidence documented by the Drug Enforcement Administration (DEA) indicates that by the latter part of 1986 more than 8,000 pounds of cocaine had been interdicted entering the United States. The DEA estimates that this represents perhaps a small fraction (approximately 10%) of the total amount of cocaine imported into this country during 1986. Despite these trends, there is also the suggestion that cocaine use per se has leveled off since 1979. According to statistics compiled by the National Institute on Drug Abuse, some 22 million Americans have used cocaine (O'Malley, Johnston, & Bachman, 1985). The number of current users or those who have taken the drug in the past 30 days has remained relatively constant at about 4.3 million since 1979.

The question does arise, however, as to what this implies for abuse problems, since use does not necessarily imply abuse. This requires some historical notation. In the early 1970s the opinion toward cocaine was that it was a safe recreational

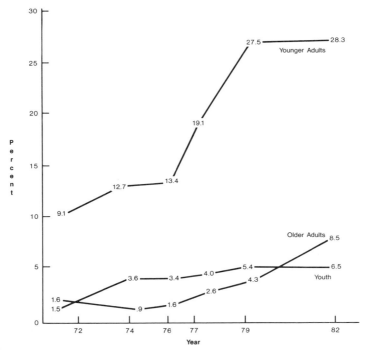

Figure 19-1 Trends in Lifetime Prevalence of Cocaine Use for Three Age Groups (1972–1982). *Source:* From "A Decade of Trends in Cocaine Use in the Household Population" by H.I. Abelson and J.D. Miller in *Cocaine Use in America: Epidemiologic and Criminal Perspectives* by N.T. Kozel and E.H. Adams (Eds.), 1985, Washington, D.C.: NIDA Research Monograph No. 61, U.S. Government Printing Office.

drug that was not particularly dangerous or associated with physical dependence. Nevertheless, research initiated at that time by Siegel (1984b), looking at longitudinal use patterns, suggests that 10 years later at least 50% of the users that began as experimental or social and recreational users at that time had escalated their usage to problem-producing levels that increase the risk of toxicity and dependency. This usage pattern further offers two observations: (1) although some individuals are capable of controlling use with no escalation to abusive patterns, a large proportion (at least half) is likely to experience difficulties with the drug requiring help with their usage patterns; and (2) a period of time (months to several years) will lapse before these problems begin to become intense enough to require intervention. This is in contrast with substances such as alcohol, where only 10% to 15% of users escalate to problem drinking or alcoholic proportions. These problems for alcohol abuse can take as long as 15 years to develop to critical levels. Therefore, even if the prevalence of cocaine use tends to remain steady (or even begins to drop), an ever-increasing number of users can be expected to seek help as their initial social and recreational patterns escalate to problematic levels. In fact, this may only be a small proportion. Looking again at epidemiology, between 1976 and 1981 there was a threefold increase in the rate of cocaine-related medical emergencies, a fourfold increase in cocaine-related deaths, and a fivefold increase in the proportion of admissions to (government-funded) drug treatment programs with cocaine as the primary drug (Adams & Durell, 1984). These trends remain unabated and are reflected in the rising number of users (see Figure 19-2) experiencing problems that follow even a steady-state rate of appearance of new users. It is important, however, to keep this problem in perspective in terms of other forms of substance abuse. The pervasiveness of substance abuse places the societal cost of alcoholism in excess of $116 billion per year, compared to only about $60 billion per year for abuse of drugs such as cocaine.

PROFILE OF INDIVIDUAL USERS

Given the epidemiological factors described above, several questions may be posed. Who is the typical cocaine user, and what is his or her demographic profile? Is it true, as the media suggest, that the use of cocaine is considerably more likely to occur among individuals of high income, education, and occupational prestige, or are problems of dependency relegated to a small dysfunctional subgroup with "addictive personalities"? Data does suggest that those with a high level of education (college and baccalaureate degrees), high employment status (managers

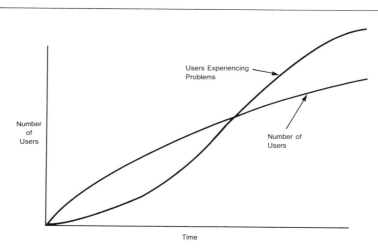

Figure 19-2 The Appearance of Users Experiencing Problems as Related to Total Number of Individuals Using Cocaine.

and professionals), and large incomes (greater than $50,000 per year) represent the largest percentage of users (Kandel, Murphy, & Karus, 1985). Nevertheless, there is no linear relationship between these variables and lifetime prevalence of use. Exhibit 19-1 presents data gathered from a random sample of 500 individuals who were among the first 100,000 callers to the 1-800 cocaine hotline in New Jersey in 1983 (Gold, 1984). About half of these users were using cocaine daily, and as a group an average of 6 g of cocaine was used per week. Overall, about 60% believed that they were addicted, and more than 70% said that they had lost control and could not limit cocaine use. This profile—which shows the typical cocaine user to be between the ages of 25 and 40, male, white, and with education and income exceeding the average—indicates that the "typical addict" portrait of the 1960s has been replaced by a portrait of a troubled part of middle-class America.

A further important determiner of who uses cocaine is related to the cost of the drug, currently $80 to $100 per gram to the consumer. A certain level of income or resources is necessary for a user to acquire adequate supplies for a long enough period to develop problems. Cost is also often cited as a rate-limiting factor in use.

The wholesale price of cocaine has dropped dramatically to less than half the price of a few years ago. Concurrent with this is a steady increase in purity. As this price-purity balance changes, society may experience an epidemic unprecedented in both magnitude and extent. That is, as a greater population segment is exposed to a purer drug because of greater availability and lower cost, the health consequences will inevitably increase, assuming that there is no reduction in demand. One manifestation of these simple economics is the growing prevalence of the more highly addictive form of cocaine known as "crack" or "rock." Crack has invaded lower socio-economic groups and ghetto areas, increasing ethnic utilization of this particular drug. Packaging practices have also changed. Formerly, the quantity of cocaine most commonly sold was 1 or ½ g, but new packaging techniques have resulted in smaller amounts of cocaine being sold in $5, $10, and $15 quantities, enough for several quick inhalations for a brief series of highs. This makes cocaine readily available to people with just a few dollars in their pockets, including those in ghettos and schoolchildren. Therefore, a popularity rise based

Exhibit 19-1 Profile of the Cocaine User

Age:	25 to 40 years
Length of use:	5 years
Sex:	3:1 male-to-female ratio
Education:	2 years of college
Ethnic background:	85% white
Income:	$25,000/year

simply on penetration of a different target market may also affect trends in cocaine use.

CLINICAL PHARMACOLOGY OF COCAINE

Cocaine is a ubiquitous drug in that it has several usage formats or routes of administration. The drug may be powdered and inhaled intranasally or dissolved and injected intravenously; it may also be converted into a free-base form and smoked with a pipe. Differences in routes of administration determine the intensity of the drug's effect, its duration of action, and to some extent its abuse liability. The most common usage route today is still insufflation, or snorting through a hollow straw or rolled-up currency. Probably 60% to 90% of use is through this route. In this form of self-administration, the crystalline substance dissolves on the nasal mucous membranes and is absorbed into the bloodstream. Although there is no intense "rush," the user experiences approximately 20 to 40 minutes of stimulation, after which insufflation is typically repeated (Van Dyke, Barash, Jatlow, & Buck, 1976). Users report euphoria and a sense of well-being along with a pleasant feeling of stimulation. Increases in talkativeness and physical activity are also observed.

The effects of cocaine, of course, depend on the amount taken at one time, the past drug experience of the user, the circumstances in which the drug is taken (the place, feelings, and activities of the user, whether it is used in the presence of other people, simultaneous use of alcohol or other drugs, and so forth), and the manner in which the drug is taken. Short-term effects are those that appear rapidly after a single dose and disappear within a few hours or days. Cocaine in low dosages produces a short-lived sensation of euphoria accompanied by feelings of increased energy, enhanced mental alertness, and greater sensory awareness. It also reduces the need for food and sleep and postpones the onset of fatigue. Large dosages intensify the user's high but may also lead to bizarre, erratic, and violent behavior (Jones, 1984). Physical symptoms include accelerated heartbeat, increased blood pressure, faster breathing, rise in body temperature, dilation of the pupils, sweating, and pallor.

THE RISE OF CRACK

Although the intranasal route remains the most common form of administration of cocaine, in recent years a rise in the popularity of free-basing or crack has resulted in a new and more addictive form of cocaine use. The insufflatable or injectable form of cocaine can be converted back into the free-base form, which can then be smoked. Steps for converting street cocaine into crack are relatively simple and can be performed either by the consumer or, as is increasingly being seen, in "crack houses," which convert the cocaine before sale. The following steps outline the simple procedure:

1. Street cocaine, actually the hydrochloride salt of cocaine, is initially dissolved in water and heated to ensure complete dissolution. It is then treated with a strong base such as sodium bicarbonate, or baking soda.
2. Once the dissolved cocaine is converted to its free-base form (free of the hydrochloride salt), the water solution is usually mixed with a volatile solution such as ether, which takes up the cocaine from the water. (This is a particularly dangerous step as ether is highly flammable and explosive and can be set off with merely a spark, a flame, or a lit cigarette.) If ether is not available, water may be boiled to the point where cocaine is no longer soluble and precipitates out in the form of hard pellets, called "rock" or "crack." The street term "crack" is derived from the sound made by pellets as they are heated during smoking. Trapped air pockets expand and make a popping sound.
3. If ether is used, it is drawn off and evaporated, leaving behind cocaine free-base crystals. Contrary to popular belief, this does not necessarily purify cocaine, because many adulterants such as lidocaine and procaine will also end up in the final product. However, some common cutting agents such as mannitol (a sugar) and inositol (vitamin B) will be extracted out, to some extent purifying the cocaine and reducing the quantity. Users complaining of "impurities" causing negative effects are usually mistaken; they are experiencing the negative effects of cocaine itself.

The final product, cocaine free-base or crack, is typically divided into quarter-gram increments, placed in vials, and sold by street dealers or from crack houses. A quarter-gram will provide three or four "hits," or inhalations, and sells for $10 to $25, depending on where it is purchased. Crack users typically return for more.

Why is crack such an intensely compelling drug? What accounts for its meteoric rise in popularity over insufflation as the preferred cocaine usage format? The answer is partially suggested in Figure 19-3, which points out that the "rush" from inhaled free-base is not only instantaneous, occurring in the first few seconds, but exceeds the high even of injected cocaine (Perez-Reyes, Ondrusek, DiGuiseppi, Jeffcoat, & Cook, 1982). The euphoric properties of the drug, and to a large extent its abuse and dependency liability, are due to how quickly the drug enters the brain and the concentration that reaches the brain. Inhaled free-base enters the brain in approximately 7 seconds, creating an immediate "rush" that exceeds even that of injected cocaine, which takes roughly twice as long to penetrate the brain. Also, unlike other drugs (such as opiates and alcohol) that are metabolized solely by the liver, cocaine is fragile and is broken down immediately

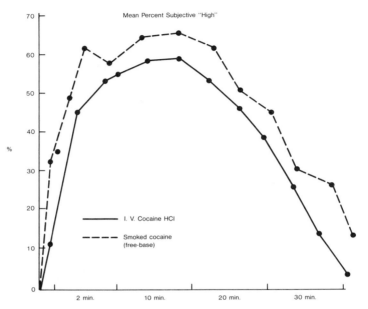

Figure 19-3 Subjective "High" for Free-Base Cocaine Compared to That for Intravenous Cocaine. *Source:* From "Free Base Cocaine Smoking" by M. Perez-Reyes, G. Ondrusek, S. DiGuiseppi et al., 1982, *Clinical Pharmacology and Therapeutics, 32*(4), pp. 459–465. Copyright 1982 by The C.V. Mosby Company. Reprinted by permission.

by enzymes in the bloodstream (Inaba, Stewart, & Kalow, 1978). Thus, the longer cocaine is in contact with the bloodstream, the more it is deactivated, effectively reducing the concentration ultimately reaching the brain. Apparently, because crack takes half the time to reach the brain required by intravenous cocaine, as much as twice the amount of a comparable dosage of the latter reaches the brain intact to produce its euphoric effect. This translates into a much larger abuse problem with this form of cocaine. In addition, the larger surface area of the lung compared to the bloodstream or the nasal mucosa allows for a greater entry factor, again increasing the concentration of cocaine and contributing to greater effects.

Another reason for the popularity of this usage format is that the limiting factor is solely the amount of crack that a user has available. People who habitually insufflate cocaine eventually experience constriction of the blood vessels of their nasal passages, so that they can no longer use the drug in this manner and achieve a reasonable effect. Similarly, users who inject the drug intravenously constantly damage veins and search for new ones. Unlike heroin, cocaine is a potent vasoconstrictor; continued use causes blood vessels to collapse, making them unusable, and ultimately damaging them beyond recovery. An intravenous cocaine user can therefore continue using the drug for a relatively short period. A free-base user, however, can inhale the drug with few discernable acute effects and without the stigma often associated with using needles. The local anesthetic properties of cocaine dull the pain from the often searingly hot cocaine vapors and allow even longer periods of use.

COCAINE TOXICITY

As a result of individual sensitivity or through intentional or inadvertent overdose, cocaine can generate a toxic reaction regardless of its route of administration. In this sense it closely resembles acute amphetamine poisoning (Jones, 1984). When this occurs, the user appears restless, agitated, and intensely anxious. There may be evidence of overactive reflexes, tremors, lack of coordination, and muscular twitching. In severe cases, delerium and hallucinations may develop along with a serious exaggeration of physical symptoms such as pain and pressure in the chest, nausea, blurred vision, fever, muscle spasms, and even convulsions and seizure activity (Siegel, 1984a). Treatment of cocaine toxicity is determined by clinical signs (Gay, 1982), but the most common treatment is 10 to 30 mg of diazepam (intramuscularly or intravenously) along with reassurance for anxiety reactions. Other pharmacological treatments include propanolol hydrochloride, which specifically antagonizes the manifestations of central cardiovascular hypermetabolism (Rappolt, Gay, & Inaba, 1977).

Although once touted as a relatively benign drug with limited toxicity, there is increasing evidence and greater numbers of incidents of its potentially fatal consequences. This is demonstrated not only by the deaths in 1986 of athletes Len Bias and Don Rogers but by increasing reports of cocaine-related fatalities from emergency room statistics across the country. The number of cocaine-related deaths has tripled since 1981 ("America's Crusade," 1986). The common mechanisms by which cocaine can have fatal results (excluding the homicides and other violence-related incidents in which cocaine often plays an indirect but significant role) are as follows.

1. Cardiopulmonary arrest: Because of the local anesthetic properties of cocaine, exceptionally large dosages may ultimately produce a marked depression of the central nervous system, ending in respiratory arrest. Death can be caused by pulmonary edema or major ventricular arrhythmia, the latter of which is the most common cause of overdose death (Benchimol, Bartall, & Dresser, 1978).
2. Status epilepticus: Repeated convulsions and seizures during cocaine use are potentially fatal.
3. Plasma cholinesterase deficiency: In individuals with congenital deficiency in the enzyme responsible for breaking down cocaine,

death can occur from even first-time low-dosage use of cocaine because the drug is not metabolized and recycles continuously throughout the body, leading rapidly to toxic levels (Jatlow, Barash, Van Dyke, Raddiny, & Byck, 1979).

4. Acute hypertensive crisis: Cocaine can create rapid increases in blood pressure that are sufficient to rupture weak blood vessels in the head, causing cerebral hemorrhage and death.

5. Hyperpyrexia (extremely high fever): Cocaine creates an elevated body temperature, potentially to lethal levels.

6. AIDS: Intravenous users can be exposed to this viral infection; AIDS has claimed a number of such individuals.

7. Paranoid delusory miscalculation: Accidental death can be caused by impaired judgment and delusions of superhuman abilities.

8. Suicide: Withdrawal-related depression can be severe enough to lead to suicide, either by common methods or by intentional overdose.

In addition to the intense addiction associated with cocaine and the possibility of death through overdose and the mechanisms outlined above, physical damage from cocaine use is also evident. There are increasing numbers of reports, both anecdotal and in the literature, concerning perforated nasal septa from cocaine insufflation in which the chronic blood vessel constriction results in tissue death (Villensky, 1982). Also, the use of any injected drugs can increase the risk for contracting hepatitis, septicimia (blood poisoning), and AIDS. Free-basing can also affect lung structure and function, as noted by several investigators (Weiss, Goldenheim, Mirin, Hales, & Mendelson, 1981; Shesser, Davis, & Edelstein, 1981). Cocaine acts as an anesthetic when applied to any body tissue, so that the effects of continuous administration of the hot searing vapor of free-basing are not felt by the user. This can result in permanent lung damage or at least impairment.

Other physical problems associated with cocaine use are as follows.

1. Runny nose, sniffling, and nosebleeds: Intranasal use of cocaine irritates the nasal lining, often resulting in a constantly runny nose, congestion (nasal vasodilation rebound after use), and sniffling. Over time, this can cause nosebleeds, sinus infections, and permanent damage to nasal tissue due to chronic nasal constriction.

2. Hoarseness, coughing, or respiratory infections: Smoking of free-base or crack can result in frequent clearing of the throat, a raspy voice, and chronic bronchitis or pulmonary infection.

3. "Bags" under the eyes and pale complexion: Heavy cocaine use leads to chronic lack of sleep and curtailment of outdoor activity; thus users become fatigued and out of shape and undergo a general decline in health, creating this appearance.

4. Weight loss: It is not uncommon for users to experience weight loss of 30 to 80 pounds as a result of the appetite-suppressant effects of cocaine. This is compounded by malnutrition.
5. Tremor, loss of coordination, and poor reflexes: Cocaine users experience a loss of fine motor control and general physical coordination due to overstimulation of the neuromuscular system (Kestenbaum, Resnick, Washton, & Lipton, 1978). They appear to be unsteady, shaky, and tense, and they often have accidents as a result of this impairment.
6. Dilated pupils: Recent use of cocaine causes a relaxation of the muscles controlling pupillary constriction. The user's pupils enlarge and do not respond to light with constriction.
7. Scratching and skin lesions: Chronic use of cocaine can cause a severe irritation and itching sensation of "bugs under the skin" known as parasitosis. Users will often scratch or pick at their skin, leaving red marks, lesions, raw spots, and even infected regions.

In addition to the physical and medical complications associated with cocaine use, psychological and behavioral changes can also occur.

1. Memory problems and forgetfulness: Chronic use of cocaine disrupts memory, concentration, and attention span. Users often lose items such as car keys and checkbooks and forget responsibilities and appointments; their ability to focus their attention and follow through on any activity is severely impaired.
2. Absenteeism and lateness: Since users often "binge" (use cocaine for as long as they can obtain it), they typically run late, miss appointments and deadlines, and shirk personal responsibilities. They become so preoccupied with the drug that they will not interrupt their use to show up for work or to meet commitments or any other responsibilities. Their excuses are often bizarre, unbelievable, and far-fetched.
3. Temper outbursts and irritability: Especially during later stages of cocaine use, particularly during withdrawal, users are extremely irritable, anxious, and short-tempered. Their preoccupation is with getting their next "hit," and anything or anybody in the way is an annoyance and is treated as such.
4. Sleepiness and fatigue: After an extended, sleepless "binge," users are "sprung" (strung out); that is, they are fatigued and will often fall asleep on the job or elsewhere.
5. Impulsive and "hyper" behavior: Using cocaine on the job creates some unpredictable results, such as bursts of extreme energy and

compulsive work characterized by high energy and high productivity. These periods are sporadic and often temporary, and work output is typically fragmented, incomplete, and of dubious quality.

6. Extreme mood swings: Often called "lability of mood," these swings from euphoria to despair are abrupt, rapid, and severe and can occur even during periods of no drug use (i.e., between binges). Mood swings can encompass minutes to hours or even days.

7. Loss of interest and engagement in outside activities: As cocaine takes over an individual's life other interests and priorities fall by the wayside, and activities that were once important, such as sports, exercise, cultural events, and family and social activities, are neglected because they interfere with cocaine use.

8. Social isolation: Cocaine users are only interested in being around other users, so that all contact is broken with nonusing friends.

Personality changes and interpersonal relationship changes are also often seen as a result of chronic cocaine use.

1. Rapid, choppy speech patterns: During conversation, cocaine users are nervous, fidgety, and constantly in motion. They are compulsive in speech patterns and difficult to interrupt.

2. Repeated or forgotten conversations: Because of memory dysfunction, users repeat the same conversation within a short time period. Conversely, ideas or projects discussed one day will be forgotten the next.

3. Rapid changes of topic and fragmented ideas: Under the effects of cocaine, it is frequently difficult to convey an idea to completion before moving on to the next. This results in the intoxicated user having problems in being understood and in accomplishing effective communication. He or she jumps from one topic to another with little continuity.

4. Paranoid ideas: During or after long bouts of cocaine use, paranoid ideation is frequent. This may involve the perception of criticism from co-workers, infidelity of a spouse, or the suspicion of being the object of a conspiracy. These ideas tend to come and go and usually do not involve true delusional systems, although this can occur with protracted use of the drug. If these delusional systems do occur, they are often exhibited in the context of a clear sensorium; that is, the person may be well oriented and coherent and have an intact mental status but rigidly adhere to a paranoid delusional system (Siegel, 1984a).

5. Family and financial problems: Cocaine users often mention that they are experiencing relationship problems at home or at work. Usually they say that the relationships are not important to them and that they would be better off if they could get away from the other person. At this stage, cocaine has become more important to them than parents, spouses, children, or friends. Often users will obsess about financial problems resulting from cocaine as well. Cocaine is an expensive habit, and regular use can wreak havoc with a user's financial status.

6. Depression: During periods when cocaine users are not using the drug, they do experience moderate to severe depression and will occasionally entertain suicidal thoughts. They often attribute these depressive feelings to unhappiness with their job, marriage, and life in general when the depressive symptoms are a direct result of cocaine withdrawal itself. The user's denial system, however, typically creates an attribution of these problems to external factors and not to drug use.

NEUROCHEMISTRY OF COCAINE ACTION

An appreciation of the basic neurochemical and neuropharmacological substrates involved in the action of cocaine in the brain can yield information concerning its euphoria-inducing properties and lay the groundwork for an understanding of why this substance has its addictive potential. Throughout most of its range of action, cocaine is a stimulant and shares properties of strong abuse liability with other drugs of abuse. What cocaine shares with opiates, barbiturates, benzodiazepines, and alcohol is a neurochemically based rewarding or reinforcing property. Cocaine interacts with the catecholaminergic system of the brain, a neurotransmitter system mediating multiple effects in the central nervous system. The adrenergic effects of cocaine (or effects on the adrenalin- and noradrenalin-mediating systems) were first reported in 1910 by Frohlich and Loewi (1966), who demonstrated enhanced sensitivity to adrenalin in tissue exposed to cocaine. It is now well established that cocaine blocks the reuptake of noradrenalin at adrenergic nerve endings in addition to facilitating noradrenalin release (Langer & Enero, 1974; Muscholl, 1961). This blockade of noradrenalin uptake by cocaine is competitive and does not appear to result from its anesthetic action. Furthermore, peripheral and central blockade of noradrenalin reuptake occurs at cocaine concentrations that are consistent with those found in human abuse of cocaine (Just, Grafenburg, & Thel, 1977).

Acute administration of cocaine causes an elevation in brain concentrations of noradrenalin within 10 minutes, which is followed by marked reductions to lower than normal levels within 20 minutes (Pradham, Roy, & Pradham, 1978). As mentioned earlier, certain physiological effects of cocaine intoxication appear to result from this sympathetic activation and can be explained by acutely potentiated central and peripheral noradrenergic transmission. These effects include tachycardia, hypertension, vasoconstriction, mydriasis (dilation of the pupils), and tremor. These same signs of autonomic activation can be produced by electrical stimulation of the locus coeruleus, which is the principal noradrenergic nucleus of the brain (Redmond, Huang, Snyder, & Maas, 1976). The dopaminergic system appears to mediate the euphoric response to cocaine; this system is therefore critical in the phenomena of cocaine self-administration and the development of addiction (Goeders & Smith, 1983). Cocaine appears to be a potent inhibitor of dopamine reuptake as well and facilitates the release of this neurotransmitter (Farnebo & Hambesger, 1971). This has the effect of acutely activating the dopaminergic system and mediating euphoria and the other positive, stimulatory effects of cocaine. However, repeated use of cocaine ultimately reduces dopamine concentrations in the brain (Taylor & Ho, 1977). When given acutely, cocaine elevates dopamine concentrations in the brain; the concentration drops to lower than normal levels several minutes later (Pradham et al., 1978).

It appears that, although acute administration of cocaine blocks dopamine reuptake and increases dopamine transmission and concentrations in the brain, a functional reduction in dopamine activity ultimately follows. Studies of dopaminergic receptors imply chronic reductions of available dopamine with compensatory supersensitivity (increased quantity) of postsynaptic receptors over time. Thus the predominant dopaminergic disruption appears to be compromised dopaminergic function. This hypothesis could explain why cocaine addicts repeatedly self-administer cocaine, often many times daily, as a way of transiently increasing synaptic dopamine. Postsynaptic dopaminergic deficiency is temporarily corrected by an acute use of cocaine. This effect is amplified by the supersensitivity of dopaminergic receptors. As cocaine's acute effects wear off, however, further depletion of dopamine may result with perpetuation of the cycle. The addict could experience this depletion of dopamine as a craving for cocaine, which explains the perceived need for a succession of dosages of cocaine throughout the day.

Cocaine-induced dopaminergic dysfunction may also be related to several other effects. The sexual excitement produced by cocaine, which is probably due to its dopaminergic effects in the limbic system (Gatz, 1966), reportedly includes spontaneous ejaculation without genital stimulation (Dimijian, 1974). Chronic cocaine use, however, can lead to impotence and frigidity (Siegel, 1982b). Acting through dopaminergic fiber tracts in the lateral hypothalamus, cocaine also appears to inhibit appetite (Groppetti & Diguilio, 1976). Finally, the psychomotor activation characteristically seen with cocaine intoxication is probably a dopaminergic effect.

Cocaine's involvement with a number of basic body systems underscores the profoundness with which cocaine affects brain functioning. Cocaine's interaction with the natural reward system, sexual activity functioning, and basic states such as hunger and thirst implies the drug's involvement with the portion of the central nervous system that governs drives and emotions. It is believed that the brain has specialized neural circuits that are activated by the various reinforcers capable of influencing behavior and also that the activation of these circuits is necessary for natural reinforcers to be effective (Wise, 1978; 1984). In other words, the brain has a built-in system to determine which activities and behaviors are intrinsically reinforcing, such as the acquisition of food and water, the completion of sexual drive activities, and the like. Just as it is reasonable to assume that opiate receptors did not evolve only to serve the need of modern humans for synthetic analgesics, so it is reasonable to assume that the neural substrates of drugs of abuse did not evolve to serve nonmedical pursuits of euphoria. Analgesics suppress pain by centrally activating endogenous pain control circuits (Mayer and Price, 1976); similarly, drugs of abuse could be expected to be reinforcing by centrally activating endogenous reward circuits.

It is from this perspective that students of drug abuse may begin to appreciate the interactions of these drugs with the basic reward circuits of the brain. Dopamine and noradrenalin, which mediate cocaine's effects, are the two basic transmitters involved in the reward sections of the brain. For instance, portions of the medial forebrain bundle, which is part of the midbrain structure, contain such reward circuits; these are activated by cocaine. In general, the circuits are designed to mediate external events in terms of their reinforcing properties. Thus peripheral input from situations such as orgasm and the satiety felt from a good meal or a long drink of water on a very hot day are all processed through these reward circuits. The brain is essentially programmed to experience these events as leading to reinforcement, thereby enhancing the probability that these events will occur in the future. Thus the brain is programmed to respond to basic survival mechanisms and activities that inherently enhance survival. Therefore, the problem with direct stimulation of these areas by cocaine is that the brain is essentially programmed to experience the administration of this drug as an event that enhances survivability, which of course is false programming. The brain responds as if the administration of this drug and the surrounding antecedent conditions are intimately involved in the basic drive mechanisms; a pattern of compulsive drug administration is thereby created in conjunction with the brain's programming that taking the drug is an event important for survival.

An appreciation of this intense neuropharmacological scheme can help explain the often bizarre and illogical behavior not only of animals given free access to cocaine but also of humans who self-administer cocaine. For instance, a recent study by Bozarth and Wise (1985) compared behaviors in self-administration of intravenous heroin and cocaine in the rat. The general findings of this study revealed that rats given continuous free access to intravenous heroin showed a stable drug self-administration pattern with a gradual increase in heroin intake over the first 2 weeks of testing. Those rats self-administering heroin maintained grooming behavior, pretest body weight, and a state of good general health. In contrast, rats self-administering cocaine tended to cease grooming behavior, to lose up to 47% of their pretest body weight, and to show a pronounced deterioration in general health. The mortality rate for 30 days of continuous testing was 36% for animals self-administering heroin and 90% for those self-administering cocaine. What this research suggests is: (1) The pattern of intake of cocaine by these rats did show periods of episodic or "bingelike" intake, that is, cycles of excessive cocaine self-administration alternating with brief periods of total abstinence, much as is seen in the human population. This administration pattern was different from that of heroin, which was stable and fairly consistent. (2) Basic survival behaviors, including eating, drinking, and so forth, were ignored by the rats self-administering cocaine to the extent that most, if not all, were severely compromised if not killed by this usage pattern.

In human behavior it is commonplace to observe individuals compulsively taking cocaine and apparently oblivious to the impact on finances, family, friends, work behavior, etc. In effect, the brain has been reprogrammed to view the administration of cocaine as something basic, something that is akin to a motivational state, although not innate, but "acquired," that carries all the strengths of the more built-in motivations such as hunger, thirst, and sexual reproduction.

THE DEVELOPMENT OF DEPENDENCE ON COCAINE: IMPLICATIONS OF LONG-TERM USE

Part of the body of misconceptions surrounding cocaine use in the early 1970s was that it was a safe recreational drug with minimal tolerance and minimal addictive properties. Experience has shown that this is not at all the case. As with most drugs of abuse, the development of tolerance is clear-cut and apparent (Fischman, 1984). Tolerance per se is defined as either the diminishing effects of a drug over time with a consistent dosage or the need for larger dosages of a drug to achieve the initial desired effect. Cocaine tolerance follows the first definition, as shown in a study of long-term use in a cohort of 99 users during a 10-year period (Siegel, 1984b). At the outset of this study, fully 100% of the participants indicated positive effects from acute use of cocaine related to euphoria, stimulation, and aphrodisiac effects. Five years into the study, this figure had dropped to only 32% of the cohort noting positive experiences from acute use and only 16% claiming elevated mood. During this same period, however, negative effects reported by users ranging from restlessness and irritation to increased fatigue and hyperexcitability were relatively constant at approximately 44%, although some indexes such as fatigue and irritability increased over the same period. This implies that the cocaine experience per se does not remain positive, as in the initial stages of use, despite what was assumed to be increased use; on the other hand, negative effects with continued use increase. This is somewhat in contrast to effects seen with other drugs such as alcohol or the opiates, in which positive experiences diminish but use remains steady. Nevertheless, use of these drugs tends also to forestall negative effects from withdrawal as long as use continues. The situation with cocaine is that, despite increased use in terms of frequency and amount, positive effects continue to diminish whereas negative effects tend to increase in intensity and amount over time (Post, 1975).

The progression of clinical symptomatology associated with cocaine use has been described by a number of investigators and clinicians in terms of the various stages of long-term effects over time. Siegel (1984b) describes a four-stage pattern with the following characteristics: Stage 1 is the positive, euphoric stage characterized by positive mood changes, vigilance, and pleasant stimulation. With chronic use a user progresses to stage 2, known as the dysphoric stage, in which the predominant mood changes are depression, fatigue, and decreased concentration. A further characteristic of stage 2 is the self-medication of these negative effects with more cocaine. This invokes the neurochemical model described earlier, whereby the dopaminergic system becomes dependent on the administration of cocaine to maintain normal mood and arousal levels. Stage 3 in this paradigm is termed the paranoid stage, which is characterized by heightened sensitivity to sounds, sights, and intrusive thoughts. This stage may be characterized by changes in the auditory threshold and peripheral vision, leading to hypervigilant behavior (constant scanning and scrutiny of the environment fed by actual changes in auditory perception and peripheral vision cues). Stage 4 is known as the psychotic stage, in which the previous cognitive and emotional changes have graduated to a schizophreniform psychosis characterized by delusions and hallucinations.

Siegel (1984a) refers to this process as the ''stoking of the fire in the brain'' (p. 335). That is, vague patterns and images, much like reflections in a window, are enhanced to a point where they take on a certain reality. Siegel distinguishes this particular state of awareness from the distorted perceptions and hallucinations resulting from LSD use. These hallucinatory and perceptional distortions are characterized by a sense of unreality and are dealt with as such. As mentioned before, the delusory and hallucinatory content consequent to chronic cocaine use provides no cues as to the unreality of the situation and the perceptions. These delusions can occur in an individual with an intact mental status and clear sensorium who is profoundly affected by the reality of a certain fixed delusional state. For instance, an abuser experiencing the sensations characterizing parasitosis may believe in the existence of bugs beneath his or her skin to the point of actually dissecting his own limbs to remove the offending creatures.

Richard Rawson (personal communication, 1984), with the Matrix Treatment Centers for Cocaine Dependency in Los Angeles, also describes a four-phase process characterizing the cognitive effects resulting from chronic cocaine use. Phase 1 in the cognitive process is termed the introductory phase. At this stage, cocaine use is seen as an intellectual and emotional choice made by a person for certain desired effects. As use progresses to phase 2, the maintenance phase, positive effects noted in phase 1 begin to diminish but the beginnings of denial and rationalization create a structure for this use whereby it still "makes sense" to the user. Continued use graduates the user to phase 3, known as disenchantment. In this phase, the positive aspects once characterizing initial use are all but missing, but a person continues to use in spite of this awareness. Users interviewed at this point often say that they are still using but that the benefits or effects that they derive from the drug do not compensate for the negative effects that are occurring. They still use, but they simply cannot provide a reason for it and, in fact, deem its use as negative. Phase 4 is known as the disaster phase. At this point the positive aspects are purely relief from a more negative and intense state of lack of cocaine. Negative aspects are increased during both use and nonuse periods. Users say that they do not like the effects, but at this point use is compulsive and continues. The user is locked into his or her use because triggers for use by now are generalized. That is, in the introductory phases triggers for use are typically situational, such as parties or social occasions where use is apparent. As the user progresses through the subsequent phases, situations and cues become much more pervasive. That is, in addition to environmental cues such as places and individuals, internal triggers grow in strength; for example, negative affective states, whether or not they are associated with cocaine deprivation, promote cravings. At this point a powerful physiological induction has been made, and the usage pattern is now overdetermined by both previous positive associations with cocaine effects and internal and external negative associations, which drive the user to more and more cocaine consumption.

This model for the development of dependency closely parallels the patterns of drug use delineated by the National Commission on Marijuana and Drug Abuse of 1973, which are as follows. The first phase is experimental use, characterized by short-term, nonpatterned trials of cocaine of varying intensity, with a maximum frequency of ten times or a total intake of less than 1 g. This usage pattern by definition is self-limiting. If use is not terminated voluntarily at this point, the pattern escalates to the next phase, known as social-recreational use. Social-recreational users engage in more regular use of cocaine than experimenters. This use generally occurs in social settings, among friends or acquaintances who wish to share an experience perceived by them as acceptable and pleasurable. These users are motivated by social factors, and their use is always voluntary; it does not tend to escalate to more individual-oriented patterns or uncontrollable use. If this usage pattern does escalate, however, users enter the circumstantial-situational stage, in which use of cocaine is task-specific and self-limited and does differ in frequency, intensity, or duration. This pattern is motivated by a perceived need or desire to achieve a known and anticipated drug effect deemed desirable to cope with a specific condition or situation. Motivations often cited by users, in order of decreasing frequency, are (1) to increase performance at work, (2) to enhance mood during periods of situational depression, and (3) to enhance performance at play (for example, sports, hiking, or sex). At this stage denial begins as a person rationalizes that drug use is necessary for tasks to be accomplished adequately and satisfactorily. This pattern may escalate to intensified drug use, which is characterized by a long-term patterned use at least once a day. This use is motivated chiefly by a perceived need to achieve relief from a persistent problem or a stressful situation or by a desire to maintain a certain self-prescribed level of performance. This is the usage pattern described previously in animal species given free access to cocaine. The final stage of drug dependence development is termed compulsive drug use, characterized by high-frequency, high-intensity levels of relatively long duration that produce some degree of both psychological and physical dependence. At this stage use patterns are locked in, and much of the user's daily life is spent either obtaining, using, or recovering from drug effects.

Two conclusions can be drawn from this review of escalating patterns of dependency on cocaine and the changing effects of cocaine as a function of long-term use. First, the use of cocaine is no longer seen as a moderate, social-recreational, controlled usage format with little liability for escalating usage patterns or the development of physical or psychological dependence. Clearly, as many as 50% of individuals show escalating patterns with increasing problematic usage resulting from this. Nevertheless, the hypothesis that long-term use of cocaine is inevitably associated with an escalating dependency marked by more frequent patterns of use is also unsupported. Many social users are capable of controlling use with no escalation to more individual-oriented patterns. Others, by escalating patterns of use, do increase the risk of dependency and toxicity. At this point in time it is impossible to tell which users will experience this phenomenon and which will minimize their use. As stated previously, as many as 50% of users may show this escalatory pattern. Further research will have to focus on the conditions, situations, or personality or genetic variables that determine into which category recreational users will ultimately fall.

WITHDRAWAL AND ABSTINENCE SYMPTOMATOLOGY

The *Diagnostic and Statistical Manual of Mental Disorders* (Third Edition) (DSM-III; American Psychiatric Association, 1980) defines withdrawal as the development of a substance-specific syndrome that follows the cessation or reduction in intake of a substance that was previously used regularly by an individual to induce the state of intoxication. Until recently, cocaine was regarded as a drug that produced only psychological and not physical dependence, with little or no discernable withdrawal reactions. The DSM-III does not contain the diagnosis of cocaine dependency because of the presupposition that tolerance and withdrawal did not occur in cocaine abuse. This reflects to a large degree that when DSM-III was field tested cocaine abuse was uncommon, and no systematically obtained data were available to refute this conclusion (Siegel, 1982a). This further promoted the misconception that cocaine was a "safe" recreational drug, free from the dramatic withdrawal syndromes seen with alcohol or the opiates. Nevertheless, even with smaller dosages and less intense routes of administration, such as orally or intranasally, a transient withdrawal syndrome of approximately 24 hours' duration is noted (Resnick & Resnick, 1984). This is similar to amphetamine withdrawal in the characteristic depressed mood, fatigue, and disturbed sleep. As use patterns have escalated and diverse routes of administration have allowed higher dosing over longer periods of time, however, a clearer picture of post-use symptomatology has emerged. These symptoms persist in some users after cessation of use and follow a regular sequence in both the immediate and prolonged periods after cessation. Gawin and Kleber (1986) divide abstinence symptomatology into three phases, which are outlined as follows.

Phase 1: The "Crash" (9 hours to 4 days post-use). Within 15 to 30 minutes of cessation of use (typically when supplies are exhausted), users report a mounting depression and intense craving for more cocaine that often leads to seeking more drug despite previous plans to limit use. Importantly, this craving dissipates if more cocaine is not obtained. The "crash" that follows is marked by extreme dysphoria consisting initially of depression, full anhedonia, insomnia, irritability, anxiety, a subjective sense of confusion, and gradually diminishing cocaine craving. Suicidal ideation and paranoid thinking also characterize this phase in a significant number of individuals. Dysphoric agitation becomes dysphoric lethargy and anergia. These symptoms persist for up to 40 hours, graduating into hypersomnolence with intermittent awakenings and hyperphagia lasting 8 to 50 hours. Interestingly, as time accumulates during the "crash" phase, craving for cocaine decreases while craving for sleep increases. Users often report ordering more cocaine during the early part of the "crash" when cravings are intense but then they do not use it, if delivered, during the latter part, when a strong abhorrence of cocaine emerges.

Phase 2: Withdrawal (1 to 10 weeks). Phase 2 begins with 1 to 5 days of nearly normal affective functioning and a normal sleep-waking cycle with minimal cocaine craving. This quiescence, however, progresses to a sporadic clinical syndrome involving substantial anhedonia, mild dysphoria, anergia, anxiety, and irritability. The intensity of these symptoms parallels cocaine craving, and users report "intense boredom" during this part of phase 2. Users feel that only more cocaine can rescue them from this combination of boredom and anhedonia, a process that continues for 1 to 10 more weeks before craving decreases.

During the first several hours to days after the initial "crash," abusers report a normal mood and ability to function. Often there is a keen awareness of the negative consequences of cocaine and a feeling of renewed control over cravings. As time progresses, however, memory of cocaine's dysphoric properties wanes and is replaced by stronger memories of the euphoric properties of the drug. This is coupled with increasingly strong cravings and anxiety, often accompanying a preoccupation to obtain more cocaine. If cocaine is used a "binge" typically results, and abusers return to phase 1. It is this return of cravings after a period of feeling normal that sabotages the user's motivation not to resume cocaine use. The methodical pattern of "binging," "crashing," normalization, resisting, and return to use can recur unchecked for many months.

Phase 3: Extinction (indefinite). If abstinence is maintained, there is a gradual return to a euthymic state. This phase is nevertheless still punctuated by an episodic return of cravings of diminished severity. This return waxes and wanes in intensity and is usually brought on by either internal or external environmental cues. Very often, being in situations or around people once associated with cocaine can evoke cravings, as can experiencing negative affective states such as depression and anxiety. Positive emotional states such as excitement or drug-induced euphorias from alcohol or marijuana can also trigger cravings. This pattern apparently represents a conditioned withdrawal phenomenon, as is seen with other addictive drugs when cravings are determined by both positive and negative events (Wikler, 1973). These conditioning factors are also an integral part of the high risk of relapse among cocaine abusers, as abstainers are often demoralized by the continued appearance of significant cravings months after cessation of use and periods of apparent control (Wikler, 1986). With continued exposure to these cues without the pairing of cocaine use, however, these cravings eventually subside as the conditioning is gradually extinguished.

Thus a withdrawal state, which is much more complicated and multiphasic than is typical with other drugs of abuse, characterizes the cessation of cocaine use. Although more pronounced with intense administration routes such as free-basing or intravenous use, this pattern can be characteristic of intranasal use as well, depending on the frequency, intensity, and duration of the habit. Craving is highest at the end of a "binge" and the beginning of the "crash." Craving diminishes afterward, only to return late in phase 2 and idiosyncratically during phase 3. Therefore, unlike general depressant or opiate withdrawal, the fully developed "crash" is usually not treated with self-administration of cocaine. This accounts for the cyclic, "binge-like" usage pattern seen with both animals and humans. That is, a return of cravings after a period of seeming quiescence and control often leads to a resumption of cocaine use, thereby delaying relapses.

Elucidation of these factors identifies phase 2 of withdrawal as crucial in the treatment of abuse and prevention of relapse. Most inpatient programs are of insufficient length or do not emphasize the development of coping skills, so that the cocaine user is not aided effectively during phase 3; this may account for the observation of better outcomes for outpatient compared to inpatient programs (Wesson & Smith, 1985; Kleber & Gawin, 1984a).

PSYCHIATRIC DIAGNOSES AND COCAINE ABUSE

It is well known that a certain population of substance abusers uses drugs in an attempt to medicate the pain and symptomatology of various psychiatric disorders. Investigators disagree as to the prevalence of this process with the cocaine-abusing population. Smith (1984) views cocaine addiction as the primary diagnostic condition in 90% of his subjects, with any specific psychiatric symptomatology disappearing after continued abstinence maintenance. Nevertheless, investigators such as Gawin and Kleber (1986), Weiss, Mirin, and Michael (1983), and Siegel (1984a) find significant psychopathology and DSM-III diagnoses in a large percentage (up to 50%) of their subjects.

Chronic symptomatology spans the gamut from dysthymic disorder and major depression to bipolar affective disorder, cyclothymia, and attention deficit disorder. In these cases, cocaine theoretically (1) reverses the dysphoria or augments the hypomanic phases of cyclothymic or bipolar disorder, (2) eases the anhedonia and dysphoria of the depressive disorder, or (3) alleviates the symptoms of attention deficit disorder, residual type. Such diagnostic issues have importance, especially if cocaine is used in a self-medicating fashion. The symptoms are more effectively treated economically and legally by conventional pharmacotherapeutic agents. Moreover, a larger problem of cocaine dependency superimposed on a pre-existing symptom disorder is eliminated. If the symptoms that sustain cocaine use can be reduced by appropriate treatment, this treatment would also facilitate abstinence in such abusing populations.

Given that the above assumptions are true, the substantiation of an Axis I diagnosis is important with regard to pharmacological treatments. The protracted withdrawal and recovery process from chronic cocaine use may lead to the erroneous assessment of major depression or bipolar disorder. This, in addition to small sample sizes, may account for the diagnostic discrepancies noted by the aforementioned investigators. Thus such diagnoses need to be deferred unless clear corroborating histories or longitudinal assessments during drug-free periods are available.

Because of the similarity of cocaine abstinence symptomatology and certain Axis I disorders, investigators have attempted to treat this phenomenon with pharmacological agents directed toward these symptoms. Data from Gawin and

Kleber (1984b) indicate that desipramine facilitates abstinence not only in depressed patients but also in patients without any Axis I diagnosis. Other investigators have suggested the value of using such tricyclic antidepressants in treating the severe depression associated with the discontinuation of chronic use (Rosecan, 1983; Tennant & Rawson, 1983). These studies suggest that tricyclics such as desipramine also decrease cocaine cravings after 2 to 3 weeks of treatment, regardless of the diagnostic status of the subject. Some subjects reported a decrease in cocaine-induced euphoria while taking tricyclics, but a complete block of euphoria was not reported. This tended to aid in attainment of abstinence, and in another study by Gawin and Kleber (1984b) five of six patients not in the sample who were taking desipramine also reported stopping cocaine use and maintaining abstinence during the course of the study. Tennant and Rawson (1983) also found a positive effect of desipramine on reduction of cravings and maintenance of abstinence.

Patients with symptoms suggesting cyclothymic disorder who were treated with lithium carbonate also became abstinent and demonstrated decreased cravings for cocaine. In contrast to the desipramine-treated subjects, however, those treated with lithium carbonate who were not so diagnosed did not appear to benefit. The same was true of patients diagnosed with attention deficit disorder, because patients not so diagnosed did not show any improvement with methylphenidate. Reports do exist, however, that substantiate improvement in cocaine users diagnosed with attention deficit disorder, residual type (Khantzian, 1983).

Nonspecific pharmacological factors also merit attention in these cases, because patients presenting with cocaine dependency are often discouraged by the lack of specific interventions other than "talking." Subjects may simply tolerate the psychotherapeutic processes in order to "get meds" that change the way they feel. This tends to contribute to the abuser's mindset, which is accustomed to the resolution of problems through pharmacological means. Despite the congruity of the known pharmacological changes induced by cocaine and agents such as the tricyclics and the seductiveness of the hypotheses that predict efficacy of treatment as a result, continued investigation with double-blind, placebo-controlled investigations is continuingly important.

TREATMENT OF COCAINE ABUSE AND DEPENDENCY

The compulsive behaviors and the intensity of the addiction process clearly evoke some pessimism regarding the ultimate rehabilitation and continued abstinence of the cocaine-dependent patient. Treatment is further hindered by the difficulty of convincing the user to seek help, the difficulty of maintaining therapeutic progress while the patient is still using, "crashing," or suffering the psychiatric sequelae of abuse, and the difficulty in establishing long-term isolation from an environment that supports and glorifies cocaine use.

The problem of cocaine dependence often exceeds the use of the drug itself because drug behaviors often constitute a way of life, with the user totally preoccupied with drug-seeking and drug-taking. Users become unaccustomed to a drug-free existence and suffer from the characteristics of an addictive disease "process." That is, the user finds it difficult to attribute his or her problems directly to cocaine use. This is denial. Thus, they are likely not to ask for help, or if they do it is for information about cocaine and its effects and how to minimize the negative aspects rather than asking for help with their drug addiction. The process of selective retention results in the user remembering and anticipating only the euphoria from cocaine. In addition, recovery from the physical and psychological effects is often so rapid that premature termination of treatment is commonplace. The greatest single reason for relapse is probably the belief that the abuser can return to controlled use of cocaine. As in any addictive disorder, once the line has been crossed into compulsive use (and in cocaine use, bingeing patterns), the individual loses the ability to return to any less abusive use pattern (Siegel, 1985b; Smith, 1984).

GOALS OF TREATMENT

As in other addictive processes, it is important to select treatment strategies that meet the unique needs of each patient, always keeping in mind that these strategies may change during the course of therapy. Initial efforts have to be focused on helping the patient end all cocaine use. It must be stressed that any other aspect of therapy will be ineffective or compromised so long as the patient continues to use the drug. After this, a support system of external controls must be set up to help the person struggling with abstinence. Finally, resolution of the issues that underlie cocaine abuse may require longer-term follow up. It is also important to establish diagnostically any underlying major psychopathology in need of treatment. Such a total recovery process requires a combination of individual and group work, education about cocaine and addictive disorders in general, and long-term follow up and relapse-prevention training. Also, enlisting the help of the family as allies through family therapy greatly enhances success. Often, lifestyle changes touching on nutrition and diet, exercise, and stress management round out the successful recovery. Recovery therefore is defined as a comfortable and responsible life without the use of psychoactive drugs. A return to "controlled use" cannot be a treatment goal.

CESSATION OF USE

The first goal of giving up cocaine is in itself difficult to accomplish. The therapist should be prepared for resistance, ambivalence, and "slips." These inconsistencies should be met with a nonjudgmental and nonpunitive attitude. Each instance should be viewed as an opportunity to identify the "triggers" that produced the "slip"—either internal negative emotional states or external environmental cues.

As noted previously, intense dysphoria and depression characterizing withdrawal are often seen by the user as intolerable and treatable only with cocaine. In this instance, a period of hospitalization may be beneficial. Some treatment specialists have utilized to good advantage clinical dosages of antidepressant medications to combat the depression associated with withdrawal. In addition, there are reports that these pharmacological adjuncts to treatment ease the craving and aid in abstinence maintenance. Other investigators, however, stress that this approach should only be used with individuals diagnosed as endogenously depressed during recovery (Smith, 1984). Clearly, such a diversity of findings illustrates the need and potential for more refined, systematic studies in the area of pharmacological treatments in cocaine dependency. At present, whether or not to use pharmacological interventions should remain a clinical decision based on the individual's particular case. In general, hospitalization or medication approaches may be used when other outpatient options have been unsuccessful or if there is evidence of (1) severe impairment of psychosocial functioning, (2) medical or psychiatric complications, or (3) concurrent dependence on other addictive drugs.

The patient experiencing difficulty with abstinence may be aided by strategies that make use of external controls, such as urinalysis, contingency contracting, or assignment of financial control to another person.

Urinalysis

Regular and random urinalysis for cocaine and cocaine metabolites as part of the treatment contract can be an effective and welcome part of therapy, especially if it is introduced early in the course of treatment. It should be explained to the patient that urinalysis is a tool to aid in maintaining abstinence and that "slips" will not be dealt with in a punitive fashion. Rather, the patient should be encouraged to explain the dynamics around the slips and to use them to aid in future abstinence attempts. Without this "insurance," it may be assumed that the patient will continue using cocaine during therapy and deny it or refuse to discuss it with the therapist. This results in the patient's losing the chance to learn coping skills and undermines the therapeutic alliance, because the patient feels that he or she has "gotten away" with something that the therapist was "not smart enough to figure out." A general drug screen may also reveal other psychoactive drug use that may be problematic or may constitute "gateways" to an impending relapse. Thus the "slips" that are revealed become opportunities to explore inner and outer antecedents to cocaine use, and they allow the therapist to model problem-solving and coping strategies that help replace a sense of failure and guilt in the client with insight and the possibility of positive change. In general, urine screening for cocaine should be sensitive, usually employing a radioimmunoassay technique. By this method, cocaine metabolites are detectable for 24 to 36 hours (Barnett, Hawks, & Resnick, 1981), therefore requiring at least two to three tests per week to cover all abuse possibilities.

Contingency Contracting

Contingency contracting provides a further source of external motivation to aid the patient in maintaining abstinence despite his or her ambivalence. A contract, drawn up between the therapist and patient, outlines the consequences or punishment that will follow any violation of abstinence or other evidence of continued use (usually revealed by urinalysis or the patient's missing a scheduled urine test).

Such controls typically involve writing a letter outlining the extent of the patient's drug abuse and the severe impact it has on the patient's ability to function, either professionally or personally. This letter is intended for the patient's employer, professional licensing agency, or other such party and can be sent by the therapist on the basis of a prearranged agreement. Contingencies may also include forfeiture of privileges or financial support, payment of fines, public disclosure, or contributions to aversive organizations (such as the Ku Klux Klan, the American Nazi Party, and the like).

Follow-up reports from one facility show that contingency contracting was a useful tool that facilitated patient compliance with treatment regimes for 66 of 70 patients who signed such contracts and adhered to them for at least 3 months (Anker & Crowley, 1982). In contrast, much greater rates of failure occurred in patients who were treated at the same time at the same clinic but did not sign contracts; all 76 of these individuals resumed use of cocaine during the first month of treatment. Although the patient's self-selection of treatment biased these results, considerable clinical evidence supports the value of this method in dealing with the extremely ambivalent attitude patients have toward giving up cocaine.

In addition to problems of long-term efficacy and possible inapplicability to more severe cocaine abuse, apparent ethical problems do exist in those cases where the procedure could have been based on positive reinforcement for abstinence maintenance or at least on less aversive techniques. That is, when negative rather than positive reinforcement procedures are applied, an obligation to use the least deleterious technique exists. Variations in contract design, such as applied contingencies graded in severity, a top contingency level with less drastic consequences, or applying positive consequences for abstinence (for example, obtaining a sum of money from the patient at the outset and returning part each week for "clean" urine) could also circumvent the problems noted. Other cases might ideally need a combination of both positive and negative reinforcement. Such variations have not yet been examined in cocaine abuse treatment. Optimal ways of applying the promising approach of contingency contracting will become clear only after further investigation (Kleber & Gawin, 1984b).

FAMILY TREATMENT

Cocaine use rarely occurs in a vacuum; an individual's abuse pattern reciprocally affects his or her family members, necessitating the inclusion of the patient's family in the treatment process. Use of the family in the initial stages of intervening in the above cycle can be the key to mobilizing some individuals toward treatment. This process, known as "intervention," capitalizes on the motivation of significant others to help the potential patient. Commonly, family members contact the treatment professional for information about how to help the abuser who at the time is unwilling or unable to seek treatment himself or herself. Intervention generally involves working with the concerned family members or other closely involved individuals to make a careful list of the abuser's problem behaviors and to educate them about the addictive disease process. This is initially done without including the person identified as the abuser. Later, the patient is invited to a therapist-led family confrontation, where each member reads from a list of his or her observations and feelings about the abuser and his or her behavior. This is accomplished in a carefully controlled fashion to minimize accusations, judgments, and extreme emotionality. The goal of this process is to make abusers aware of the effect that their problem has on themselves and their families and to elicit an agreement to seek help. This process can be effective in "generating" the crisis that typically precedes seeking therapy, without the abuser having to "hit bottom" and feeling totally helpless and hopeless.

On the other hand, it is also common for family members to deny the abuser's self-destructive addictive behaviors and to try to minimize the problem. They will accept rationalizations for drug-related behaviors and continually "rescue" the patient and prevent him or her from suffering the negative consequences of drug use. This is a process known as "enabling," whereby the family actually colludes in the patient's continued use of drugs, thereby removing an important source of external motivation for seeking treatment. Part of the educational process of intervention is to break through this denial pattern and to help the family allow the patient to experience the suffering necessary for him or her to request professional help. By participating in treatment, family members can learn to identify and change their own destructive and counterproductive behaviors and to recognize the signs of cocaine use or an impending relapse in their significant other (Resnick & Resnick, 1984).

Family therapy is important not only in the initial stages of intervention and abstinence maintenance but in the later stages of recovery as well. The protracted process of helping the abuser establishes family members as caregivers. In essence, family members are rewarded for enabling behaviors because they feel that they are actually helping the person to survive. Their self-esteem comes to depend on their status as caregivers and is then consequently threatened when the abuser is not maintaining abstinence. Nevertheless, family members often feel increasingly unneeded or useless as the user maintains recovery and may try, unconsciously, to sabotage the entire process. They may feel that the person is still using or dealing drugs and may assign treatment failure cues to minor events. On the basis of all the past failures and past feelings, they often develop an inability to see success in the person or refuse to acknowledge recovery. Often, they may want to revenge themselves on the person and will become hostile. It is important, therefore, to identify these dynamics to families in treatment and to help them balance their roles.

INDIVIDUAL TREATMENT

Individual therapy approaches form an integral part of the mixture of treatment components necessary in the recovery process. Such approaches make up the basis for newer treatment programs such as New Horizons and Matrix Treatment Associates. The efficacy of these programs has yet to be scientifically established, but reports from these groups are encouraging. As mentioned previously, attempts at psychodynamic therapy are probably not fruitful early in the recovery process because a person's cognitive functioning is still impaired. Later in treatment, however, it is important to bring the abuser to an understanding of the function that cocaine has played in his or her life and to help him or her serve this function without drugs. For example, cocaine can serve narcissistic needs through the glamour associated with its use (or by direct pharmacological effects) or through the social networks and drug-using subculture associated with it. Also, dependency needs can be met through potential facilitation of interpersonal interactions, with the drug as a catalyst. Sexual functioning and interpersonal interactions are greatly affected by cocaine abuse, and the restoration of these functions without cocaine should also gain focus in recovery.

In terms of the various therapeutic orientations characterizing cocaine treatment, the above constitutes the psychodynamic orientation. Individual treatment early in the recovery process is aligned with cognitive-behavioral and supportive orientations. Thus one-to-one therapy in the initial stages of recovery is more educative and didactic, during which the abuser is made aware of the aspects of his or her addiction and the process of recovery as it relates specifically to cocaine effects. This facet is particularly important, since the abuser seeking treatment needs to know that the therapist has an understanding of the problem, a knowledge of cocaine and its effects, and an appreciation of what the abuser is experiencing. The process of educating the abuser about what cocaine does, why he or she is out of control, and what to expect during recovery is known as "forecasting" (Richard Rawson, personal communication, 1984). When done effectively, this enhances transference and aids in the patient's compliance with and continuity in treatment. Thus it behooves the therapist to gain as much knowledge as possible about this addiction and to learn to communicate effectively when working with this population.

Conditioning factors play a powerful role in producing cravings for drugs and in compulsive or impulsive use (Wikler, 1973). The patient needs to gain an understanding of what happens when he or she is confronted with cues from the environment that have been repeatedly paired with the effects of cocaine in the past. For instance, the dysphoric symptoms that occur during "crashing" can be linked to both external and internal environmental events (including situation, person or place, intense emotional arousal, and depression) and create an intense craving. It is important to include opportunities for the patient to extinguish the conditioned aspects of cocaine use. The patient can be taught to identify individual cues that trigger each episode of craving and to develop competing thoughts and behaviors, thereby obtaining more awareness of his or her choices and how to make more adaptive ones. A therapist can induce such a dysphoric state in the office to teach the person behavioral techniques that promote deep relaxation, thereby extinguishing the craving response. For example, tetracaine powder simulating cocaine can be placed in front of the patient to elicit craving responses, which can then be eliminated by breathing exercises and relaxation training (Resnick & Resnick, 1984). These practice sessions help extinguish the conditioned responses and allow the abuser to develop a sense of control over these urges.

Even though most abusers eventually experience only a minimal "high" from cocaine, they persist in using the drug to try to reproduce the euphoria that they initially experienced. The reason is that they do not anticipate feeling bad. When imagining using cocaine, most patients report a sense of euphoria and repress their awareness of the subsequent stronger and more protracted dysphoria. By consciously including dysphoria as part of their anticipatory feelings about cocaine, patients learn cognitively to relabel their use as a negative experience. This cognitive-behavioral approach is combined with other behavioral techniques involving situational, environmental, and person-specific changes to give the client a set of relapse-prevention skills to aid in recovery maintenance. This process must be repeated on several different occasions for it to be effective. This positive approach to recovery incorporates ways of dealing with cravings by skills building and is a preferable alternative to "white-knuckle sobriety," but nonetheless it requires a long-term educational and re-educational process.

All these orientations are necessary in the treatment of cocaine abusers, and their mixture should be determined by taking into account the individual needs of the cocaine abuser at the outset of treatment. Choice of primary therapeutic orientation will obviously shift from cognitive-behavioral to psychodynamic to supportive as severity of abuse increases. Also, as therapy progresses different orientations are adopted (or overlapped) as appropriate. This is the art of therapeutic intervention with cocaine abusers and requires therapists who are facile in their ability to switch orientations when necessary.

GROUP TREATMENT

The efficacy of self-help groups, such as Alcoholics Anonymous and Narcotics Anonymous for those individuals participating in them, points to the importance of such an approach in long-term maintenance of sobriety from chemical dependency. Cocaine Anonymous, an offspring of these more generic addictive disease groups, provides such a process for cocaine abusers. In these groups, which use the disease model of addictive disorders, recovering cocaine abusers discover how others resist hunger and maintain their recovery. Whether or not such support groups are linked to the 12-step program of Alcoholics Anonymous, they do form an important part of recovery. The Cocaine Recovery Support Group in San Francisco has increased the number of individuals entering into recovery after drug crisis and detoxification (Smith, 1984). Great emphasis is placed on discussing the emotions and thoughts that precede a cocaine relapse. In such a group, silence is viewed as the "enemy of recovery," and recovering cocaine abusers discuss cocaine dreams, drug hunger, addictive thinking, and high-risk situations that precipitate relapse. Discussion of positive experiences with drugs is discouraged. Some groups are led by professional group facilitators who discuss alternatives to specific situations, thoughts, and feelings to prevent relapse. Others have no "leader" and are composed of recovering cocaine abusers who share their stories and ideas about success and failure. Clearly, the advantage gained from identification with other abusers and the support network that the group process offers are integral factors in making this an important adjunct to treatment modality.

ADJUNCTIVE THERAPIES

Exercise

Another important aspect of therapy may involve an exercise program, in which a recovering abuser uses exercise to improve overall health and physical condition to replace drug use and to make a direct attempt to deal with cocaine cravings. Exercise that produces sufficient cardiopulmonary stimulation for longer than 20 minutes can increase the release of endogenous endorphins with a subsequent reduction in craving, anxiety, and depression. This process also emphasizes that the recovery program is a positive health- and image-enhancing process that is part of a general life-style change that promotes good health and increases wellness (Siegel, 1982a; 1984a).

Nutrition

Cocaine abusers have notoriously poor nutritional and dietary habits that are based to a large extent on the anorectic properties of cocaine. Abusers go for extended periods without food during "binges," often using alcohol as their only source of caloric input. This is often followed during the "crash" by rebound hunger, where the abuser is hyperphagic and consumes considerable amounts of food, usually junk foods with poor nutritional content. Severe weight loss and malnutrition can result, which potentially compromise any therapeutic efforts and produce symptoms and conditions that further complicate treatment. If a patient is hospitalized, a dietary consultation should be requested to ensure that the patient receives adequate and appropriate nutrition. Outpatients should have some basic dietary and nutritional information; inquiry into their eating habits and weight status periodically is also important. Vitamin and mineral supplements can be considered in cases of severe nutritional deficit. Daily logs of nutritional intake for various periods of time (perhaps 3 or 4 days during recovery) can be enlightening to the recovering abuser and the therapist alike.

Implications of the neuropharmacology of cocaine point to the existence of depleted catecholamines (noradrenalin and dopamine) and serotonin after long periods of cocaine abuse. This exhausted supply of necessary neurotransmitters and the subsequent altering of receptor populations is theoretically linked to the symptoms of depression, fatigue, and anhedonia that characterize this phase. Oral administration of precursors to these neurotransmitters, notably tyrosine (for dopamine and noradrenalin) and tryptophan (for serotonin) have been shown to elevate brain concentrations of these transmitters (Gold, Pottash, & Annitto, 1983; Mandell & Knapp, 1977). Clinical investigators have augmented diets with dosages of these precursors and have found encouraging results with respect to changes in mood, affect, and sedation (Gold et al., 1983; Rosecan, 1983). As tyrosine and tryptophan compete for uptake, recommendations are for alternate-day dosing with tyrosine (0.1 g/kg) and tryptophan (2000 mg four times a day and 4000 mg at bedtime).

REFERENCES

Abelson, H.I., & Miller, J.D. (1985). A decade of trends in cocaine use in the household population. In N.T. Kozel and E.H. Adams (Eds.), *Cocaine use in America: Epidemiologic and criminal perspectives* (NIDA Research Monograph No. 61). Washington, DC: U.S. Government Printing Office.

Adams, E.H., & Durell, T. (1984) Cocaine: A growing public health problem. In J. Grabowski (Ed.), *Cocaine: Pharmacology, effects and treatment of abuse* (NIDA Research Monograph No. 50, pp. 9–15). Washington, DC: U.S. Government Printing Office.

American Psychiatric Association. *Diagnostic and statistical manual of mental disorders* (3rd ed.). (1980). Washington, DC: Author.

"America's Crusade." (15 September 1986). *Time*, pp. 60–68.

Anker, A.L., & Crowley, T.J. (1982). Use of contingency contracts in specialty clinics for cocaine abuse. In L.S. Harris (Ed.), *Problems of drug dependence, 1981* (NIDA Monograph Series No. 41, pp. 452–459). Washington, DC: U.S. Government Printing Office.

Barnett, G., Hawks, R., & Resnick, R. (1981). Cocaine pharmacokinetics in humans. *Journal of Ethnopharmacology, 3*(2), 353–366.

Benchimol, A., Bartall, H., & Dresser, K.B. (1978). Accelerated ventricular rhythm and cocaine abuse. *Annals of Internal Medicine, 88*, 519–520.

Bozarth, M.A., & Wise, R.A. (1985). Toxicity associated with long-term intravenous heroin and cocaine self-administration in the rat. *Journal of the American Medical Association, 254*, 81–83.

Carroll, E. (1977). Coca: The plant and its use. In R.C. Petersen & R.C. Stillman (Eds.), *Cocaine: 1977* (NIDA Research Monograph No. 13, pp. 35–47). Washington, DC: U.S. Government Printing Office.

Dimijian, G.G. (1974). Contemporary drug abuse. In A. Goth (Ed.), *Medical pharmacology: Principles and concepts* (p. 313). St. Louis: C.V. Mosby.

Farnebo, L.O., & Hambesger, B. (1971). Drug-induced changes in the release of ^{3}H-monoamines from field-stimulated rat brain slices. *Acta Physiologica Scandinavia, 371*(Suppl.), 35–44.

Fischman, M.W. (1984). The behavioral pharmacology of cocaine. In J. Grabowski (Ed.), *Cocaine: Pharmacology, effects, and treatment of abuse* (NIDA Research Monograph No. 50, pp. 72–91). Washington, DC: U.S. Government Printing Office.

Frohlich, A., & Loewi, O. (1910). Uber eine Steigerung der Adrenalinemp-findlichkeitdurch Cocain. *Archives of Experimental and Pathological Pharmacology 62*, 159–169.

Gatz, A.T. (1966). *Menter's essentials of clinical neuroanatomy and neurophysiology*. Philadelphia: Davis.

Gawin, F.H., & Kleber, H.D. (1984). Cocaine abuse treatment: Open pilot trial with desipramine and lithium carbonate. *Archives of General Psychiatry, 41*, 903–909.

Gawin, F.H., & Kleber, H.D. (1986). Abstinence symptomatology and psychiatric diagnosis in cocaine abusers. *Archives of General Psychiatry, 43*, 107–113.

Gay, G.R. (1982). Clinical management of acute and toxic cocaine poisoning. *Annals of Emergency Medicine, 11*(10), 562–572.

Goeders, N.E., & Smith, J.E. (1983). Critical dopaminergic involvement in cocaine reinforcement. *Science, 221*, 773–775.

Gold, M. (1984). *1-800–COCAINE*. New York: Bantam.

Gold, M.S., Pottash, A.L.C., & Annitto, W.J. (1983). Cocaine withdrawal: Efficacy of tyrosine. *Journal of the Society of Neuroscience, 157*.

Cocaine 233

Groppetti, A., & Diguilio, A.M. (1976). Cocaine and its effects on biogenic amines. In S.T. Mile (Ed.), *Cocaine: Chemical, biological, clinical, social, and treatment aspects* (p. 97). Ohio: CRC Press.

Inaba, T., Stewart, D.T., & Kalow, W. (1978). Metabolism of cocaine in man. *Clinical Pharmacology and Therapeutics, 23*, 547–552.

Jatlow, P., Barash, P.G., Van Dyke, C., Raddiny, J., & Byck, R. (1979). Cocaine and succinylcholine sensitivity: A new caution. *Anesthesia and Analgesia, 58*, 235–238.

Jones, R.T. (1984). The pharmacology of cocaine. In J. Grabowski (Ed.), *Cocaine: Pharmacology, effects and treatment of abuse* (NIDA Research Monograph No. 50, pp. 34–54). Washington, DC: U.S. Government Printing Office.

Just, W.W., Grafenburg, L., & Thel, S. (1977). Comparative metabolic autoradiographic and pharmacologic studies of cocaine and its metabolite norcocaine. *Naunyn-Schmiedeberg's Archives of Pharmacology, 293*(Suppl.), 56.

Kandel, D.B., Murphy, D., & Karus, D. (1985). Cocaine use in young adulthood: Patterns of use and psychosocial correlates. In N.J. Kozel & E.H. Adams (Eds.), *Cocaine use in America: Epidemiologic and clinical perspectives* (NIDA Research Monograph No. 61). Washington, DC: U.S. Government Printing Office.

Kestenbaum, R.S., Resnick, R., Washton, A., & Lipton, J. (1978, June). *Cocaine effects on psychomotor performance*. Paper presented at the Annual Meeting of the Committee on Problems of Drug Dependence, Baltimore, MD.

Khantzian, E.T. (1983). An extreme case of cocaine dependence and marked improvement with methylphenidate treatment. *American Journal of Psychiatry, 140*, 784–785.

Kleber, H.D., & Gawin, F.H. (1984a). The spectrum of cocaine abuse and its treatment. *Journal of Clinical Psychiatry, 45*(12), 18–23.

Kleber, H.D., & Gawin, F.H. (1984b). Cocaine abuse: A review of current and experimental treatments. In J. Grabowski (Ed.), *Cocaine: Pharmacology, effects, and treatment of abuse* (NIDA Research Monograph No. 50). Washington, DC: U.S. Government Printing Office.

Langer, S.Z., & Enero, M.A. (1974). Cocaine: Effect of *in vivo* administration of synaptosomal uptake of norepinephrine. *Journal of Pharmacological and Experimental Therapy 191*, 431.

Mandell, A.J., & Knapp, S. (1977). Regulation of serotonin biosynthesis in brain: Role of the high-affinity uptake of tryptophan into serotonergic neurons. *Federation Proceedings, 36*, 2142–2148.

Mayer, P.T., & Price, D.D. (1976). Central nervous system mechanisms of analgesia. *Pain, 2*, 379–404.

Muscholl, E. (1961). Effect of cocaine and related drugs on the uptake of noradrenalin by heart and spleen. *British Journal of Pharmacology and Chemotherapy 16*, 352–359.

O'Malley, P.M., Johnston, L.D., & Bachman, J.G. (1985). Cocaine use among American adolescents and young adults. In N.J. Kozel and E.H. Adams (Eds.), *Cocaine use in America; Epidemiologic and clinical perspectives* (NIDA Research Monograph No. 61, pp. 50–75). Washington, DC: U.S. Government Printing Office.

Perez-Reyes, M., Ondrusek, G., DiGuiseppi, S., Jeffcoat, A.R., & Cook, C.E. (1982). Free-base cocaine smoking. *Clinical Pharmacology and Therapeutics, 32*, 459–465.

Post, R.M. (1975). Cocaine psychoses: A continuum model. *American Journal of Psychiatry, 132*(3), 225–231.

Pradham, S., Roy, S.N., & Pradham, S.N. (1978). Correlation of behavioral and neurochemical effects of acute administration of cocaine in rats. *Life Science, 22*, 1737–1744.

Rappolt, R.T., Gay, G.R., & Inaba, D.S. (1977). Propanolol: A specific antagonist to cocaine. *Clinical Toxicology, 10*(3), 265–271.

Rawson, R. (1984). Personal communication.

Redmond, D.E., Huang, Y.H., Snyder, D.R., & Maas, J.W. (1976). Behavioral effects of stimulation of the locus coeruleus in the stumptail monkey. *Brain Research, 116*, 502–510.

Resnick, R.B., & Resnick, E.B. (1984). Cocaine abuse and its treatment. *Symposium on Clinical Psychopharmacology. II: Psychiatric Clinics of North America, 7*, 713–728.

Rosecan, J.S. (1983, July). The treatment of cocaine abuse with imipramine, L-tyrosine, and L-tryptophan. Paper presented at the Seventh World Congress of Psychiatry, Vienna.

Shesser, R., Davis, C., & Edelstein, S. (1981). Pneumomediastinum and pneumothorax after inhaling alkaloidal cocaine. *Annals of Emergency Medicine, 10*(4), 213–215.

Siegel, R.K. (1982a). Cocaine smoking disorders. *Journal of Psychoactive Drugs, 14*(4), 332–337.

Siegel, R.K. (1982b). Cocaine and sexual dysfunction: The curse of mama coca. *Journal of Psychoactive Drugs, 14*, 71.

Siegel, R.K. (1984a). Cocaine smoking disorders: Diagnosis and treatment. *Psychiatric Annals, 14*(10), 728–732.

Siegel, R.K. (1984b). Changing patterns of cocaine use: Longitudinal observations, consequences, and treatment. In J. Grabowski (Ed.), *Cocaine: Pharmacology, effects and treatment of abuse* (NIDA Research Monograph No. 50, pp. 92–110). Washington, DC: U.S. Government Printing Office.

Siegel, R.K. (1985a). Treatment of cocaine abuse: Historical and contemporary perspectives. *Journal of Psychoactive Drugs, 17*(1), 1–9.

Siegel, R.K. (1985b). New patterns of cocaine use: Changing doses and routes. In N.J. Kozel & E.H. Adams (Eds.), *Cocaine use in America: Epidemiologic and clinical perspectives* (NIDA Research Monograph No. 61). Washington, DC: U.S. Government Printing Office.

Smith, D.E. (1984). Diagnostic, treatment, and aftercare approaches to cocaine abuse. *Journal of Substance Abuse Treatment, 1*, 5–9.

Taylor, D., & Ho, B.T. (1977). Neurochemical effects of cocaine following acute and repeated injection. *Journal of Neuroscience Research, 3*, 95–101.

Tennant, F.S., & Rawson, R.A. (1983). Cocaine and amphetamine dependence treated with desipramine. In L.S. Harris (Ed.), *Problems of drug dependence, 1982* (NIDA Research Monograph No. 43, pp. 351–355). Washington, DC: U.S. Government Printing Office.

Van Dyke, C., Barash, P.G., Jatlow, P., & Buck, R. (1976). Cocaine: Plasma concentrations after intranasal application in man. *Science, 191*, 859–861.

Villensky, W. (1982). Illicit and licit drugs causing perforation of the nasal septum. *Journal of Forensic Science, 27*, 958–962.

Wesson, D.R., & Smith, D.E. (1985). Cocaine: Treatment perspectives. In N.J. Kozel & E.H. Adams (Eds.), *Cocaine use in America: Epidemiologic and clinical perspectives* (NIDA Research Monograph No. 61, pp. 193–203). Washington, DC: U.S. Government Printing Office.

Weiss, R.D., Goldenheim, P.D., Mirin, S.M., Hales, C.A., & Mendelson, J.H. (1981). Pulmonary dysfunction in cocaine smokers. *American Journal of Psychiatry, 138*, 1110–1112.

Weiss, R.D., Mirin, S.M., & Michael, J.L. (1983, May). *Psychopathology in chronic cocaine abusers*. Paper read before the 136th Annual Meeting of the American Psychiatric Association, New York.

Wikler, A. (1973). Dynamics of drug dependence: Implications of conditioning theory for research and treatment. *Archives of General Psychiatry, 28*, 611–616.

Wikler, A. (1986). Conditioning processes in dependence and relapse. In *Opiate dependence: Mechanisms and treatment* (p. 120). New York: Plenum.

Wise, R.A. (1978). Catecholamine theories of reward: A critical review. *Brain Research, 152,* 215–247.

Wise, R.A. (1984). Neural mechanisms of the reinforcing actions of cocaine. In J. Grabowski (Ed.), *Cocaine: Pharmacology, effects and treatment of abuse* (NIDA Research Monograph No. 50, pp. 15–33). Washington, DC: U.S. Government Printing Office.

Chapter 20

Heroin

Gary R. Lewis and Gary W. Lawson

PHARMACODYNAMICS OF HEROIN AND OPIATE DRUGS

Opium and its alkaloid constituents (morphine and codeine), its semisynthetic (heroin), and the purely synthetic opiatelike agents (methadone and meperidine [Demerol]) are the most effective analgesics in use today; these drugs are known as narcotic analgesics. Even with the considerable research that went into the development of these drugs, the mechanisms by which they reduce pain only began to emerge in the mid-1970s. Tolerance develops rapidly to each of these drugs, and the dosage must be repeatedly increased to maintain a constant physiological effect. Concomitant with the tolerance is the establishment of a physiological dependency. These drugs also have the capacity to induce a sense of euphoria in many people. The euphoria appears to be more than simply the reduction of anxiety or pain.

Although there are a number of analgesics on the market, they offer little advantage over morphine; therefore, morphine remains the standard by which other narcotics are judged (Eddy & May, 1973) (see Table 20-1). Raw opium contains only approximately 10% by weight of morphine and an even smaller

Table 20-1 Peak Action and Analgesic Length of the Major Opium-like Drugs

	Doses in mg.	Time to Peak Action (in minutes post S.Q. injection)	Duration of Analgesic Action (in hours)
Morphine	10	30–60	4–5
Codeine	120		2–4
Heroin	3–4	15	4–5
Methadone	8–10	30	4–6
Meperidine	80–100	10	2–4

amount of codeine. The addition of two acetyl groups to the morphine molecule gives diacetylmorphine (heroin) (Figure 20-1). The acetyl groups allow heroin to penetrate the blood-brain barrier more readily than morphine; heroin is therefore two to three times more potent than morphine (see Table 20-1). Medicinal chemists have worked to produce compounds that would be effective analgesics and have attempted without success to separate the analgesic effect of narcotics from their dependence-producing effects. As a result, there are many sympathetic narcotics sold as prescription pain relievers. Especially noteworthy is Fentanyl, which is approximately 100 times more potent than morphine.

Pharmacological research during the 1970s revealed the interaction between narcotics and the central nervous system. A pharmacologist at Stanford University, Avram Goldstein, developed a technique in which opiate receptors could be measured by means of radioactively labeled molecules. In 1973 Pert and Snyder at Johns Hopkins University used naloxone to measure opiate receptors in rat brain tissue, allowing the mapping of the brain areas that contained opiate receptors (Foldes, 1969). In 1974, laboratories in both England and Sweden succeeded in isolating leucine enkephalin and methionine enkephalin from brain extracts. The enkephalins act like morphine and are many times more potent. This then led to the discovery of endorphins (endogenous morphinelike substances) that are also found in brain tissue and have substantial opiate effects.

PROFILE OF THE HEROIN ADDICT

Today, the typical heroin addict is male, a member of a minority population (most often Black), and in his early twenties. Demographically, he is indistinguishable from his nonaddict peer and neighbor. In a study by Duberstein and Kaufman (1971), 33% of the heroin-overdose patients in a large metropolitan hospital emergency room were confirmed addicts, 46% were intermittent users, and 21% were addicts who had undergone a recent period of abstinence. The same study also pointed out that there appears to be a seasonal pattern to both heroin

```
                 R1                               R2

Morphine         ______OH                                       ______OH
Codeine          ______O ___CH3               ______OH
Heroin           ______O _____C _____CH3 _____O _____C _____CH3
                              II                          II
                              O                           O
```

Figure 20-1 Narcotic Agents Isolated or Derived from Opium overdose and heroin deaths. The peak activity is between the months of May and October.

Sociological and personality factors contribute to heroin addiction. In examining past histories of heroin addicts, Chein (1964) describes not an addictive personality but rather an underdeveloped personality, one that is determined during development by pathological social conditions. This may account for the high incidence of drug use in urban ghettos, which are places of high anxiety and frustration with few options as to how to cope with this environment. Individuals who grow up in ghettos are often seen as unteachable, and an aimless, delinquent subculture develops as the only sympathetic diversion to a hostile home and school environment.

Although it is unambiguous that the complexion of the social setting has much to do with initial experimentation with heroin and other drugs, sociological factors do not entirely explain lifelong addiction (Dole & Nyswander, 1966). It is also difficult to imagine that an individual consciously embraces such a precarious and impairing lifestyle unless that individual has a serious psychosocial affliction that allows the drug to meet his or her unfulfilled needs. To addicts, heroin is both adaptive and functional because it helps them overcome the anxiety of facing life without proper preparation (McAuliffe & Gorden, 1974). In this context, the heroin addict is regarded as being abnormally high in externalization and abnormally low in ego development. The result is a particular susceptibility to social and environmental reinforcers and influences. In the case of addicts, drugs as well as many other environmental influences become powerful determinants of behavior.

The destructive nature of heroin and the hazards to which long-term heroin users are subjected led Khantzian (1977) to a theory of self-disregard associated with impairments of the ego functions of self-care and self-regulation. There is little evidence of the addict's fear, anxiety, or realistic assessment of the dangers inherent in his or her lifestyle.

MISCONCEPTIONS ABOUT HEROIN

Much has been written about heroin and its use, and many misconceptions have been taken as fact. One of the most common misconceptions is that "mainlining" heroin or morphine induces in everyone an intense pleasure unequaled by any other experience. Addicts describe in glowing terms the "rush" or "kick" they frequently experience (Balster & Harris, 1982). Often, it is described as similar to a whole-body "orgasm" that persists for 5 minutes or more. Some addicts report that they try with every injection to re-experience the extreme euphoria of the first injection but that they always experience less of an effect. There are studies, however, as well as clinical and street reports that some people experience only nausea and discomfort after the initial intravenous administration of morphine or heroin (Isbell & White, 1953). For whatever reasons some of these users persist, and the discomfort decreases. Under these conditions the injections soon result primarily in pleasant effects. To maintain these pleasurable feelings, however, the addict must gradually increase the dosage as tolerance develops. There is no way to predict what type of individual readily experiences pleasure or what type experiences unpleasant effects. Goldstein (1972) refers to the two "powerfully pleasurable effects"—the initial brief rush and then the longer period of tranquility. "This sequence of events occurs with virtually every non-tolerant person, although the first few experiences may be accompanied by vomiting. Even so, the sensations are often pleasurable ('You don't mind vomiting behind smack')" (p. 295).

The withdrawal symptoms of heroin addiction are also misunderstood (see Table 20-2). The addict undergoing withdrawal without medication is always portrayed as being in excruciating pain. With a long-term habit withdrawal without medical can induce extreme suffering, but with short-term use withdrawal is not so difficult. Most addicts of the 1960s and 1970s were described as having "ice cream habits," or low daily dosages.

Perhaps the most common misconception about heroin is that after one trial a user is addicted for life. In actuality, becoming addicted takes some time, perhaps a week if the beginner is persistent. Regular use of the drug seems to be more important in establishing psychological addiction than the amount used.

DANGERS OF HEROIN USE

Heroin addiction continues to appear in various groups in each new generation. In the mid-1980s "low-class" junkies were joined by a group of young, wealthy,

Table 20-2 Sequence of Appearance of Heroin Withdrawal Symptoms

	Time after Last Dosage (hours)	
Signs	Heroin	Morphine
Craving for drugs; anxiety	6	24
Yawning; perspiration; running nose; teary eyes	14	34–48
Increase in pupil dilation; goose bumps; tremors; hot and cold flashes; aching bones and muscles	16	48–72
Increased intensity of above; insomnia; elevated blood pressure; increased temperature, pulse rate, and respiratory rate; restlessness; nausea	24–36	
Increased intensity of above; fetal positioning; vomiting; diarrhea; weight loss; spontaneous ejaculation; hemoconcentration; increased blood sugar levels	36–48	

"respectable" heroin users both in the United States and Europe. A new and very pure form of heroin called black tar began in 1986 to appear on the streets of many of the major metropolitan cities of this country. The availability of heroin has become further complicated by the presence of various synthetic drugs; illicit chemists have developed derivatives of Fentamyl that are sold as "China white" or "synthetic heroin." These "designer drugs" are especially interesting in that the chemists are able to alter the basic molecule to produce drugs that are not yet listed as controlled substances.

Another synthetic heroin, MPTP, is a derivative of meperidine that has been produced by several illicit laboratories. There is a substantial danger of trace amounts of the impurity MPTP being included if the chemist applies too much heat in the reaction. This highly toxic substance was responsible for permanent brain damage in several users in the 1980s. MPTP destroys dopamine neurons, leading to a form of Parkinson's disease.

A new danger for intravenous users of heroin is exposure to the AIDS virus. This virus does not survive well on its own and is transmitted by an infected person's body fluids, primarily blood and semen. Because intravenous drug users often share needles, there is a high risk of contracting AIDS among the group.

TREATMENT

Just about every form of psychotherapy, psychosocial intervention, or psychotropic medication has been used at one time or another for the treatment of drug dependence. Heroin and other opium-based natural and synthetic derivatives are among the most addicting of all drugs, and there have been many attempts to treat users addicted to these drugs. Perhaps the most important aspect of treatment for opiate users is the medical treatment of overdose. An overdose can easily end in death for the heroin user, and treatment requires trained personnel, equipment, and an environment in which life-saving procedures can be performed. Nonmedical psychotherapists should always defer treatment of overdose and detoxification to their medical counterparts. For a review of various treatment approaches for heroin addiction, see Milby (1981). For information about the use of drugs such as methadone for the treatment of heroin addiction, see Chapter 8 of this text.

REFERENCES

Balster, R.L., & Harris, L.S. (1982). Drugs as reinforcers in animals and humans: Symposium. *Federation Proceedings, 41*(2), 209–246.

Chein, I. (1964). *The road to narcotics. Delinquency and social policy.* New York: Basic Books.

Dole, V.P., & Nyswander, M.E. (1966). Narcotic blockade. *Archives of Internal Medicine, 118,* 204–209.

Duberstein, J.L., & Kaufman, D.M. (1971). A clinical study of an epidemic of heroin intoxication and heroin-induced pulmonary edema. *American Journal of Medicine, 51*, 704.

Eddy, N.B., & May, E.L. (1973). The search for a better analgesic. *Science, 181*, 407–414.

Foldes, F.F., Duncalf, D., & Kuwabara, S. (1969). The respiratory, circulatory, and narcotic antagonistic effects of nalorphine, levallorphan, and naloxone in anesthetized subjects. *Canadian Anesthesia Society Journal, 16*, 151–161.

Goldstein, A. (1972). Heroin addiction and the role of methadone in its treatment. *Archives of General Psychiatry, 26*, 291–297.

Isbell, H., & White, W.M. (1953). Clinical characteristics of addictions. *American Journal of Medicine, 14*, 558–565.

Khantzian, E.J. (1977). The ego, the self, and opiate addictions: Theoretical and treatment considerations. In *Psychodynamics of Drug Dependence* (NIDA Research Monograph No. 12). Washington, DC: U.S. Government Printing Office.

McAuliffe, W.E., & Gorden, R.A. (1974). A test of Lindesmith's theory of addiction: The frequency of euphoria among long-term addicts. *American Journal of Sociology, 79*(4), 795–840.

Milby, J.B. (1981). *Addictive behavior and its treatment.* New York: Springer.

Chapter 21

Marijuana

John McCaig and Gary W. Lawson

The use and abuse of cannabis (marijuana) in 1986 became a less highlighted issue than other popular controversies surrounding certain illegal drugs, particularly cocaine. Its popularity has nonetheless remained. Next to cigarettes and alcohol, cannabis is North America's most frequently used drug. Epidemiological studies vary somewhat with respect to the frequency of cannabis use, but at least 17% of the general population of the United States has tried cannabis one or more times. Such a large percentage is still more impressive when very young children and the elderly are excluded from the statistics. To be sure, cannabis users cut across many facets of society. The highest concentrations are found among school dropouts, people younger than 25 years of age, males, military personnel, criminal offenders, venereal disease patients, psychiatric patients, and users of alcohol and other types of drugs (Blum, 1984). That cannabis is not now as much a public concern as it was during the 1970s is probably partly because it is generally less damaging in its effects than alcohol, cigarettes, or cocaine. A more subtle reason may lie in the fact that cannabis has come to be adopted, with reservations and some measure of tolerance, by the liberal majority. Society is ambivalent with respect to cannabis, refusing to condone its use and at the same time refusing to lend support to the kind of police and judicial action that might effectively curtail it. This ambivalence is reflected in a significant decrease in the number of scientific studies that deal with the social and psychological problems associated with cannabis abuse, a trend that appears to have begun in 1982.

PHARMACOLOGY OF CANNABIS

Cannabis contains 421 compounds, 61 of which have a cannabinoid structure. Only one of these compounds, tetrahydrocannabinol (THC), has an effect on mental functions. Cannabis sold on the street may have a THC content ranging from 1% to 10%. Hashish, which is produced from the resins and flowers of the cannabis plant, may contain up to 15% THC. Hash oil, which consists of solvent extracts of the leaf, flower, and resins of cannabis, may contain up to 60% THC. In the past 10 years growers have produced plants with progressively higher levels of THC, so that cannabis now sold on the street is frequently five to ten times more powerful than that sold a decade ago. Other constituents of cannabis include phenols, cresols, and polynuclear aromatic nucleotides that are thought to be carcinogenic.

The primary locus of action of THC is probably the hypothalamus. The effects of THC can be stopped by introducing agents that effectively block pituitary andrenocorticotropic hormone (ACTH) production. THC stimulates the hypothalamus, which in turn stimulates the pituitary's production of ACTH. The neocortex (or outermost layer) of the adrenal gland is stimulated by ACTH to produce cortisones. Cortisone is responsible for regulating, among other actions, the metabolism of fats and carbohydrates. An excess of cortisone results in a decrease in this metabolism, and as a consequence the individual may experience lethargy. This mechanism accounts in part for the sluggishness often associated with use of cannabis. It may also account for the ''munchies'' or increase in appetite, as the body craves fats and carbohydrates to provide quick food energy. While this action in the body accounts for some of the symptoms associated with cannabis use, little else is understood about its effect on the brain.

The adverse effects of cannabis use fall into three general categories: biological, behavioral, and social. The perception of adversity itself is in many instances a subjective judgment; this is particularly true of psychological and social symptomatology. For example, persons who use cannabis commonly report a lowered capacity for concentration. Some report this reaction as a pleasant and relaxing experience; others become afraid that they will not understand what is going on around them, be misunderstood by others, or be thought of as stupid. Social withdrawal is another frequent reaction to cannabis (which is probably not unrelated to waning concentration); some interpret this behavior as impolite and inappropriate, while others consider it a sign of self-assured reserve. Even some of the biological (as opposed to psychophysiological) reactions to cannabis are subject to interpretation. Sleepiness (which is not unrelated to waning concentration and social withdrawal) is a frequent effect of cannabis and may or may not result in anxiety, depending, for example, on whether the individual has strong beliefs about what he or she should feel.

The toxic effects of cannabis have been studied in a wide variety of animal and human studies. Studies that have attempted to find the lethal dosages in animals have shown that death generally occurs from cardiac arrest and respiratory failure (profound hyponia) that does not respond to artificial respiration. Lethal dosages range from 40 mg/kg in the rat to 128 mg/kg in the monkey. In these studies it was found that potency is inversely related to body size, so that rats are more resistant than rabbits, rabbits more so than monkeys, and so on (Rosenkrantz, 1981). If the lethal dosage applied to monkeys is used as a basis for extrapolation, a lethal dosage for a 70-kg man (154 lbs.) is equivalent to the amount of THC that could be extracted from a pound of high-quality marijuana.

The general toxic effects of cannabis on humans cannot be determined on the basis of animal studies alone, principally because the cerebral cortex is so much more highly developed in humans. It is probable that reactions affecting higher-level biochemical functions in humans do not occur or go undetected in animals. Further, human society presents not only psychological and psychophysiological factors completely unrelated to the laboratory but biological conditions that are unique and extremely varied.

Of the social factors, perhaps none is so confounding as the fact that cannabis is illegal. Illegal drugs present many methodological problems for the clinical investigator. Most drug users use many different drugs, a fact that they may often deny even to clinical investigators. When these drugs are used in combination, their effects may be synergistic rather than additive. The use of a number of drugs at the same time is called "polydrug abuse," and its results can be extremely unpredictable.

Toxicological field studies of humans have been particularly difficult to perform because dosages cannot be readily controlled, adulterants are often present, and cannabis is frequently taken with other drugs, perhaps most commonly alcohol (Grant, Reed, Adams, & Carlin, 1979). Since neurological impairment in alcoholics is well established (Bolter & Hannon, 1980), nondrinkers must be used in such studies. It is difficult, however, to find subjects who smoke marijuana who do not also drink alcohol or use other illegal drugs.

Pre-existing physiological problems also complicate the task of determining the toxicological effects of cannabis on the body. In studies of acute reactions in humans (Belleville, Swanson, & Agieh, 1985), chronic bronchitis, pulmonary disease, and cancer have been found as well as more minor conditions such as rhinitis, sinusitis, and acute bronchitis. The pre-existing health conditions of subjects may well contribute significantly to these outcomes. Similar problems confound the results of studies of cardiovascular and gastrointestinal toxicity (Halikas, Goodwin, & Guze, 1981; Tennant, 1980). Subjects in these studies were shown to suffer acute reactions including tachycardia, hypertension, vasomotor constriction, vomiting, diarrhea, and abdominal distress. No direct toxic effect on the heart could be discerned, however. The gastrointestinal problems found in users were thought to be the result of a decrease in the production of gastric acid secretions, which in turn leaves the intestinal tract more susceptible to infections.

In humans, preexisting neurological conditions may account for all reported cases of neurological damage said to be caused directly by cannabis. Neurotoxicity is defined as a "functional aberration that appears to be qualitatively distinct from those which are characteristic of reversible acute and chronic effects" (Fehr

& Kalant, 1976, p. 26). In animal studies this kind of damage has been established with respect to cannabis. Rats exposed to a prolonged high dosage of THC developed irreversible jumping "popcorn reactions" believed to be the result of seizure activity. Abnormally spiked electroencephalographic measures supported the seizure theory. The neurological damage was determined in part through behavioral experiments. Maze learning, operant conditioning involving time discrimination, and open-area exploration behaviors were found to be impaired. Because these tasks entail good spatial orientation and response inhibition, it was believed that the damage occurred in the hippocampus (Radouco-Thomas, Magnan, & Radouco-Thomas, 1976; Fehr, Kalant, LeBlanc, & Knox, 1976; Stiglick & Kalant, 1981). Other studies did not differentiate long-term damage from the withdrawal phase of recovery, during which abnormalities in electroencephalographic patterns would not be considered evidence of neuronal damage (Barratt & Adams, 1972; Heath, 1976).

NEUROPSYCHOLOGICAL STUDIES

Neurological and neuropsychological studies on the effects of cannabis abuse in humans have been extensively reviewed (Wert & Raulin, 1986). Neurological impairment has been assessed in these studies by means of the traditional medical tests: neurological examination; mental status examination (neuropsychiatry); laboratory tests on blood, urine, or cerebrospinal fluid; electroencephalography; evoked potentials; echoencephalography (ultrasound); angiography, pneumoencephalography; neuroradiological techniques; computerized axial tomography; and radionuclide brain scanning and flow studies. Neuropsychological examinations employed in this research have included the Ammons Full Range Vocabulary Test, Raven's Progressive Matrices, Wechsler Intelligence Scale for Children (revised), Wechsler Adult Intelligence Scale, Halstead-Reitan Neuropsychological Test Battery, tests of abstract reasoning, memory scales, fine-motor scales, sensory-perceptual tests, and many others. It was concluded that "the current research does not support the contention that cannabis use results in chronic cerebral impairment" (Wert & Raulin, 1986, p. 639).

Although permanent neuronal damage does not appear to be a problem associated with cannabis abuse, functional neuropsychiatric disorders are listed in the *Diagnostic and Statistical Manual of Mental Disorders* (Third Edition) (DSM-III; American Psychiatric Association, 1980). Cannabis intoxication, cannabis delusional disorder, cannabis abuse, and cannabis dependence are defined as follows.

1. Diagnostic criteria for cannabis abuse
   A. *Pattern of pathological use:* Intoxication throughout the day; use of cannabis nearly every day for at least a month; episodes of cannabis

delusional disorder; impairment in social or occupational functioning, including marked loss of interest in activities previously engaged in, loss of friends, absence from work, loss of job, or legal difficulties (other than a single arrest due to possession, purchase, or sale of an illegal substance).

   B. *Tolerance:* Need for markedly increased amounts of cannabis to achieve the desired effect or markedly diminished effect with regular use of the same amount.

2. Diagnostic criteria for cannabis intoxication
   A. Recent use of cannabis.
   B. Tachycardia.
   C. At least one of the following psychological symptoms within 2 hours of use: euphoria, subjective intensification of perceptions, sensation of slowed time, or apathy.
   D. At least one of the following physical symptoms within 2 hours of substance use: conjunctival injection, increased appetite, or dry mouth.
   E. Maladaptive behavior effects, such as excessive anxiety, suspiciousness or paranoid ideation, impaired judgment, or impaired social or occupational functioning.
   F. Not due to any other physical or mental disorder.

3. Diagnostic criteria for cannabis delusional disorder
   A. Recent use of cannabis.
   B. An organic delusional syndrome within 2 hours of substance use.
   C. The disturbance does not persist beyond 6 hours after cessation of substance use.
   D. Not due to any other physical or mental disorder.

Cannabis abuse disorder roughly corresponds to the now-discarded label of "amotivational syndrome." The amotivational syndrome was described by a host of symptoms that are similar to those found of depressed patients and patients who abuse sedative-hypnotic drugs. These symptoms include apathy, impaired ability to carry out complex tasks, failure to pursue long-term goals, diminished communication skills, sluggishness of mental responses, and neglect of personal appearance. The syndrome was believed to clear after several weeks of discontinued use. Documentation of the disorder is sketchy, and it is not at all clear whether these patients were experiencing the effects of cannabis or whether they were experiencing another psychiatric disturbance such as depression that in turn resulted in substance abuse. This is equally true of the more current and specific disorder cannabis abuse, since the caveat "not due to any other physical or mental disorder" never has been satisfactorily determined in the research (Negrete, 1981).

Cannabis delusional syndrome roughly corresponds to a cannabis-induced psychosis (Negrete, 1981) reportedly characterized by mental confusion, impulsive behavior, delusional formations, memory impairment, and sensory-perception distortions. In cannabis delusional syndrome there are no prominent sensory-perception distortions (hallucinations) evident. There exists no DSM-III category of cannabis hallucinosis. The validity of cannabis-induced psychosis as a disorder involving psychotic sensory-perception disorders is highly suspect. Where this has been reported, the presence of adulterants, particularly phencyclidine (PCP), is suspected. Alternatively, a predisposed premorbid condition is commonly reported and suggests that such psychotic disturbances are not the consequence of long-term cannabis abuse.

Acute panic and paranoid states (without psychosis) are also reported in the literature (Negrete, 1981), but epidemiological studies have found a significant decline in the frequency with which these have been reported in the past 10 years. The incidence of these states has always been less frequent in India, where cannabis has been used popularly for centuries, than in Europe and North America, where it is a relatively new drug. Explanations for these epidemiological findings vary. Societal reactions to cannabis abuse are believed to account for the "paranoia attacks," wherein users find themselves simply afraid of being caught. A lack of experience in handling the drug may also account for the phenomenon. Alternatively, physicians may no longer find attacks unique and may not report their occurrence as frequently. Finally, those who have made use of medical and psychological help in the past may now choose to "ride out" a paranoia attack; many frequent users acknowledge feelings of self-consciousness, anxiety, and mild paranoia, although these feelings rarely overwhelm them to the point of an attack (Negrete, 1981).

PHYSIOLOGICAL EFFECTS

The physiological hazards of smoking cannabis probably significantly outweigh the psychological damage that occurs from prolonged use. In animal studies, cannabis smoke has been shown to have carcinogenic properties. Tar, a smoke condensate, has been shown to be mutagenic. Alterations in cell development called metaplasia have taken place in the sebaceous glands in animals whose skin was painted with the substance (Magus & Harris, 1971). Tumor formations have also been demonstrated (Hoffman, Brunnerman, Gori, & Wynder, 1975). Particularly carcinogenic substances such as benzopyrene are known to be significantly less abundant in the tar of tobacco than in the tar of cannabis (Novotny, Lee, & Bartle, 1976). Precancerous changes have been noted in rodents that were made to inhale cannabis smoke over a prolonged period.

In humans, heavy users show histopathological changes that are generally considered to be characteristic of much older tobacco smokers who were judged to be prone to cancer of the lung (Tennant, 1980). The possible synergistic effects of smoking cannabis and tobacco have yet to be fully determined, but it is suggested that such patients are at high risk for developing lung cancer.

There are no hard data that establish a causal relation between cannabis use and cancer, although strong correlations have been calculated. Research evidence of this kind no doubt will be as difficult to compile as the evidence against smoking. Designing studies to examine the detrimental psychological effects of cannabis use is a still more difficult task for the methodological reasons alluded to earlier. When all the data are in, the implications for social change are likely to remain controversial and problematic. Cannabis appears to have become somewhat entrenched in the moral center and is probably here to stay. Even if cannabis remains illegal, society may continue to tolerate its use. Indeed, society may never come to examine its impact with a trenchant and introspective eye. Like cigarettes, alcohol, and coffee, cannabis is, or may soon become, a "hidden drug."

REFERENCES

Barratt, E.S., & Adams, P. (1972). The effects of chronic marijuana administration on brain functioning in cats. In J.M. Singh, L. Miller, & H. Lal (Eds.), *Drug addiction: Experimental pharmacology* (pp. 145–157). New York: Futura.

Belleville, J.W., Swanson, G.D., & Agieh, K.A. (1985). Respiratory effects of delta-9-tetrahydrocannobinol. *Clinical Pharmacological Therapy, 17*, 541–548.

Blum, K. (1984). *Handbook of abusable drugs* (pp. 447–513). New York: Gardner Press.

Bolter, J.F., & Hannon, R. (1980). Cerebral damage associated with alcoholism: A reexamination. *Psychological Records, 30*, 165–179.

Fehr, K.A., Kalant, H., LeBlanc, A.E., & Knox, G.V. (1976). Permanent learning impairment after chronic heavy exposure to cannabis or ethanol in the rat. In G.G. Nahas (Ed.), *Marihuana: Chemistry, biochemistry, and cellular effects* (pp. 495–505). New York: Springer-Verlag.

Fehr, K.O., & Kalant, H. (1982). Long-term effects of cannabis on cerebral function: A review of the clinical and experimental literature. In K.O. Fehr & H. Kalant (Eds.), *Adverse health and behavioral consequences of cannabis use*. Working papers for the ARF/WHO Scientific Meeting, Toronto.

Grant, I., Reed, R., Adams, K., & Carlin, A. (1979). Neuropsychological functioning in young alcoholics and polydrug abusers. *Journal of Clinical Neuropsychology, 1*, 39–47.

Halikas, J.A., Goodwin, D.W., & Guze, S.B. (1979). Marijuana effects: A survey of regular users. *Journal of the American Medical Association, 217*, 692–694.

Heath, R.G. (1976). Marihuana and delta-tetrahydrocannabinol: Acute and chronic effects on brain function of monkeys. In M.C. Braude & S. Szara (Eds.), *Pharmacology of marihuana, (Vol. 1)* (pp. 345–356). New York: Raven Press.

Hoffman, D., Brunnermann, K.D., Gori, G.B., & Wynder, E.L. (1975). On the carcinogenicity of marijuana smoke. *Recent Advances in Phytochemistry, 9*, 63–81.

Magus, R.D., & Harris, L.S. (1971). Carcinogenic potential of marijuana smoke condensate. *Federation Proceedings, 30*, 279 Abs.

Negrete, J.C. (1982). Psychiatric effects of cannabis use. In K.O. Fehr & H. Kalant (Eds.), *Adverse health and behavioral consequences of cannabis use*. Working papers for the ARF/WHO Scientific Meeting, Toronto.

Novotny, M., Lee, M.L., & Bartle, K.D. (1976). A possible chemical base for the higher mutagenicity of marijuana smoke as compared to tobacco smoke. *Experientia, 32*, 280–282.

Radouco-Thomas, S., Magnan, F., & Radouco-Thomas, C. (1976). Pharmacogenetic studies on cannabis and narcotics: Effects of delta-tetrahydrocannabinol and morphine in developing mice. In G.G. Nahas (Ed.), *Marihuana: Chemistry, biochemistry, and cellular effects* (pp. 481–494). New York: Springer-Verlag.

Rosenkrantz, H. (1982). Cannabis, marijuana and cannabinoid toxicological manifestations in man and animals. In K.O. Fehr & H. Kalant (Eds.), *Adverse health and behavioral consequences of cannabis use*. Working papers for the ARF/WHO Scientific Meeting, Toronto.

Stiglick, A., & Kalant, H. (1981). Learning impairment in the radial-arm maze following prolonged cannabis treatment in rats. Working papers for the ARF/WHO Scientific Meeting, Toronto.

Tennant, F.S. (1980). Histopathologic and clinical abnormalities of the respiratory system in chronic hashish smokers. In L.S. Harris (Ed.), *Problems of drug dependence, 1979* (Vol. 27, pp. 309–315). Rockville, MD: National Institute on Drug Abuse.

Wert, R.C., & Raulin, M.L. (1986). The chronic cerebral effects of cannabis use. I. Methodological issues and neurological findings. *International Journal of the Addictions, 21*, 6.

Chapter 22

Voluntary Inhalation of Volatile Substances*

Thomas Young and Gary W. Lawson

The voluntary inhalation of commercial solvents for mind-altering purposes probably began in California during the 1950s (Cohen, 1977a). Today, recreational use of volatile substances is not only found in the United States but among the Australian aborigines (Nurcombe, Bianchi, Money, & Cante, 1970) and the natives of arctic Manitoba (Boecks & Coodin, 1976). The major volatile solvents include aliphatic hydrocarbons (hexane), aromatic hydrocarbons (benzene, toluene, zylene, styrene, and naphthalene), mixed aliphatic-aromatic hydrocarbons (gasoline), aliphatic nitrates (amyl nitrite), esters (methyl acetate, ethyl acetate, *n*-propylacetate, *n*-butylacetate, methyl formate, and ethyl formate), ketones (acetone, methylethyl ketone, methylhexyl ketone, disubutyl ketone, and methylamyl ketone), and halogenated solvents and propellants.

Although the practice of inhaling volatile substances is often dismissed as "childish behavior," its serious nature is illustrated by the fact that most of the 700 aerosol-related deaths during the 1970s "seem to be attributable to inhalant abuse" (Sharp & Korman, 1981, p. 236). Furthermore, depending on the specific agent, chronic toxicity can include bone marrow depression (Louria, 1969), leukemia (Aksoy & Erdem, 1978; Goldstein, 1977; Infante, Rimsky, Wagoner, & Young, 1977), anemia (Sokol, 1965), encephalopathy (Knox & Nelson, 1966), lead poisoning (Durden & Chipman, 1967; Law & Nelson, 1968), liver, kidney, cerebellar, and chromosomal damage (Grabski, 1961; Malcolm, 1969; O'Brien, Yeoman, & Hobby, 1971), and neuropathy (Berry, Heaton, & Kirby, 1978).

There is a lack of reliable data on the prevalence of inhalant use. For example, it has been estimated that 12 percent of the nation's high school seniors have tried

*From "Voluntary Inhalation of Volatile Substances: A Clinical Review" by Thomas Young and Gary W. Lawson, 1986, *Corrective and Social Psychiatry and Journal of Behavior Technology Methods and Therapy, 32*(3), pp. 49–54. Copyright April 1986 by Martin Psychiatric Research Foundation, Inc. Adapted by permission.

inhalants (Johnston, Bachman, & O'Malley, 1979). Available statistics, how-ever, are marked by various methodological problems and probably underestimate the actual incidence of inhalant use. The data also appear to be conservative in terms of the prevalence of inhalant use among adults. It has been reported that 2% of adults have tried volatile inhalants for recreational purposes (Wallace, 1974), but Cohen (1977b) has speculated "there are greater numbers of users in the 21 to 30 year old age group than previously reported" (p. 9).

Nevertheless, national survey figures for inhalant use report levels of use roughly comparable to those for the major hallucinogens and for cocaine (Abelson, Fishburne, & Cisin, 1977; Carroll, 1977; Johnston et al., 1979). In spite of this, much less attention has been devoted to the voluntary inhalation of volatile substances (Sharp, 1977). This is obviously an unfortunate situation in view of the clinical problems associated with inhalant use.

PSYCHOSOCIAL ASPECTS

The heaviest incidence of inhalant use occurs among adolescents in their midteens. Several factors account for the popularity of volatile substances among this age group. First, commercial solvents are the easiest mind-altering drug for teenagers to obtain; in very remote rural areas gasoline is often the only available intoxicant. Second, for many adolescents inhalants are simply more cost-effective and convenient than alcohol or marijuana. Third, their effect is quickly felt and their impact dissipates rapidly, allowing many "highs" (Cohen, 1973, 1975, 1977b).

Although inhalant use is still predominately among males, the ratio of male users to female users has declined over the past decade from ten to one to two to one. This is consistent with the sociological trend of increased involvement of females with illicit drugs in general (Cohen, 1977b; Sharp & Korman, 1981). Furthermore, it was once believed that inhalant use was primarily among the poor, but today it is spread fairly heterogeneously across all socioeconomic strata (Grossett, Lewis, & Phillips, 1971; Sharp & Korman, 1981). In terms of race, Hispanics are slightly overrepresented among inhalant users, blacks are slightly underrepresented, and non-Hispanic whites are close to their base rate (Korman, Price, Weis, Semler, & North, 1977; Medida & Cruz, 1972; Stybel, Allen, & Lewis, 1976). Differential preferences for specific agents also exist by race. Specifically, spray paints appear to be preferred by Hispanics, and liquid paper and cements are more frequently used by blacks. In contrast, gasoline, shoe polish, and amyl nitrates are popular inhalants among non-Hispanic whites (Sharp & Korman, 1981).

Usually, an adolescent is introduced to inhalant use through peers or significant others (Ackerly & Gibson, 1964; Korman, Semler, & Trimboli, 1980). Thus the principal part of learning inhalant use occurs within intimate personal groups. Furthermore, the learning not only includes techniques but specific attitudes; hence, much of the research on inhalant use appears to lend at least some support to Sutherland's (1947) differential association theory.

Personality factors, however, also seem to play a role in the use of inhalants. Press and Done (1967), for example, studied 16 inhalant users and found the subjects to be marked by feelings of inadequacy, bashfulness, and frustration. Similar findings have been reported by Meloff (1970) and by Richek, Angle, McAdams, and D'Angelo (1975). Apparently inhalant users are often troubled by poor self-esteem and feelings of powerlessness.

Volatile substances are also frequently used as a means of coping with stressful life events. Problems in acculturation (Chaze, 1985; Cohen, 1973), existential boredom (Medina-Mora, Schnaas, Rerroba, Isoard, & Suarez, 1978; Stybel et al., 1976), and school adjustment (Barker & Adams, 1973; Korman et al., 1977; Meloff, 1970; Nurcombe et al., 1970) have been widely cited as environmental pressures in the initiation of inhalant use. Familial pathology and disorganization have also been implicated by several investigators. Ackerly and Gibson (1964), for example, discovered that most of the families in their sample were "multiple problem families" that had gone through periods of considerable turmoil. Other studies have reported that a parent is often missing through abandonment or death (De la Garza, Mendiola, & Rabago, 1978; Jackson, Thornhill, & Gonzalez, 1967; Massengale, Glaser, & Lelievre, 1963). Press and Done (1967) point out that it is not uncommon for one or both of the parents to be marked by alcoholism. Consequently the inhalant user is often an "identified patient" with a need for family therapy (for example, see Haley, 1980).

CLINICAL EFFECTS

Pollack (1976) notes that intoxication is "a clinical condition that is defined by clinical signs and symptoms, ranging from mild, moderate, to severe, with coma and eventual death" (p. 258). As a clinical condition, intoxication is influenced by a number of important variables related to the drug and to the user. The former involves variables such as pharmacology and dosage, and the latter involves factors such as age, medical history, drug history, behavioral history, and personality (Siegel, 1978). This multivariate perspective helps explain why commercial solvents can produce a mental state that ranges from euphoria to frank ego dysfunction.

In general, "alteration in consciousness may be achieved by high concentrations of gas or vapor in air within one to two minutes, while lower concentrations may require five to ten minutes to achieve the desired effects" (Comstock & Comstock, 1977, p. 54). The clinical manifestations of solvent inebriation are similar to those of the early phase of alcohol-induced intoxication or the second stage of anesthesia. These symptoms are largely due to progressive, generalized central nervous system depression with early signs of cortical disinhibition (Cohen, 1977a). The psychological state is typical of a delirium and includes mental confusion, impaired perception and cognitive skills, psychomotor clumsiness, and emotional disinhibition. Other symptoms consist of dizziness, ataxia, slurred speech, partial or total amnesia, drowsiness, and a euphoric, dreamy reverie. Feelings of numbness, weightlessness, and omnipotence are also common. Hyperactivity and impulsiveness are occasionally seen in the early phase of solvent intoxication as well. As the intoxication intensifies, illusions, pseudohallucinations, hallucinations, and delusions may occur (Cohen, 1973, 1975, 1977b; Done, 1973; Wyse, 1973).

During the euphoric stage of intoxication, the inhalant user may pose a danger to self and others. Accident proneness, antisocial behavior, and self-destructive acts are part of the clinical picture of solvent abuse. Since inhalants diminish behavioral control before they affect motor activity, users frequently come to the attention of legal authorities (Friedman & Friedman, 1973; Korman et al., 1980; Press & Done, 1967; Tinklenberg & Woodrow, 1974).

The period of intoxication is relatively short, lasting a few minutes to 1 to 2 hours. The user gradually returns to a normal state of consciousness as the depressant effect diminishes. Although solvent use can result in a "hangover," it is said to be less bothersome than that induced by alcohol. Solvent hangovers typically feature headache and pain in the extremities (Cohen, 1977a). Other residual side effects may include photophobia, diplopia, tinnitus, menstrual disorders, depression, anxiety, difficulty in concentrating, frequent cough, angina, night sweats, shortness of breath, extreme tiredness or weakness, abnormal thirst, indigestion, constipation, and diarrhea (Comstock & Comstock, 1977).

Death in most cases of acute toxicity is due to cardiac arrest and various cardiac dysrhythmias (Bass, 1970; Taylor & Harris, 1970). Suffocation is another common cause of death during solvent inhalation. This may result when the user covers his or her head or entire body in a plastic bag. A similar situation may occur when toxic substances are inhaled in a sealed closet or when the user loses consciousness and falls on the bag or rag containing the volatile material (Cohen, 1977a). Suffocation due to laryngospasm has also been reported with the use of aerosols (Chapel & Thomas, 1970).

Psychological dependence is common among inhalant users. One study reported a case in which a user inhaled up to 25 tubes of glue (21 ml each) daily (Press & Done, 1967). There is disagreement, however, with regard to the existence of physical dependence. Some investigators have reported a syndrome resembling delirium tremens (De la Garza et al., 1978; Lindstrom, 1973; Nylander, 1962; Satran & Dodson, 1963), but others have argued that such manifestations may be psychological in origin (Done, 1973). Cohen (1977a) has concluded "if physical dependence develops at all from inhalant sniffing, it is very mild" (p. 2971).

TREATMENT

A number of investigators have reported on the use of learning paradizing in the treatment of inhalant users. Skoricova and Molcan (1972), for example, treated 22 adolescents and 10 adults with aversive therapy and reported a 50% success rate. Mecir (1971) treated a 17-year-old inhaler by pairing inhalation of a cleaning liquid containing trichloroethylene with discomfort produced by an injection of apomorphine. Kolvin (1967) used relaxation and aversive imagery techniques in the treatment of a 15-year-old gasoline sniffer, and Blanchard, Libet, and Young (1973) treated a spray paint inhaler through covert sensitization and apneic aversion.

DeAngelis and Goldstein (1978), however, note that drug users frequently present their substance use as the therapeutic focus in order to prevent the therapist from dealing with underlying conflicts and issues. Consequently, they suggest that the psychotherapeutic process should focus on internal and external conflicts rather than the presenting problem. Following this logic, Laury (1972) emphasizes the importance of family therapy. Chevaili (1978) also stresses the need to work with the family and significant others at home, school, and work. Silberberg & Silberberg (1974) discuss the need to improve the inhalant user's concept of self-worth, especially within the context of the school. Logotherapy may be useful in cases marked by existential boredom, frustration, or despair (Crumbaugh, Wood, & Wood, 1980).

Inhalant use is obviously a complex, multivariate problem requiring multiple therapeutic approaches (Lawson, 1984). Thus therapeutic decisions always should be based on a professional evaluation of the user's biological, psychological, and sociological profile (Lawson, Petersen, & Lawson, 1983).

CONCLUSION

Inhalant use is not only a clinical problem but a sociological dilemma, particularly among adolescents. From a social-psychiatric perspective, volatile substances are used as both an alloplastic and an autoplastic response to alienation, especially feelings of helplessness (for example, see Freud, 1959) and powerlessness (for example, see Marx, 1939; Mills, 1957). Since adolescents are typically characterized by social, political, and economic marginality (Keniston, 1960; Kvaraceus, 1972; Goodman, 1960; Greenberg, 1978; Vexler, 1972), it is not surprising that many enjoy the feeling of omnipotence that inhalants can induce. Consequently, inhalant use is not only the clinical manifestation of intrapersonal and interpersonal oppression but of sociological oppression as well.

REFERENCES

Abelson, H.I. Fishburne, P.M., & Cisin, I. (1977). *National survey on drug abuse* (Vol. 1), Washington, DC: U.S. Government Printing Office.

Ackerly, W., & Gibson, G. (1964). Lighter fluid sniffing. *American Journal of Psychiatry, 9*, 1056–1061.

Aksoy, M., & Erdem, S. (1978). Followup study on the mortality and the development of leukemia in 44 pancytopenic patients with chronic exposure to benzene. *Blood, 52*, 258.

Barker, G., & Adams, W. (1973). Glue sniffing. *Sociology and Research, 47*, 289–310.

Bass, M. (1970). Sudden sniffing death. *Journal of the American Medical Association, 212*(12), 2075–2079.

Berry, G., Heaton, R.K., & Kirby, M.W. (1978). Neuropsychological assessment of solvent inhalers. In C.W. Sharp & L.T. Carroll (Eds.), *Voluntary inhalation of industrial solvents*. Rockville, MD: National Institute on Drug Abuse.

Blanchard, E., Libet, J., & Young, L. (1973). Apneic aversion and covert sensitization in the treatment of hydrocarbon inhalation addiction: A case study. *Journal of Behavior Therapy and Experimental Psychiatry, 4*(4), 383–387.

Boecks, R., & Coodin, F. (1976). *An epidemic of gasoline sniffing*. Paper presented at the First International Symposium on the Deliberate Inhalation of Industrial Solvents, Mexico City.

Carroll, E. (1977). Notes on the epidemiology of inhalants. In C.W. Sharp & M.L. Brehm (Eds.), *Review of inhalants: Euphoria to dysfunction*. Rockville, MD: National Institute on Drug Abuse.

Chapel, J., & Thomas, G. (1970). Aerosol inhalation for "kicks." *Missouri Medicine, 67*(6), 378–380.

Chaze, W.L. (1985). Alcohol, poverty—The killing fields of rosebud. *U.S. News and World Report*, 2 September, 52–53.

Chevaili. A. (1978). Is the inhalant user incurable? In C.W. Sharp & L.T. Carroll (Eds.), *Voluntary inhalation of industrial solvents*. Rockville, MD: National Institute on Drug Abuse.

Cohen, S. (1973). The volatile solvents. *Public Health Review, 2*, 185–213.

Cohen, S. (1975). Inhalant abuse. *Drug Abuse Alcohol Newsletter, 4*(9), 3.

Cohen, S. (1977a). Abuse of inhalants. In S.N. Pradhan & S.N. Dutta (Eds.), *Drug abuse: Clinical and basic aspects*. St Louis: C.V. Mosby.

Cohen S. (1977b). Inhalant abuse: An overview of the problem. In C.W. Sharp & M.L. Brehm (Eds.), *Review of inhalants: Euphoria to dysfunction*. Rockville, MD: National Institute on Drug Abuse.

Comstock, E.G., & Comstock, B.S. (1977). Medical evaluation of inhalant abusers. In C.W. Sharp & M.L. Brehm (Eds.), *Review of inhalants: Euphoria to dysfunction*. Rockville, MD: National Institute on Drug Abuse.

Crumbaugh, J.C., Wood, W.M., & Wood, W.C. (1980). *Logotherapy: New help for problem drinkers*. Chicago: Nelson-Hall.

DeAngelis, G.G., & Goldstein, E. (1978). Long-term treatment of adolescent PCP abusers. In R.C. Petersen & R.C. Stillman (Eds.), *Phencyclidine (PCP) abuse: An appraisal*. Rockville, MD: National Institute on Drug Abuse.

De la Garza, F., Mendiola, I., & Rabago, S. (1978). Psychological, familial and social study of 32 patients using inhalants. In C.W. Sharp & L.T. Carroll (Eds.), *Voluntary inhalation of industrial solvents*. Rockville, MD: National Institute on Drug Abuse.

Done, A. (1973). Inhalants. *The technical papers of the second report of the National Commission on Marijuana and Drug Abuse*. Washington, DC: U.S. Government Printing Office.

Durden, W.D., & Chipman, D.W. (1967). Gasoline sniffing complicated by acute carbon tetrachloride poisoning. *Archives of Internal Medicine, 119*, 371–374.

Freud, S. (1959). Inhibitions, symptoms, and anxiety. In J. Strachey (Ed.), *Standard edition of the complete psychological works of Sigmund Freud* (Vol. 20). London: Hogarth Press.

Friedman, C., & Friedman, A. (1973). Drug abuse and delinquency. *The technical papers of the second report of the National Commission on Marijuana and Drug Abuse*. Washington, DC: U.S. Government Printing Office.

Goldstein, B.D. (1977). Hematotoxicity in humans. *Journal of Toxicology and Environmental Health, 2*, 69.

Goodman, P. (1960). *Growing up absurd*. New York: Random House.

Grabski, D. (1961). Toluene sniffing producing cerebellar degeneration. *American Journal of Psychiatry, 118*, 461–462.

Greenberg, D.P. (1978). Delinquency and the age structure of society. In P. Wierkman & P. Whitten (Eds.), *Readings in criminology*. Lexington, MA: D.C. Heath.

Grossett, J.T., Lewis, J.M., & Phillips, V.A. (1971). Extent and prevalence of illicit drug use as reported by 56,745 students. *Journal of the American Medical Association, 216*, 1464.

Haley, J. (1980). *Leaving home*. New York: McGraw-Hill.

Infante, P.F., Rimsky, R.A., Wagoner, J.K., & Young, R.J. (1977). Leukemia in benzene workers. *Lancet, 2*, 76.

Jackson, R., Thornhill, E., & Gonzalez, R. (1967). Glue sniffing—Brief flight from reality. *Journal of the Louisiana State Medical Society, 119*, 451–454.

Johnston, L.D., Bachman, J.G., & O'Malley, P.M. (1979). *Drugs and the class of '78: Behaviors, attitudes, and recent national trends*. Rockville, MD: National Institute on Drug Abuse.

Keniston, K. (1960). *The uncommitted*. New York: Dell.

Knox, J., & Nelson, J. (1966). Permanent encephalopathy from toluene inhalation. *New England Journal of Medicine, 275*, 1494–1496.

Kolvin, I. (1967). Aversive imagery treatment in adolescents. *Behavior Research and Therapy, 5*, 245–248.

Korman, M., Price, G., Weis, C., Semler, I., & North, A. (1977). *A psychosocial and neuropsychological study of young inhalant users: Preliminary findings*. Dallas: University of Texas Health Science Center.

Korman, M., Semler, I., & Trimboli, F. (1980). A psychiatric emergency room study of 162 inhalant users. *Addictive Behaviors, 5*, 143.

Kravaceus, W.C. (1972). Alienation as a phenomenon in youth. In W.C. Bier (Ed.), *Alienation*. New York: Fordham Univ. Press.

Laury, G. (1972). Psychotherapy with glue sniffers. *International Journal of Child Psychotherapy, 1*(2), 98–110.

Law, W., & Nelson, E. (1968). Gasoline sniffing by an adult. *Journal of the American Medical Association, 204*, 1002–1004.

Lawson, G., Petersen, J.S., & Lawson, A. (1983). *Alcoholism and the family*. Rockville, MD: Aspen Publishers.

Lawson, G. (1984). Characterizing clients and assessing their needs. In G. Lawson, D. Ellis, & P.C. Rivers (Eds.), *Essentials of chemical dependency counseling*. Rockville, MD: Aspen Publishers.

Lindstrom, K. (1973). Psychological performances of workers exposed to various solvents. *Work Environment Health, 10*, 151–155.

Louria, D.B. (1969). Medical complications of pleasure-giving drugs. *Archives of Internal Medicine, 123*, 82.

Malcolm, A. (1969). Sniffers get break . . . in chromosomes. *Medical World News, 10*, 41.

Marx, K. (1939). *The German ideology*. New York: International Publishers.

Massengale, O., Glaser, H., & Lelievre, R. (1963). Physical and psychological factors in glue sniffing. *New England Journal of Medicine, 269*, 1340–1344.

Mecir, J. (1971). Therapeutic measurements in the addiction of minors to inhalation of volatile compounds affecting activity of CNS. *Ceskoslovenska Psychiatric, 67*(4), 224–229.

Medida, M., & Cruz, A. (1972). *A survey of paint and glue inhalation among Phoenix inner-city youth*. Phoenix, AZ: Valle Del Sol.

Medina-Mora, I.M.E., Schnaas, A.A.L., Rerroba, G.G., Isoard, V.Y., & Suarez, U.C. (1978). Epidemiology of inhalant use in Mexico. In C.W. Sharp & L.T. Carroll (Eds.), *Voluntary inhalation of industrial solvents*. Rockville, MD: National Institute on Drug Abuse.

Meloff, W. (1970). An exploratory study of adolescent glue sniffers. *Dissertation Abstracts International, 31*, 1391.

Mills, C.W. (1957). *White collar*. New York: Oxford Univ. Press.

Nurcombe, B., Bianchi, G., Money, J., & Cante, J. (1970). A hunger for stimuli: The psychosocial background of petrol inhalation. *British Journal of Medical Psychology, 43*(4), 367–374.

Nylander, I. (1962). Thinner addiction in children and adolescents. *Acta Paedopsychiatrica, 29*, 73.

O'Brien, E.T., Yeoman, W.B., & Hobby, J.A.E. (1971). Hepatorenal damage from toluene in a "glue sniffer." *British Medical Journal, 2*, 29–30.

Pollack, S. (1976). *Forensic psychiatry in the defense of diminished capacity*. Los Angeles: University of Southern California Press.

Press, E., & Done, A. (1967). Solvent sniffing: Psychologic effects and community control measures for intoxication from the intentional inhalation of organic solvents. *Pediatrics, 39*(3), 451–461.

Richek, H., Angle, J., McAdams, W., & D'Angelo, J. (1975). Personality/mental health correlates of drug use by high school students. *Journal of Nervous and Mental Disorders, 160*, 435–442.

Satran, R., & Dodson, V. (1963). Toluene habituation: Report of a case. *New England Journal of Medicine, 268*, 1034–1035.

Sharp, C.W. (1977). Preface in C.W. Sharp & M.I. Brehm (Eds.), *Review of inhalants: Euphoria to dysfunction*. Rockville, MD: National Institute on Drug Abuse.

Sharp, C.W., & Korman, M. (1981). Volatile substances. In J.H. Lowinson & P. Ruiz (Eds.), *Substance abuse: Clinical problems and perspectives*. Baltimore: Williams & Wilkins.

Siegel, R.K. (1978). Phencyclidine and ketamine intoxication: A study of four populations of recreational users. In R.C. Petersen & R.C. Stillman (Eds.), *Phencyclidine (PCP) abuse: An appraisal*. Rockville, MD: National Institute on Drug Abuse.

Silberberg, N., & Silberberg, M. (1974). Glue sniffing in children: A position paper. *Journal of Drug Education, 4*, 301–308.

Skoricova, M., & Molcan, J. (1972). Catamnestic study of volatile solvent addiction. *Acta Nerv Super (Praha) 14*, 116.

Sokol, J. (1965). Glue sniffing among juveniles. *American Journal of Corrections, 26*, 18.

Stybel, J., Allen, P., & Lewis, F. (1976). Deliberate hydrocarbon inhalation among low-socioeconomic adolescents not necessarily apprehended by the police. *International Journal of Addictions, 11*, 345–361.

Sutherland, E. (1947). *Principles of criminology*. Philadelphia: Lippincott.

Taylor, G., & Harris, W. (1970). Glue sniffing causes heart block in mice. *Science, 170*, 866–868.

Tinklenberg, J., & Woodrow, K. (1974). Drug use among youthful assaultive and sexual offenders. In C. Frazier (Ed.), *Aggression*. Baltimore: Williams & Wilkins.

Vexler, S. (1972). General alienation of youth. In W.C. Bier (Ed.), *Alienation*. New York: Fordham Univ. Press.

Wallace, B.C. (1974). *Education and the drug scene*. Lincoln, NE: Professional Educators Publications.

Wyse, D. (1973). Deliberate inhalation of volatile hydrocarbons: A review. *Canadian Medical Association Journal, 108*, 71–74.

Chapter 23

Nicotine and Caffeine: The Silent Drug Problems

Gary W. Lawson and Michael Nanko

Two of the most commonly used drugs in Western society are nicotine and caffeine. It is important for the nonmedical psychotherapist to know the effects and side effects of these drugs, because they often complicate the clinical picture of a patient. Also, there may be times when a patient will seek the assistance of a therapist to stop using or at least to cut down on the use of these powerful drugs.

TOBACCO AND NICOTINE

Depending on the measure used to determine the cost to society, tobacco could be the number one drug problem in the United States. One of the most addicting drugs is nicotine, the active ingredient of tobacco. Dr. William Polin, director of the National Institute on Drug Abuse, terms cigarette smoking "the most widespread drug dependence in our country" (Whelan, 1986, pp. 91–97). The average smoker consumes 30 cigarettes a day. Each inhaled puff provides a dosage of drug that goes directly to the brain, resulting in 50,000 to 70,000 such dosages per person each year. No other form of drug use occurs with such frequency and regularity.

The addictive nature of smoking is evident in national surveys, which indicate that almost 90% of smokers would like to quit and that 85% have tried to quit but failed (Whelan, 1986). Repeated studies indicate the addictive nature of tobacco. Cigarette smokers are physically and psychologically tied to the effects of tobacco. They must have nicotine for their bodies to function efficiently. Cigarette withdrawal symptoms include significant body changes leading to decreases in heart rate, increases in appetite, disturbances in sleep patterns, anxiety, irritability, and aggressiveness.

This section examines the pharmacology of nicotine and the medical and health problems related to the use of tobacco. Trends in the use of tobacco and the complexities that make tobacco the ignored drug in American society are reviewed. Treatment approaches and the role of the nonmedical psychotherapist in the elimination of this drug problem are also addressed.

Psychopharmacology of Nicotine

Nicotine is a naturally occurring liquid alkaloid that is colorless and volatile. On oxidation it turns brown and smells much like burning tobacco. Both tolerance and dependency are among the effects of the continued use of nicotine. About 60 mg is a lethal dosage for a nonsmoking adult, although tolerance does build up rapidly. The average cigarette delivers 0.05 to 2.5 mg nicotine; low tar and nicotine cigarettes deliver less. Nicotine is an unusual drug in that it first stimulates and then depresses the nervous system. The stimulatory effect is due to the release of norepinephrine and to the fact that nicotine mimics the action of acetylcholine. Nicotine thus stimulates cholinergic nerves first, but because it is removed only slowly from the receptors the subsequent effect is depression, caused by blocked nerve activity.

The biologic half-life of nicotine in humans is approximately 20 to 30 minutes. Most of the consumed nicotine is metabolized in the liver and eliminated through the kidneys. The rate of urinary excretion is faster when the urine is acidic. Up to 90% of the nicotine is absorbed into the bloodstream when tobacco smoke is inhaled. The physiological effects of smoking one cigarette have been mimicked by injecting about 1 mg of nicotine intravenously. Low-level nicotine poisoning causes nausea, dizziness, and general weakness; these symptoms are often experienced by the first-time smoker. In acute poisoning, nicotine causes tremors that develop into convulsions and frequently end in death.

Medical Effects of Tobacco Use

The short-term effects of cigarette smoking include increased pulse rate, increased blood pressure, decreased skin temperature, feeling of relaxation (in regular smokers), increased acid in the stomach, reduced urine formation, and loss of appetite and physical endurance. Additionally, the use of tobacco stimulates and then reduces brain and nervous system activity. The long-term effects of smoking include narrowing or hardening of the blood vessels in the heart, brain, and other organs, shortness of breath, coughing, increase in respiratory infections, chronic bronchitis, emphysema, and stomach ulcers. Regular smokers increase their risk of death from lung cancer by more than 700% while simultaneously exposing themselves to other staggeringly elevated risks of cancer of the larynx (500%), mouth (300%), esophagus (400%), and bladder (100%) as well as emphysema (1300%) and coronary heart disease (100%). Moreover, all these risks are assumed at the same time. When the heavy use of alcohol is included with smoking, these risk rates more than double.

The risk of premature death is significantly higher (about 70%) for men who smoke cigarettes than men who do not. A 30-year-old male who smokes two packs a day has a life expectancy 8.1 years shorter than his nonsmoking counterpart. The risk for premature death for women would be equally as high were it not for the fact that they begin smoking later. The death rate increases with the amount smoked, and the mortality rate is greater for those who smoke longer.

Cigarette smoking during pregnancy has a significantly harmful effect on the fetus, the survival of the newborn infant, and the continued development of the child. The father's smoking, even when the mother does not smoke, may affect the fetus through secondhand smoke or through an effect on the sperm.

The use of tobacco in forms other than cigarettes is also harmful. For those who chew tobacco there is an increased risk of cancer of the oral cavity, pharynx, and esophagus. This is especially alarming because of an increase in the number of boys using chewing tobacco and snuff.

Trends in Tobacco Use

In 1964 a distinct drop in cigarette smoking occurred, and since then it has continued to decrease for adults (from 52% to 39% for males and from 32% to 29% for females). A 1975 study revealed that the number of physicians still smoking had decreased from 30% in 1967 to 21%; dentists, from 34% to 23%; and pharmacists, from 35% to 28%. In contrast, smoking by girls between the ages of 12 and 18 nearly doubled between 1968 and 1974. The age at which children begin regular smoking is down to 11 to 12 years. This is particularly alarming considering that early drug use (smoking) is often predictive of the use of stronger drugs later in life (Blum, 1984).

In 1984 the U.S. Surgeon General called for a smoke-free society. At that time, about 40% of the adult population smoked. Today 29.9% of the adult population smokes, and 87% of that population wants to quit. Nearly 25% smoke one pack a day. Although the total population that smokes is decreasing, some age groups show an increase. At present, nearly 1 million teenagers start smoking each year. A survey concerning adolescent smoking behavior in a rural school that included 82% of the entire 8th and 11th grades showed no differences between smokers and nonsmokers in knowledge of smoking effects, athletic self-perception, or exposure to smoking behavior of teachers, physicians, dentists, or clergy. Significant differences were found with respect to exposure to smoking behavior of parents, siblings, and peers. A significant association between smoking males and depression was also noted (Malkin & Allen, 1980).

Diagnosis, Treatment, and the Role of the Nonmedical Psychotherapist

The *Diagnostic and Statistical Manual of Mental Disorders* (Third Edition) (DSM-III; American Psychiatric Association, 1980) lists the following as the diagnostic criteria for tobacco dependence.

1. Continuous use of tobacco for at least 1 month.
2. At least one of the following:
   —serious attempts to stop smoking or significantly reduce the amount of tobacco use on a permanent basis have been unsuccessful;
   —attempts to stop smoking have led to the development of tobacco withdrawal;
   —the individual continues to use tobacco despite a serious physical disorder (such as respiratory or cardiovascular disease) that he or she knows is exacerbated by tobacco use. (p. 178)

Many people want to quit smoking, and many people have already stopped. Smoking is a hard habit to break, but there are ways to quit and ways for a therapist to help those individuals who want to stop.

Among the nonchemical approaches used to stop smoking are contingency contracting, relaxation exercises, acupuncture, hypnosis, and biofeedback. For most people abrupt discontinuance of smoking is preferable to cutting gradually. The withdrawal symptoms from smoking tobacco are unpleasant and uncomfortable, but they can be ameliorated by symptomatic management. Like heroin addiction, treatment of smokers should go on for months or even years after abstinence has been achieved.

The use of nicotine chewing gum as an aid to quit smoking has been reported to be effective. As in the treatment of any addiction, a combination of treatments including supportive counseling is often the most effective intervention.

Perhaps the first step for psychotherapists to take is to be role models for their patients by not smoking in the first place or by quitting if they do in fact smoke. Second, therapists could work for legislation that would keep nonsmokers from having to breathe secondhand smoke and that would make it illegal for tobacco companies to advertise to recruit new smokers. If drug abuse is ever to be dealt with effectively in this country, the most preventable drug problem, tobacco, must be addressed first.

CONSUMPTION OF CAFFEINE: CONCERNS FOR THE MENTAL HEALTH PRACTITIONER

Caffeine is a central nervous system stimulant. Although moderate use of caffeine appears in general to be a relatively benign practice, heavy and long-term use has been found to produce an array of deleterious effects on physical and mental health. Much attention has been directed toward the possible side effects of caffeine abuse (Wells, 1984). Excessively high dosages of caffeine have been associated with a whole constellation of physical ailments as well as a host of psychopathological symptoms, such as hallucinations, delusions, confused states, and, less dramatically, anxiety, agitation, and depression (Stillner, Popkin, & Pierce, 1978).

Caffeine is found naturally in coffee, tea, and cocoa. It is also a food additive that is added principally to soft drinks. One survey estimated that 2 million pounds of caffeine are added to food each year (National Research Council, 1977). As a drug, caffeine is used as a stimulant, a headache remedy, and a diuretic, and it is an ingredient in many over-the-counter medications as either the principal constituent or as an additive. In cold remedies, for example, caffeine is included to counteract the drowsiness induced by other ingredients.

Since 1946 the percentage of people who drink coffee has declined and the percentage of those who drink soft drinks has risen (Ray, 1978). In one reputable nationwide food consumption survey, the average caffeine intake of children 5 to 18 years of age was determined to be 37.4 mg per day (Morgan, Stults, & Zabik, 1982). Tea accounted for 34.2% of the total caffeine consumption, followed by soft drinks (26.4%), coffee (22.1%), and chocolate (17.3%). Coffee is still the drink of choice for adults and more so in the United States than in any other country.

Data on consumption of caffeine in over-the-counter drugs are more difficult to study. Drug companies usually do not disclose information about their sales of stimulants. Nevertheless, two investigators have reported that 15.3% of college students studied had used cold remedies in the week before their survey and that 41% had used analgesics. There is no way to determine the dosage of caffeine in these over-the-counter drugs, however (Wells, 1984). Another survey reported by Wells (1984) found that the primary source of caffeine for their subjects (college women) was from over-the-counter medications, including appetite suppressants.

The total amount of caffeine consumed is only a rough indicator of actual dosage. A more accurate measure is the milligrams of caffeine consumed per kilogram of body weight. For example, a cup of coffee at 74 mg/cup yields a dosage of 1.1 mg/kg for a 154-pound individual.

Physiology of Caffeine Use

Caffeine acts on the central nervous system in ways that are not completely known. Gilbert (1976) has done an extensive review of the literature on the physiology and biochemistry of caffeine. Briefly, caffeine acts on smooth and skeletal muscles, cardiovascular functioning, respiration, circadian rhythm, and gastrointestinal system. Ingestion of caffeine and theophylline can lead to decreased drowsiness, increased vigor, and more rapid thought. In large dosages there may be restlessness, insomnia, tremors, vomiting, and seizures. Signs of toxicity may also be headache, tachycardia, hypotension, precordial pain, and convulsions. There is variability among individuals as to sensitivity to caffeine. For example, one cup of coffee may cause tremors in some people but barely elevate the central nervous system in others. Caffeine has also been linked to birth defects in rats. Some research examined the pregnancy outcomes of women who drank more than four cups of coffee per day but did not find an association.

Metabolism

Caffeine is absorbed rapidly after oral ingestion. It appears in virtually all tissue after about 5 minutes, and peak blood plasma levels are reached within 30 minutes. Caffeine in colas is absorbed more slowly than that in coffee and tea. The half-life of caffeine in the plasma is 2.5 to 4.5 hours.

Drug Interactions

The toxic effects of caffeine can be enhanced through drug interaction. Monoamine oxidase inhibitors, for example, when taken in combination with caffeine, may lose their effectiveness by causing increased excitability or agitation. Caffeine inhibits the effects of Valium, increases central nervous system activity in combination with Darvon, and combats the depressant effects of alcohol (although it does not affect the loss of judgment or motor coordination in alcohol intoxication) (Wells, 1984).

Caffeine has been found to enhance the analgesic efficacy of acetaminophen, aspirin, or their combination. Beaver (1984), in a review of 30 clinical caffeine studies, confirms the statistically significant effect of caffeine as an analgesic adjuvant. Caffeine seems to be a safe and useful way to extend the efficacy of over-the-counter analgesics. The adjuvant effect of caffeine is not limited to pain of a particular cause. Most of the research suggests that the adjuvancy of caffeine is most reliable in combination with both aspirin and acetaminophen compared to aspirin alone.

In a comprehensive analysis of existing research, Istvan and Matarazzo (1984) found little research on combined caffeine and tobacco consumption and   myriad problems in the few studies that were done (dosage issues, coffee drinkers compared to tea drinkers, and the like). To summarize the essence of the research, there is a strong correlation beween heavy coffee drinking and smoking (heavy drinking corresponds to six or more cups per day; level of smoking not specified) and a stronger correlation in males. There was little if any correlation with tea drinking.

Tolerance, Withdrawal, and Dependence

The general consensus of the medical community is that there is usually less tolerance to caffeine's stimulant effect on the central nervous system than to most of its other effects. Interestingly, tolerance to caffeine can be eliminated by increasing the dosage (by two to four times) and by complete abstinence. Dependency on caffeine is real, and one withdrawal symptom that is well substantiated is headache, which generally develops in habitual users (five cups or more per day) after about 18 hours of abstinence. Some reports suggest that nausea and lethargy may precede the headache. This effect has been experimentally documented in several double-blind and placebo studies (Blum, 1984).

Caffeinism

Habitual high caffeine consumption has been associated with a characteristic symptom constellation known as "caffeinism," and prolonged use has been identified as a possible etiological factor in the development of a number of disease states.

The DSM-III lists maladaptive conditions related to caffeine under the diagnostic category caffeine organic mental disorder. Organic mental disorder is differentiated from organic brain disorder in that the latter refers to a constellation of psychological or behavioral symptoms and signs without reference to etiology, whereas the former designates a particular organic brain syndrome in which etiology is known or presumed. Although organic mental disorder comprises a heterogeneous group of abnormalities, the basic feature of disorders in this category is a psychological or behavioral abnormality associated with transient or permanent dysfunction of the brain.

Organic mental disorders are diagnosed by the presence of (1) one of the organic brain syndromes and (2) a specific organic factor, determined on the basis of history, physical examination, or laboratory tests, that is judged to be etiologically related to the abnormal mental state. Differentiation of organic mental disorder as a separate class does not imply that nonorganic (functional) mental disorders are somehow independent of brain processes. Rather, differentiation points out the fact that it is plainly impossible at times to determine whether a given mental disorder in an individual should be considered an organic mental disorder (because it is due to brain dysfunction of known organic etiology) or whether it should be diagnosed otherwise (because it is more adequately accounted for as a response to psychological or social factors, as in adjustment disorder, or because the presence of a specific organic factor has not been established, as in schizophrenia). The organic factor responsible for the organic mental disorder may be a primary disease of the brain or a systematic illness that secondarily affects the brain. It may also be a substance or toxic agent (caffeine) that is either currently disturbing brain function or has left some long-lasting effect.

Diagnosis

It has been projected that caffeinism affects as many as one person in ten of the general population (Kaplan & Shadock, 1981). By definition, caffeinism is a diagnosable dependence. Ingestion of caffeine is habitual, occurring in daily patterns over time. It is used primarily as a stimulant to increase alertness and reduce fatigue and is generally ingested in the form of coffee, tea, cola drinks, and over-the-counter antifatigue agents. The DSM-III is concerned with the short-term effects of excess consumption; it describes the state of caffeine intoxication as follows.

1. Recent consumption of caffeine, usually in excess of 250 mg.
2. At least five of the following:
    —restlessness
    —nervousness
    —excitement
    —insomnia
    —flushed face
    —diuresis
    —gastrointestinal complaints
    —muscle twitching
    —rambling flow of speech and thought
    —cardiac dysrhythmia
    —periods of inexhaustibility
    —psychomotor agitation

3. Not due to any other mental disorder, such as anxiety disorder

Other symptoms not listed in the DSM-III include headache, agitation, tinnitus, light-headedness, and perception of light flashes.

Diagnosis should include long-term ingestion of excessive amounts of caffeine. What constitutes an excessive amount, however, is obscured by the complexity (or the absence) of research and by the variation in habits of brewing coffee and tea. The 250 mg amount is roughly equivalent to three cups of coffee (at 74 mg/cup) with no additional medications, candy, or caffeine drinks. It is more likely that extreme symptomatology occurs at much higher levels. An intake of 1000 mg per day is cause for concern. Diagnostic inquiries of patients should therefore include reference to tea, chocolate, over-the-counter medications, and soft drinks as well as coffee. This information could be helpful in conjunction with knowledge of other drug consumption and previous medical and psychological history.

Making a positive diagnosis of caffeinism is difficult because of its interactions with various drugs and its unknown relation to anxiety and depression. Considering the estimated frequency of caffeinism and the relative infrequency with which the diagnosis is applied, it is not surprising that individuals exhibiting the effects of excessive caffeine intake are at risk of being misdiagnosed. Indeed, the symptomatology of caffeinism has been reported as a significant diagnostic dilemma because the syndrome is essentially indistinguishable from anxiety neurosis (Greden, 1974).

Presumably, routine questioning about caffeine intake would suffice to permit adequate differential diagnosis, but this questioning appears to be atypical. Attention to diet should be an important component of diagnosis and treatment. In fact, differential diagnosis may be made by first intervening in food and drug consumption and then following symptoms over the period of withdrawal.

Caffeine: A Factor in Disease States

Caffeine is also suspected of being a contributing factor in the development of a number of physical disease states. Scores of research reports conclude that hospital patients (general and psychiatric) with a daily intake of 500 to 750 mg of caffeine reported higher frequencies of psychiatric symptoms and poorer physical health.

Cardiovascular Disease

Caffeine and acute psychologic stress produce elevations in plasma epinephrine and norepinephrine paralleled by elevations in blood pressure and heart rate, in addition to other effects. The similarity of these two patterns of cardiovascular and hormonal responses suggests that stress and caffeine could interact or, more specifically, that caffeine may intensify the cardiovascular and hormonal effects produced by stress (Lane, 1983). Since caffeine consumption and stress are both common features of daily life, a caffeine-related potentiation of these harmful effects of stress could have especially important implications for the development of cardiovascular disease.

In a well-designed double-blind study by Lane (1983) on caffeine and cardiovascular responses to stress, two to three cups of coffee were found to elevate the blood pressure in healthy young men during times of both rest and stress. Blood pressure was much higher during stress conditions after caffeine had been consumed (the subjects did not normally include caffeine in their daily diet).

Studies of thousands of hospitalized patients have shown that the risk of acute myocardial infarction is 1.6 times greater than the expected rate among those drinking one to five cups of coffee per day and 2.2 times greater for those drinking six or more cups per day (Miettman, Neff, Shapiro, Heinonen, & Sloan, 1973). It appears, however, that most other studies have not been able to provide a clear association of caffeine consumption and cardiovascular disease.

Cancer

Cancer of the pancreas, one of the most fatal forms of cancer, has been found to be associated with high coffee intake. Specifically, the drinking of one to two cups per day was associated with a 1.8 increase in risk of pancreatic cancer, and drinking three or more cups per day was associated with a 2.7 increase (MacMahon, Yen, Trichopoulos, Warren, & Nardi, 1981). Overall, it appeared that more than 50% of observed pancreatic cancers may be attributable to the consumption of coffee. Less consistent data are presently available regarding the possible causal roles of tea and coffee drinking in the development of cancers at sites other than the pancreas.

Birth Defects and Pregnancy Outcomes

Much of the current concern over possible teratogenic effects of caffeine in humans stems from the demonstration of such effects in a number of animal studies (James & Stirling, 1983). Evidence from human studies is equivocal; that is, the most comprehensive examination undertaken to date of the relation between caffeine consumption and human birth defects has not revealed any evidence of such an association (Rosenberg, Mitchell, Shapiro, & Shore, 1982). It is nonetheless prudent to advise expectant mothers to abstain or limit caffeine consumption during pregnancy. Many of the studies only analyzed caffeine consumption during pregnancy. There is some evidence that pregnant women spontaneously reduce caffeine consumption for the duration of pregnancy. Therefore, pregnant women need to be studied with regard to their caffeine intake before conception to get a clearer picture as to whether any birth defects might be related.

Clinical Considerations

Many surveys have demonstrated that psychiatric inpatients (and outpatients to a somewhat lesser degree), drink significantly more coffee than nonpatients matched for age and sex. One investigation found that psychiatric patients drank twice as much as nonpatients and that the number of cups of coffee correlated with a diagnosis of personality disorder (Furlong, 1975). A study of military psychiatric inpatients revealed that the high-caffeine consumption group contained a greater proportion of psychotic patients (Winstead, 1976). Greden (1974) conducted a series of studies of psychiatric patients and caffeine intake and found that half the high users experienced serious depression and that others experienced high-state anxiety. These investigators tend to support the position that anxiety and depression can be regarded as a symptom of caffeine abuse.

The medical and psychological literature is replete with case histories of patients with no previous psychiatric history who had to be hospitalized for hallucinations after consuming large amounts of caffeine in one sitting or over longer periods of time. Typically the hallucination abated after 48 hours, and normal functioning resumed about 1 week after abstinence from caffeine (Wells, 1984).

Treatment

The treatment of caffeine addiction is not unlike the treatment of any other addiction. There are many approaches that can be used. Behavioral, cognitive behavioral, and social learning therapies have all been mentioned in the literature. It is important to manage the adverse effects of caffeine withdrawal while focusing on the health advantages that the person will gain from reducing or eliminating caffeine intake. For many people the coffee habit is connected with the cigarette smoking habit. If possible patients should be encouraged to give up both at once, since this should increase their chances of success for both. Furthermore, if exercise is included in the treatment plan the chances of success should be greatly increased.

CONCLUSION

As is the case in most areas of scientific work, the clinical and experimental research in habitual and short-term use of caffeine and nicotine is not clear-cut, and there are many methodological problems and interpretation issues. Nevertheless, both caffeine and nicotine are drugs with potentially harmful effects and, along with other drugs, should be of concern to the nonmedical psychotherapist.

REFERENCES

American Psychiatric Association. (1980). *Diagnostic and statistical manual of mental disorders* (3rd Ed.). Washington, DC: Author.

Beaver, W. (1984). Caffeine revisited. *Journal of the American Medical Association, 251*, 1732–1733.

Blum, K. (Ed.). (1984). *Handbook of abusable drugs*. New York: Gardner.

Furlong, F. (1975). Possible psychiatric significance of excessive coffee consumption. *Canadian Psychiatric Association Journal, 20*(8), 577–583.

Gilbert, R. (1976). Caffeine as a drug of abuse. In R.J. Gibbons, et al., (Ed.), *Research advances in alcohol and drug problems* (Vol. 3, pp. 49–176). New York: Wiley.

Greden, J. (1974). Anxiety or caffeinism: A diagnostic dilemma. *American Journal of Psychiatry, 131*, 1089–1092.

Istvan, J., & Matarazzo, J. (1984). Tobacco, alcohol, and caffeine use: A review of their relationships. *Psychological Bulletin, 95*(2), 301–326.

James, J., & Stirling, K. (1983). Caffeine: A survey of some of the known and suspected deleterious effects of habitual use. *British Journal of Addiction, 78*, 251–258.

Kaplan, H., & Shadock, B. (1981). *Modern synopsis of the comprehensive textbook of psychiatry* (3rd ed.). Baltimore: Williams & Wilkins.

Lane, J. (1983). Caffeine and cardiovascular responses to stress. *Psychosomatic Medicine, 45*(5), 447–451.

MacMahon, B., Yen, S., Trichopoulos, D., Warren, K., & Nardi, G. (1981). Coffee and cancer of the pancreas. *New England Journal of Medicine, 304*, 630–633.

Malkin, S., & Allen, D. (1980). Differential characteristics of adolescent smokers and non-smokers. *Journal of Family Practice, 10*(3), 437–440.

Miettman, J., Neff, O., Shapiro, R., Heinonen, S., & Sloan, D. (1973). Coffee and myocardial infarction. *New England Journal of Medicine, 289*, 63–67.

Morgan, K., Stults, V., & Zabik, M. (1982). Amount of dietary intake of caffeine and saccharin by individuals aged 5 to 18 years. *Regulatory Toxicology Pharmacology, 2*, 296–307.

National Research Council. (1977). *Estimating distribution of daily intakes of caffeine: Phase III*. Washington, DC: National Academy of Sciences.

Ray, O. (1978). Caffeine: Drugs, society and human behavior. St. Louis, MO: C.V. Mosby.

Rosenberg, L., Mitchell, A., Shapiro, S., & Shore, D. (1982). Selected birth defects in relation to caffeine-containing beverages. *Journal of the American Medical Association, 247*, 1429–1432.

Stillner, V., Popkin, M., & Pierce, C. (1978). Caffeine-induced delirium during prolonged competitive stress. *American Journal of Psychiatry, 135*(7), 855–856.

Wells, S. (1984). Caffeine: Implications of recent research for clinical practice. *American Journal of Orthopsychiatry, 54*(3), 375–389.

Whelan, E.M. (1986). Big business vs. public health: The cigarette dilemma. In W. Rucker & M. Rucker (Eds.), *Drugs, society and behavior*, 86/87 (pp. 91–97). Guilford, CT: Dushkin.

Winstead, D. (1976). Coffee consumption among psychiatric patients. *American Journal of Psychiatry, 133*(12), 1447–1450.

Part VI

Considerations for the Practitioner

The chapters in this section reflect the contents of psychopharmacology courses taught by the authors. The information presented is the result of questionnaires and discussions that revealed what the important issues were for therapists in training and will be equally useful for the practicing psychotherapist.

Chapter 24

Adverse Reactions to Drugs

Gary W. Lawson

A nonmedical psychotherapist who sees patients taking psychotropic medications must be aware of the probable adverse reactions and side effects that the patient may experience. Although the prescribing physician has ultimate responsibility for the patient's use of prescription drugs, it is often the nonmedical psychotherapist who has the most contact with the patient. A physician often prescribes medication and then does not see a patient for weeks or even months, whereas it is likely that a nonmedical psychotherapist may see the same patient several times a week or at least once a week, depending on the treatment plan for the disorder. This chapter provides a review of the adverse reactions to the major medications used in the treatment of mental disorders. (The many adverse reactions to drugs of abuse are discussed in Section V.) Therapists' sensitivity to reports of side effects is essential to the welfare of patients. In collaborating with a physician, the nonmedical psychotherapist will often have more of an opportunity to discuss these side effects with a patient than with the physician. This chapter provides the background information necessary to elicit and evaluate patients' reports of side effects.

All psychoactive drugs are capable of producing side effects. There are four major steps that may be taken to control or eliminate these effects (Honigfeld & Howard, 1978): (1) dosage reduction, (2) drug discontinuation, (3) drug change, and (4) adjunctive medication. For each of these steps, the patient must contact the prescribing physician. It would be unwise for a nonmedical practitioner to give a patient advice on taking medication other than to contact his or her physician.

For many relatively mild side effects, no special steps are necessary. Mild side effects are expected and will dissipate as the body accommodates to the drug. Thus mild effects (e.g., dry mouth or headache), which often accompany the introduction of a new psychoactive drug, can be ignored as they should disappear in a short time. Other effects such as orthostatic hypotension (feeling dizzy and light-headed upon standing because of a drop in blood pressure) are for the most part well tolerated by the patient if he or she is assured that they are normal and will go away. In such cases the physician should evaluate the potential benefits of continued use of the drug in comparison to the patient's discomfort. Often, temporary dosage reduction will eliminate side effects, and after a short while the dosage can be increased without further side effects.

Only on occasion will the medication have to be discontinued altogether. Certain rare reactions, such as those involving the liver, cardiac abnormalities, or certain blood reactions, may be life threatening, in which case the drug must be discontinued. After the condition has been treated, a psychotropic medication, perhaps of another class, can be tried.

When evaluating a patient's side effects it should be remembered that what is thought to be a side effect may in fact be a symptom of the psychiatric disorder. For example, depressed patients often report vague pains, constipation, anorexia, or loss of sexual ability, all of which are symptoms that could be expected from a depressed patient even if he or she was not taking medication. The somatic delusions of schizophrenics are also often reported as side effects of antipsychotic medications. Conversely, some unwanted drug effects can be mistaken for symptoms of psychiatric disorders. Phenothiazines often induce psychomotor slowing that can be mistaken for depression, and imipramine (Tofranil) can cause patterned visual images that can be mistaken for spontaneous hallucinations. Thus knowledge of side effects for commonly used medications can be an invaluable help in a clinical evaluation or in assessing patient reports of side effects. The nonmedical practitioner can be of assistance to both the physician and the patient when he or she is knowledgeable in this area; such knowledge can also give the patient confidence in drug therapy.

There is strong experimental evidence to indicate that the physician prescribing psychoactive drugs will achieve better results for the patient by expressing a positive attitude toward drug therapy, by telling the patient that he or she may expect relief and indicating in general the areas in which this may occur, and by telling the patient that he or she may experience common side effects such as dry mouth or drowsiness but interpreting these ahead of time in a positive manner— that is, as perhaps irritating but readily managed and a good sign that the drug is working (Fisher, Cole, Rikles, & Unlenhuth, 1964). It could be argued that such an attitude on the part of the nonmedical practitioner toward a patient's drug use could be equally as helpful toward encouraging a positive outcome.

Before presenting the side effects of each class of drugs the following overview of some of the major side effects observed in patients receiving psychotropic drugs will be presented.

DRUG SIDE EFFECTS ON THE CENTRAL NERVOUS SYSTEM

The primary side effects of psychoactive drugs on the central nervous system include parkinsonian syndrome, dystonia, akathisia, dyskinesia, and drowsiness.

These side effects are produced by all known antipsychotic drugs. Most tend to appear within the first month or so of drug treatment. The dystonias and dyskinesias can develop within 1 hour of the first administration. Some of these effects are quite dramatic and should be reported to the prescribing physician immediately.

Parkinsonian Syndrome

Symptoms of parkinsonian syndrome include muscular rigidity, tremor, postural alterations, and akinesia (decrease in spontaneous movements). Also associated with this syndrome are a fixed, masklike facial expression, shuffling gait, drooling, and loss of associated movements (free swing of arms when walking).

Dystonia

Dystonia means increasing muscular rigidity, which limits the ability to move the affected area. This condition may affect certain muscles only, resulting in asymmetric, distorted movements. An acute dystonic reaction is a sudden onset of muscle cramping.

Akathisia

Akathisia manifests itself in involuntary motor restlessness, inability to sit still, or constant fidgeting. Patients have described this as a strong feeling of inner tension and a feeling of wanting to ''jump out of their skin.'' It may be difficult to distinguish this from the primary symptom of anxiety or agitation.

Dyskinesia

Involuntary, repetitive, stereotyped movements mark the condition known as dyskinesia.

Drowsiness

Drowsiness is a common side effect of all psychotropic medications. Perhaps the two drugs that produce more sedation than any other psychotropics are chlorpromazine (Thorazine) and thioredazine (Mellaril). Many patients develop a tolerance to this effect, however, after using the drugs for a short time.

DRUG SIDE EFFECTS ON THE AUTONOMIC NERVOUS SYSTEM

There are many annoying effects to the autonomic nervous system with the use of psychotropic drugs, but most often the patient adapts to these early in treatment. These effects include blurred vision, constipation, diarrhea, dizziness, dry mouth, faintness, nasal congestion, nausea, orthostatic hypotension (faintness on rising), and urinary retention (slow-starting stream).

EFFECTS ON THE ENDOCRINE SYSTEM

Endocrine system changes may include rare but reversible effects, including galactorrhea (discharge from the nipple), gynecomastia (breast growth), and menstrual changes and amenorrhea. These effects are completely reversible on drug discontinuation and may lessen with continued use of the drug.

Two other side effects are agranulocytosis and hepatitis. The first is a blood disorder involving a drastic drop in the white blood cell count. The second is a problem associated with the liver. Both are rare and require immediate medical care.

SIDE EFFECTS OF THE MAJOR DRUG CLASSES

Antipsychotic Drugs

There are likely to be side effects with any antipsychotic drug used at therapeutic dosages. Many of these reactions, such as dry mouth, are annoying but relatively minor in nature. A number of these effects may occur at the same time, for example dry mouth, blurred vision, and dizziness. A soporific effect (drowsiness) can also be expected. This effect can be useful for patients who cannot sleep or who are only able to get a small amount of sleep. Extrapyramidal effects and dystonic reactions are common side effects with the use of antipsychotic drugs.

The long-term side effects of antipsychotic drugs, particularly the phenothiazines, include skin and eye problems and tardive dyskinesia. Eye problems include excessive pigmentation of the cornea and lens. Associated effects on skin pigmentation are due to high total drug intake. The most common skin lesion, a maculopapular rash on the upper torso and face, occurs 14 to 60 days after the onset of treatment. Other skin problems include photosensitivity reactions, which occur in about 3% of all patients. This condition can be avoided if the patient stays out of the sun or uses a sun screen lotion.

There is controversy in the literature about every aspect of tardive dyskinesia, including prevalence, etiology, and outcome. Some investigators have estimated that 3% to 5% of patients taking chlorpromazine in dosages of 500 mg/day will develop the syndrome after 1 year of treatment. It is generally agreed that it occurs most often in patients older than 60 years of age and in females twice as often as in males.

Tardive dyskinesia is characterized by stereotyped, repetitive, involuntary movements such as licking, sucking, chewing, and smacking. The muscles most commonly involved are facial, mandibular, and lingual. This condition may improve upon suspending use of the drug, although paradoxically in other cases it first appears when drug therapy is discontinued. The disorder may be permanent, but some patients do improve over time. Several medications have been used to treat the disorder, including antiparkinsonian drugs, dopamine-depleting agents, and dopamine-blocking agents. None of these has been effective in controlling the symptoms over the long term, however.

Antidepressant Drugs

Because most depressed patients require treatment at the upper end of the indicated therapeutic dosage ranges before benefits are seen, the likelihood of unwanted side effects is increased with antidepressant drugs. The two major drug groups used for the treatment of depression are the tricyclics and the monoamine oxidase inhibitors (MAOIs).

Tricyclics

The side effects of the tricyclic antidepressants are similar to those of the phenothiazines. Notable exceptions are the absence of ectodermal pigmentary alterations, amenorrhea, ejaculatory inhibition, and tardive dyskinesia. Those side effects that often occur with the use of tricyclics include blurred vision, dryness of the mouth, sweating, constipation, and urinary retention. Tolerance to these effects typically develops within a few days, however. The tricyclics are also cardiotoxic, producing such cardiovascular symptoms as orthostatic hypotension, tachycardia (rapid heart rate), and palpitations. Thus, these drugs must be prescribed with caution for individuals with heart disease. Other side effects include sedation, paresthesias (a prickling or burning sensation on the skin), tremors, confusion, anxiety, restlessness, weight gain, and insomnia. Many of these reactions can be eliminated or reduced by adjusting the dosage level. Finally, toxic effects include ataxia, delirium, seizures, cardiac dysrhythmias, and coma. Because they are toxic, these drugs should be administered with caution to suicidal patients.

MAOIs

MAOIs present special problems because of their interactions with certain foods. These foods, which are high in tyramine (a fermentation by-product), include red wine, aged cheeses, some nuts, and pickled fish. Patients on MAOIs should obtain a complete list of these foods from their physicians. They should also be alert to signs of increased blood pressure, which include severe, atypical throbbing headaches; heart palpitations; neck stiffness; sweating; cold, clammy skin; dilated pupils; chest pain; and rapid or slow heart rate.

The MAOIs are also incompatible with certain drugs, especially meperidine (Demerol), stimulants, cold tablets, and appetite suppressors. Novocaine usually contains epinephrine (Adrenalin) and is another drug that should be avoided. It is important that the patient be made aware of these hazards, and it is worth the time of the nonmedical psychotherapist to ensure that their patients who are taking MAOIs have this information.

Antimanic Drugs (Lithium)

The most common features associated with mild lithium toxicity and slightly elevated plasma lithium levels are anorexia, gastric discomfort, diarrhea, vomiting, thirst, polyurea, and hand tremor. Some of the more long-term effects include a diabetes insipidus–like syndrome, elevation of blood sugar, thyroid disturbances, and elevated white blood cell levels. Although lithium can have serious side effects if blood levels are not monitored properly, there is a progression of side effects that provide ample warning that dosage levels should be reduced. If any of the symptoms listed above should occur, the patient should be referred to the attending physician for a lithium blood level check.

Antianxiety Drugs

Antianxiety medications, or so-called minor tranquilizers, have fewer side effects than most other psychotropics. Nevertheless, there are some problems that the nonmedical psychotherapist should be aware of when a patient uses these drugs. The most common of these is the hangover effect. When these drugs are given at bedtime in dosages large enough to help the patient sleep, grogginess, drowsiness, and restlessness may occur the next morning. Laboratory studies have demonstrated that after a poor night of sleep without a drug of this type, subjects are less intellectually and motor impaired than those subjects who had a satisfactory night of sleep with the drug. This type of side effect is increased in elderly patients.

Other considerations for patients using antianxiety agents include tolerance and addiction. Patients should be warned of these problems, and the nonmedical therapist should be on the lookout for patients who seem to be less alert than could be expected. Overuse and dependence are always issues with these medications. Alcoholics may substitute these drugs for alcohol or take them in combination with alcohol. Withdrawal from these drugs always should be medically supervised.

EVALUATING MEDICAL PRACTITIONERS

All practitioners, medical and nonmedical, are likely to make errors in judgment on occasion. The nonmedical therapist is not expected to police the medical profession, but the patient's interest should always come first and if a medical practitioner makes errors the nonmedical therapist should at least advise the patient to seek a second opinion. Some of the more common errors as given by Honigfeld and Howard (1978) include the following.

(1) *Inattention to the patient's medical condition.* It is important to consider the patient's general medical condition and specific medical problems when prescribing psychotropic medications. Many of the side effects can be fatal if serious medical problems exist in conjunction with the patient taking a drug. High blood pressure and liver, kidney, or heart problems as well as prior alcoholism or drug addiction are examples of problems that a prescribing physician must be aware of to make the best clinical judgments.

(2) *Failure to perform supporting laboratory work.* In certain cases, routine blood tests and electrocardiograms are necessary to ensure that the patient is not at special risk if he or she is to receive drug therapy. Certain drugs must be monitored to be certain that the dosage is not more or less than the appropriate therapeutic dosage. For example, it is essential to check the blood levels of lithium regularly.

(3) *Prescribing too low a dosage.* Perhaps the most common error made in the prescription of psychiatric drugs is inadequate dosage. Withholding antidepressant medication in optimal amounts from the seriously depressed patient or lithium from the manic patient is analogous to withholding insulin from the diabetic patient. Where indicated, psychotropic drugs are an essential part of treatment. Although they may only be

part of an overall treatment plan that includes nonmedical psychotherapy, one portion of the treatment will not work without the other.

(4) *Inadequate drug trial*. Besides the dosage level of drugs, it is important to continue the use of the drug for a sufficient length of time to determine whether it is producing the desired effect. The antidepressants, for example, need a minimum trial period of 3 to 4 weeks.

(5) *Overreacting to changes in the patient's condition*. Another common therapeutic error is the tendency among some medical doctors to raise or lower dosage with every complaint from the patient. To many patients, medication is a reminder of past problems and signifies that they require a "crutch" to handle their problems. The physician who bends too readily to the wishes of the patient to discontinue medication is doing the patient a disservice.

(6) *Inept use of many drugs rather than skillful use of a few*. Most physicians develop some "preferred" drugs in each major classification and become familiar with the proper dosage and indications for those drugs. This is proper medical procedure, because there is little difference among the various drugs in the same class. Most physicians, for good reason, are reluctant to prescribe drugs with whose action they are unfamiliar. This keeps the patient from acting as a "guinea pig" for the physician.

(7) *Prescribing several different drugs at one time*. Prescribing two drugs simultaneously is usually unwarranted because of the difficulties in evaluating therapeutic benefits or side effects of either. This practice should be reserved for situations in which the patient exhibits only a partial effect from the highest tolerated dosage of one drug alone. A second drug may be added tentatively, if the patient is monitored closely for additional gains or side effects.

(8) *Daytime use of soporific drugs*. When soporific drugs are used, the total daily dosage should be taken at bedtime or in unequal daily dosages with the largest at night. A significant exception is lithium, which must be given in equal dosages to ensure stable blood levels.

(9) *Failure to monitor drug use*. It cannot be assumed that because a drug is prescribed the patient is taking it. Any deterioration in a patient's condition observed by the nonmedical therapist or the physician is cause for consideration as to whether the patient is taking the prescribed medication. Unless the physician has regular contact with the patient or the patient's nonmedical therapist, there will be no way of knowing whether or not the medication is being taken.

(10) *Failure to evaluate patients periodically*. When the patient has been stabilized, the physician may discontinue all drugs or place the patient on a maintenance dosage. The nonmedical therapist then must monitor the

clinical status of the patient and refer him or her to the physician if there are signs of deterioration or toxicity.

(11) *Insensitivity to risk of overdose.* In sufficiently large dosages, most psychotropic medications can be fatal. This risk varies widely among different drug classes, so that the possibility of a potential overdose should be kept in mind. Even if the patient does not appear to be suicidal, it is wise to stipulate frequent refilling of the prescription rather than a long-term supply.

(12) *Abrupt withdrawal from drugs.* The use of psychotropic drugs involves some physiological habituation. Therefore, withdrawal symptoms can be expected on abrupt discontinuation. Minor withdrawal symptoms include malaise, nausea, headache, and diarrhea; serious symptoms such as seizures are also possible. To minimize the patient's discomfort, gradual rather than abrupt discontinuation of drug use should be used.

(13) *Failure to counsel patients about drug effects.* The physician should always tell patients what they can expect from the use of a drug, including the side effects and necessary precautions for use. For example, patients taking MAOI should be provided with a list of restricted foods or cautioned against drinking alcohol.

(14) *Overuse or misuse of drugs.* The more the nonmedical therapist reads and works in the area of pharmacology, the more likely he or she is to notice if a physician is prescribing the wrong medication. For example, if a physician prescribing low dosages of antipsychotic agents for anxiety states has not tried antianxiety medications first, the nonmedical therapist should ask the patient to seek a second medical opinion unless the physician has a rationale that he or she is willing to discuss. If a close working relationship and respect have been established between the physician and the nonmedical therapist, this type of confrontation or questioning can be a learning experience for all those involved.

THE NONMEDICAL PRACTITIONER'S ROLE IN MONITORING SIDE EFFECTS

The nonmedical psychotherapist should report any adverse reactions that a patient experiences to the attending physician. The physician is accustomed to evaluating side effects and weighing therapeutic effectiveness against them. Side effects can be annoying and uncomfortable, sometimes serious, and occasionally critical. They should never be ignored.

If there is reason to believe that a physician is ignoring side effects, is unwilling to talk about side effects with the patient, or has made other errors in judgment, these concerns should be discussed openly with him or her. The physician may have an appropriate rationale for his or her actions, or the patient may have distorted the facts. Regardless, a free and open discussion of such problems should be a part of any collaborative therapeutic effort. If this is not the case, the nonmedical therapist should not hesitate to seek further medical collaboration with another physician.

REFERENCES

Fisher, S., Cole, J.O., Rikles, D., & Unlenhuth, E.H. (1964). Drug-set interaction—The effect of expectations on drug response in outpatients. In P.B. Bradley, F. Flugel, & P. Hoch (Eds.), *Neuropsychopharmacology* (Vol. 3, pp. 149–156). Amsterdam: Elsevier.

Honigfeld, G., & Howard, A. (1978). *Psychiatric drugs: A desk reference.* New York: Academic Press.

Chapter 25

Drug Therapy or Psychotherapy: A Comparison of Outcomes

Gary W. Lawson

The possibilities and combinations of types of drugs and the types of psycho-therapies or psychosocial therapies used to treat the different disorders in various combinations seem endless. Nevertheless, the outcomes are limited to the follow-ing.

1. psychotherapy does not enhance drug therapy
2. drug therapy does not enhance psychotherapy
3. psychotherapy reduces the effectiveness of drug therapy
4. drug therapy reduces the effectiveness of psychotherapy
5. drug therapy and psychotherapy complement each other

For medical or nonmedical practitioners, the most important questions are: Which will achieve the best results, drug therapy or psychotherapy? Should both be used in combination, and with which disorders? Is it possible to predict which patients will respond to a particular treatment method? The research in this area, which is flawed and conflicting, only gives information about the average patient. It is the individual patient for whom the decision is made; the right treatment for most is not necessarily right for all.

This picture is complicated by the possibility that the primary treatment profes-sional will be influenced in his or her clinical judgment by the specific training he or she has had. To assume that treatment must be aimed at either the relief of symptoms (through medication) or the resolution of problems (through psycho-therapy) is not consistent with reality and constitutes an erroneous conceptual dichotomy. A sensitive therapist must consider whether both medication and psychotherapy are called for, what the balance should be, and how that balance might change during the course of treatment. The use of medication, in addition to its physical effects, has meaning for both the therapist and the patient that can positively or negatively affect the course of treatment. Not to prescribe medication is also meaningful to the patient.

Three primary groups of clinicians are involved in making treatment decisions regarding drug therapy or psychotherapy for the mentally ill or emotionally disturbed: the nonmedical psychotherapist, the nonpsychiatric physician, and the psychiatrist. Each of these groups has its problems where such decisions are concerned. The nonmedical psychotherapist often lacks information about the use of drugs, and the nonpsychiatric physician may lack information about psychotherapy and its usefulness. These physicians also have problems placing psychotropic medications in a proper perspective. Haggerty, Evans, McCarthey, and Raft (1982) report that nonpsychiatric physicians still consider psychotropic medications general supportive measures, like laxatives and minor analgesics, rather than specific treatments for diagnosable illnesses. Ketai and Hull (1978) also demonstrate that nonpsychiatric physicians are usually poorly informed about current dosage recommendations for antidepressants.

Psychiatrists are often seen as indiscriminate drug prescribers who have little or no commitment to psychotherapy. Nonetheless, unpublished data from the preliminary analysis of the American Psychiatric Association's 1983 *Professional Activities Survey* of its members disputes this. Approximately 21,000 responses were tabulated: 65.2% of psychiatrists doing any clinical work reported that psychotherapy is the primary treatment modality for half or more of their patients. Only 5.2% reported not having any patients who received psychotherapy.

The nonmedical psychotherapist must understand as much as possible about what drugs are available for what conditions. In addition, if a medical referral is made, the therapist must be aware of the medical practitioner's views concerning drugs and psychotherapy. It is important to structure drug therapy in such a way that the patient believes that he or she is taking the responsibility for controlling his or her behavior—at the beginning, for example, by making the decision to take the drug; later on, perhaps by participating in decisions on dosage; still later on, by deciding when the medication should be discontinued; and in the end, by feeling that he or she is controlling himself or herself without any drug at all.

PROBLEMS IN RESEARCH

Several types of research can be performed: studies that measure the treatment effectiveness of a certain drug for a certain disorder, studies that measure the treatment effectiveness of a certain type of psychotherapy for a certain disorder, and studies that compare drugs and psychotherapy or various combinations of these in their usefulness with certain disorders. The data obtained from an experiment are only as good as the experimental design allows them to be. The design must control the conditions of the study as carefully as possible. Only by achieving careful control of the experimental conditions is it possible to determine whether or not the variations in treatment response are due to differences in therapeutic regimen.

Some of the obvious methodological problems include the following.

(1) *The heterogeneity of patient population.* It is important to ensure that the participants in a study are as much alike as possible, in both experimental and control groups. Variables such as environmental background, family history, degree of mental illness, and emotional problems are all important in the outcome of the study, just as variables such as body weight, diet, physical illness, and normal drug response are important in drug tests. It is difficult to control for these variables, and many studies are flawed because the investigator was unable to do so effectively.

(2) *Heterogeneity of the investigators.* In general it is wrong to assume that all therapists or all therapies are the same. This problem has plagued investigators since the beginning of scientific research on psychotherapy.

(3) *The criteria for the determination of success or failure.* How a researcher determines significance of outcome is important in a study and if done inappropriately can render the research meaningless. For example, the only criterion for success in many outcome studies for alcoholism treatment is sobriety or cessation of drinking. Sober alcoholics, however, are not always in the best psychological condition, and as a group they have a much higher suicide and divorce rate than the population in general. Studies that look at various outcomes, such as quality of life, family relationships, job satisfaction, and the like, are perhaps the most useful.

(4) *Length of treatment.* When drug therapy is compared to psychotherapy, the length of treatment becomes a major issue. For example, if a medication relieves a patient of symptoms of anxiety shortly after the patient takes it, can that be compared to a psychotherapeutic intervention that may take months but eliminates the cause of the patient's anxiety?

(5) *The placebo effect.* Many patients improve just because they think that they are taking something for their condition. Placebos, when compared to antianxiety medications, have had as high as 50% of the patients taking it reporting significant improvement in their symptoms. This effect continues to be difficult to account for and makes this type of research suspect.

There are many other problems with this type of research, including poor control groups or lack of controls, patients who get better without treatment, contamination by the effects of treatments other than the one under study, and deficient statistical presentation.

SCHIZOPHRENIA: DRUG THERAPY COMPARED TO PSYCHOTHERAPY

The effectiveness of psychotropic medication in the symptomatic treatment of schizophrenia cannot be doubted. The introduction of these powerful drugs represented such a decisive advance in the treatment of schizophrenia that the question of possible individual psychotherapy with schizophrenics seemed almost obsolete. Many of the studies that compared psychotherapy with drug treatment were done in the years shortly after the introduction of these drugs. These early studies were conclusive in their findings that neuroleptics represented a considerably more effective treatment for acute forms of schizophrenia than various types of psychotherapy; few investigators after that time looked into the question further. May (1968) summarizes the comparative studies available at the time as follows.

> *Neuroleptics versus psychotherapy* (two studies): Both studies covered large, statistically equivalent groups of patients with productive symptoms; one study compared group psychotherapy and neuroleptics, the other analytically oriented individual psychotherapy and neuroleptics. The results were similar and both trials showed the neuroleptic treatment to be markedly superior in almost all clinically relevant characteristics and symptoms.
>
> *Neuroleptics versus combined neuroleptic therapy and psychotherapy* (five studies): The results were clear here as well. There were virtually no relevant differences between patients receiving neuroleptics alone and those treated with both neuroleptics and psychotherapy. Three of the five studies involved group therapy and the other two individual psychotherapy. Neither of the two forms of therapy augmented the effect of the simultaneously administered drugs to any extent.
>
> *Psychotherapy versus combined psychotherapy and drug therapy* (two studies): In both of these studies the patients received analytically oriented individual therapy with the results that the effect of the combined therapies was vastly superior to that of psychotherapy alone. It was found in both studies that the administration of drugs certainly had no unfavorable effect on the course of the psychotherapy which had been under way for up to two years.

The conclusion of this analysis was clear: "If one were faced with the hypothetical choice of using one and only one form of treatment in addition to the usual hospital care, the objective evidence would indicate that, for the average *hospitalized* schizophrenic patient, drug therapy would at present, generally speaking and on the average, be the treatment of choice over other physical and non-physical forms of treatment" (pp. 1170–1171).

May's survey of the research related almost exclusively to hospitalized inpatients, who have a prognosis quite different from that of patients seen on an outpatient basis. In a study conducted by Hogarty and Goldberg (1973), schizophrenic patients who had been discharged after showing marked improvement and had been adjusted to outpatient treatment with a neuroleptic for 2 months were divided into four different treatment groups: chlorpromazine alone, chlor-promazine plus psychotherapy, placebo alone, and psychotherapy plus placebo.

The psychotherapy consisted of regular individual sessions covering the family, social, and professional problems affecting the patients, the number of relapses during the following 12 months being the criterion of therapeutic success. The results were as follows:

- chlorpromazine plus psychotherapy: 26% relapse
- chlorpromazine without psychotherapy: 33% relapse
- placebo plus psychotherapy: 63% relapse
- placebo without psychotherapy: 73% relapse

The results clearly confirm the efficacy of neuroleptics in preventing new schizo-phrenic attacks, whereas the protective benefit of psychotherapeutic efforts was demonstrable but quantitatively not impressive.

More recent studies (Malm, 1982) have in general provided a clear indication of the value of combined drug-based and psychotherapeutic measures in the treat-ment of schizophrenia, contradicting many of the older studies. A study of particular interest in this area was by Leff, Kuipers, Berdowitz, Eberlein-Vries, and Sturgeon (1982), which involved influencing the family living with the schizophrenic patient. By vigorously breaking down the excessively critical and over-involved behavior on the part of the spouse or parents of such patients, it was possible to reduce the relapse rate (with simultaneous administration of mainte-nance neuroleptics) from 50% in the control group to 9% in the experimental group within 9 months. The importance of the role of the family in the treatment of most psychological and emotional disorders has yet to be realized by most clinicians, and the use of the family in treatment warrants further study (Lawson, Peterson, & Lawson, 1983).

The conclusions that can be drawn from the research to date on the use of drug therapy and psychotherapy in the treatment of schizophrenia are these. (1) Neu-roleptics are far superior to psychotherapy alone as a treatment for schizophrenia (clearly, potential long-term side effects must be weighed against drug benefits); (2) the combination of neuroleptics and psychotherapy can help to prevent relapse in schizophrenia better than the use of drugs alone; and (3) interventions that involve the family and the use of maintenance dosages of neuroleptics seem to have the greatest potential.

As suggested earlier, the nonmedical therapist who works with this population should keep current on the research in this area and should maintain a positive working relationship with a medical practitioner who will be able to monitor the medication that patients of this type are likely to be taking. It is also beneficial for the nonmedical therapist to know as much as possible about the drugs used for these disorders, including the expected action and the probable side effects.

DEPRESSION: DRUG THERAPY COMPARED TO PSYCHOTHERAPY

Authorities estimate that at least 12% of the adult population has had or will have an episode of depression of sufficient clinical severity to warrant treatment (Schuyler & Katz, 1973). Although there have been advances in the chemotherapy of depression, there is no evidence that the prevalence of depression has diminished. Moreover, the suicide rate, which has generally been regarded as an index of the prevalence of depression, has not decreased and in fact has shown an increase over the past several years. The teenage suicide rate in particular seems to be rising at an alarming rate. The lack of response of the suicide rate is all the more significant in view of the enormous output of effort devoted to the setting up and maintenance of suicide prevention centers and crisis hotlines.

Therapy for depression differs in a number of critical ways from therapy for schizophrenia. Depressions usually occur in phases, and in many cases there are spontaneous remissions after several months; this makes it difficult to investigate whether the treatment was a factor in the patient's improvement. Most depressive individuals can receive ambulant treatment, which explains why the illness generally does not have a severe impact on the family and others surrounding the individual. Between acute phases, more depressives are inconspicuous and do not disrupt those around them.

The research in the area of depression includes studies that examine the value of antidepressant drugs, studies that look at various types of psychotherapy in the treatment of depression, studies that compare drug treatment with psychotherapy, and studies that examine various combinations of these interventions. It is not always easy to assess the success of antidepressant treatment accurately since, as mentioned above, depression often tends to remit spontaneously. The best estimates, based on a review of numerous controlled studies of the chemotherapy of depression, indicate that about 60% to 65% of patients studied show a definite improvement as a result of treatment with a common tricylic drug (see Beck, 1973, p. 86). This leaves 35% to 40% of patients under study who do not respond to drugs. Those investigators who support psychotherapy as a treatment for depression point out that it is the only alternate method of treatment and that it must be considered for those who do not respond to drugs. They also point out that many of those who might respond to drugs refuse to take their medication because of personal objections or side effects. These same investigators point out that, although drugs are obviously less expensive than psychotherapy, it is possible that in the long run the reliance on chemotherapy might indirectly undermine patients' utilization of their own psychological methods of coping with depression (Beck, Rush, Shaw, & Emery, 1979). The literature on "attribution" suggests the possibility that patients treated with drugs will attribute their problem to a chemical imbalance and will attribute their improvement to the drug effects (Shapiro & Morris, 1978). Therefore, as social-psychological research indicates, patients may be less likely to draw on or develop their own mechanisms to deal with the depression. The relatively high relapse rate of patients previously treated with drugs (as high as 50% in the year after the termination of drug treatment) suggests that this theory might be correct.

Beck and associates (1979) have suggested that conventional wisdom indicates that an effective course of psychotherapy might be more beneficial than chemotherapy in the long run because the patient can learn from his or her psychotherapeutic experience. Such patients might be expected to cope with subsequent depressions more effectively, to abort incipient depressions, and conceivably might even prevent subsequent depressions. They further point out that the absence of a decline in the suicide rate despite the widespread use of antidepressant drugs suggests that, even though chemotherapy may temporarily resolve a suicidal crisis, it has no sustaining effect that will inoculate the patient against making a suicide attempt at some future time. Research indicates that there is a central psychological core in the suicidal patient—namely, hopelessness (or generalized negative expectancies). Positive results from using a direct approach to the hopelessness in depressed patients suggests that cognitive psychotherapy might have longer-range antisuicidal effects than the use of drugs in the treatment of depression.

Others believe that psychotherapy may be furthered by appropriate use of medication. Mogul (1985) notes that women who are offered relief from troublesome symptoms by medication may experience the offer of medication and its effects as a manifestation of their psychiatrist's alliance with them, and their increased functional effectiveness often extends to work in psychotherapy. Several controlled studies by Weissman (1978) specifically of depressed patients show that maintenance therapy with antidepressants prevents relapse and symptom recurrence more effectively than psychotherapy alone but does not lead to much improvement in social and interpersonal functioning. These problems of living are significantly better addressed by psychotherapy, but only for patients in whom relapse is prevented. Weissman concludes that "symptom relief produced more readily by drugs rendered the patient more accessible to psychotherapy."

In each individual case it is often difficult to distinguish whether the antidepressive agent contributed to the shortening of the depressive phase or whether it would have subsided spontaneously. Psychogenic depression may subside when the exterior (social or familial) and internal (psychodynamic) surroundings of the patient change, whereas somatic depression is generally also relieved when the physical cause is eliminated. These difficulties are reflected in the results of comparative trials between antidepressants and placebo or other psychotropic medications. The number of reports showing antidepressants to be significantly superior to placebo is higher than that of studies finding no significant differences; placebo was found in 31 of 88 studies (35%) to have a therapeutic effect that was more or less equivalent to that of the antidepressant drug (Morris & Beck, 1974).

A similar conclusion is reached in an analysis by Rogers and Clay (1975). Data collected in the course of 30 comparative trials between imipramine and placebo, covering a total of 1,300 patients, yielded the following average success rates: after imipramine the condition of 62% of the patients improved ''clearly'' or ''moderately,'' while only 31% of the patients on placebo similarly improved. Outpatients and hospitalized patients with acute depression showed particularly favorable results, whereas success was only modest in patients with chronic depression who had been hospitalized for several years. Since the period covered by most of these studies was 4 to 6 weeks, it may be concluded that roughly two thirds of patients with endogenous depression showed a positive response to imipramine within approximately 1 month, while one third of those on placebo showed similar results.

There have been a number of studies that have compared drug therapy and psychotherapy (Klerman, DiMascio, Weissman, Prusoff, & Paykel, 1974; Weissman, Klerman, Paykel, Prusoff, & Hanson, 1974; Paykel, DiMascio, Klerman, Prusoff, & Weissman, 1976). In general, the investigators' evaluations of the results were as follows. Drug therapy was clearly superior to psychotherapy with regard to the prevention of relapse, although social adjustment—and hence also long-term prognosis—was improved in those patients receiving psychotherapy. Further, there was a striking difference in the effect between the two forms of treatment over time; amitriptyline worked more rapidly and strongly on the actual depressive symptoms, whereas psychotherapy acted more slowly and on different mental aspects. The two therapies were additive, as seen in the group that had drugs and high-contact psychotherapy: ''Psychotherapy is not an alternative to antidepressant treatment and does not prevent relapse or the recurrence of symptoms. Alternatively, maintenance amitriptyline has no effect on social adjustment and is no better or worse than a placebo or no pill'' (Weissman et al., 1974, p. 778). Various authors, however, have criticized these studies for design flaws and sampling errors (Spitzer, 1976).

Other studies comparing drug therapy and psychotherapy have had different results. Unlike the studies discussed above, which examined separate and possible additive effect of drug therapy and psychotherapy, a study was designed to make a direct comparison between cognitive therapy and the administration of imipramine (Rush, Beck, Kovacs, Weissenburger, & Hollon, 1982). Cognitive therapy is based on the premise that depressive patients see themselves, their world, and their future in a negative light and that this arises from various logical and conceptual errors such as arbitrary inference, selective abstraction, overgeneralization, magnification and minimization, and personalization. It is aimed at revealing to the patient his or her cognitive errors through examples and at enabling the patient to amend incorrect attitudes (Rush & Beck, 1978).

This investigation examined 41 depressed patients (26 female and 15 male) between 18 and 65 years of age, some 40% of whom had suffered from depression for more than 1 year (nine having attempted suicide). The patients were suffering from depression of moderate severity, classified as nonpsychotic, unipolar major depressive disorders (Rush et al., 1982). Treatment lasted 12 weeks and consisted of a maximum of 20 sessions of therapy lasting 50 minutes each, or alternatively 12 sessions during which pharmacotherapy was discussed. The imipramine dosage in the drug group was raised from 75 to 150 mg and finally to 200 and 250 mg. Two weeks before the final session the dosage was reduced and finally discontinued. The results were as follows. Eight patients withdrew from the imipramine group, significantly more than those who withdrew from the psychotherapy group (one patient). Both forms of therapy led to highly significant improvements in all rating scales, although the psychotherapy was more effective than the drug therapy. The final evaluation, based on the Beck depression scale, is shown in Table 25-1.

The investigators concluded from these results that cognitive therapy was superior to treatment with imipramine, a claim that was further supported by the observation that after the end of the trial more patients from the imipramine group had to undergo additional treatment than was the case in the psychotherapy group. A follow-up examination 6 months after the conclusion of the study showed, however, that the difference between the treatment groups was no longer significant.

The study by Rush and co-workers (1982) is occasionally taken as proof that psychotherapy is superior to drug therapy in treatment of depressive states. Nevertheless, there are those who point out several criticisms of the study, not the least of which is the decision to withdraw the drug 2 weeks before the end of the study (Spiegel & Aebi, 1983, p. 209).

Some 10% to 15% of all affective illnesses are manic-depressive or bipolar. In these patients, lithium prevents the reappearance of the manic phase, although its efficacy is somewhat less pronounced in the case of depressive phases. In controlled studies of between 5 and 28 months' duration involving patients with

Table 25-1 Results of Comparison between Cognitive and Pharmacological Therapies

Outcome	Cognitive Therapy	Imipramine
Significantly improved or cured	15 patients	5 patients
Partially improved	2 patients	6 patients
Not improved	1 patient	3 patients
Withdrew	1 patient	8 patients

bipolar depression, the relapse rate was an average of 79% with placebo and 35% with lithium (Prien & Caffey, 1977). (For more information about the effectiveness of lithium, see Chapters 5 and 11.)

Even with conflicting findings, in many of these studies the following conclusions can be made with regard to the treatment of depression: (1) a number of treatment methods can lead to the final goal; (2) different treatment approaches are not necessarily mutually exclusive; (3) psychotherapy can mitigate problem areas that do not respond to drugs; and (4) maintenance drug therapy is useful for those patients whose acute depression has already abated under the effects of antidepressant drugs.

Again it is recommended that a therapist who sees depressed patients on a routine basis keep abreast of the newest developments not only in drug therapy but in approaches to psychotherapy in the treatment of depression. The possible advantages of family therapy for the treatment of depression should not be overlooked.

NEUROTIC ANXIETY DISORDERS: DRUG THERAPY COMPARED TO PSYCHOTHERAPY

Anxiety and tension are commonly encountered in all forms of clinical practice, but the classification of these disorders is not entirely agreed upon. It is important for the therapist to understand the differences between the various disorders so that clinically accurate decisions can be made related to the use of psychotherapy, drug therapy, or a combination of the two. It is characteristic for anxious patients to demand treatment in various ways and on repeated occasions, thus putting pressure on the therapist. If the patient's first contact is with a medical general practitioner, as is often the case, this pressure is generally met with a prescription for a tranquilizer (Rose, 1983). Although education and counseling are probably the best solution for most forms of anxiety (when they are successful), failure is common. This does not encourage medical general practitioners to commit the large amounts of time required to deal with these patients. Questions of when to use drugs and when to use psychotherapy or a combination are best answered where an in-depth diagnosis is available to guide the practitioner. Often the nonmedical practitioner is in the best position in terms of time and training to provide this diagnosis.

The *Diagnostic and Statistical Manual of Mental Disorders* (Third Edition) (DSM-III; American Psychiatric Association, 1980) separates stress and adjustment reactions with predominant anxiety from anxiety neurosis. It also separates anxiety disorders into panic disorder, generalized anxiety disorder, and agoraphobia, the last of which is also subdivided into two groups depending on the presence or absence of panic attacks. Decisions concerning treatment of these conditions should be made separately.

Acute Stress Reactions

Stress reactions (otherwise known as posttraumatic stress disorder) are transient disorders of mood occurring in apparently normal individuals in response to exceptional physical and mental stress. The more the clinician knows about the patient and the specific personal impact of the stress, the more appropriate the treatment decisions will be. Whether and how long to use drugs are particularly important issues. Drug therapy may be ill advised if the stress has important personal implications that need to be worked through. There is a body of literature that indicates the need for grief and other emotions to be experienced openly after a major loss if subsequent depressive illness is to be avoided (Freud, 1917; Lindemann, 1944; Bowlby, 1973). If drugs are prescribed to alleviate the distress that immediately follows an unexpected bereavement, it would probably help in the short term; if such a drug also aids the process of denial, it could create long-term pathology. Research is scanty in this area because of the unpredictability and emergency nature of the disorder.

If drug therapy is chosen, benzodiazepines are probably the drugs of choice. Their dosage can be flexible in both quantity and frequency, which is preferable in this instance to a fixed dosage. A maximum daily dosage should be prescribed at a low level. Severe insomnia occurring in response to stress may also be treated with these drugs. It is unusual to continue drug therapy for longer than a few days and certainly no longer than a week. The danger of continuing beyond this point is that the pleasurable antianxiety qualities of benzodiazepines may so impress the patient that further prescriptions are requested long after the initial stress has been overcome (Rose, 1983).

Anxiety States

Anxiety states are different from stress reaction and adjustment reaction in that they tend to be precipitated by less serious events and occur in individuals who are less prone to anxiety. Anxiety presents with the psychological symptoms of irritability, apprehension, awareness of threat, and restlessness and the somatic symptoms of muscular tension, trembling, palpitations, sweating, nausea, and giddiness. Anxiety may be seen on a continuum, with most psychological symptoms on one end and most somatic symptoms on the other. These two conditions have been labeled anxiety hysteria and conversion reaction, respectively, although these terms are somewhat outdated. Minor tranquilizers are probably the drug treatment of choice unless secondary depressive symptoms are present, in which case an antidepressant may be preferred. It is important for the nonmedical practitioner to assess the level of depression and pass this information on to the prescribing physician.

Panic Disorder

In the DSM-III, panic disorder is described as a disorder manifested by the sudden onset of intense apprehension, fear, or terror often associated with feelings of impending doom. If such attacks occur in patients with generalized anxiety, the diagnosis is still panic disorder. The main reason for this diagnostic separation is the apparent differential response to behavior therapy and drug therapy. Klein (1964) argues that panic disorder should not be treated with benzodiazepines and is more responsive to antidepressant drug therapy. In studies conducted in Great Britain, however, panic was not normally considered a contraindication to benzodiazepine therapy (Rose, 1983).

Phobic Disorders

Agoraphobia and social phobias are appropriately treated with minor tranquilizers, but monosymptomatic phobias—such as those of dogs, snakes, and heights—are best treated by behavioral techniques that expose the patient to the feared object. When minor tranquilizers are not effective, as is the case with many chronic phobic disorders, it may be appropriate to try a monoamine oxidase inhibitor (Lipsedge et al., 1973).

Differing viewpoints concerning the etiology of anxiety often reflect no more than the training of the individual making the observation. Neurophysiologists emphasize the importance of the ascending reticular formation and the limbic system. Psychobiologically trained therapists stress the importance of inherited and developmental factors, and psychoanalysts concentrate on internal psychic conflict. Nonmedical psychotherapists who treat anxiety with psychological methods are no different, and they pay a great deal of attention to whether or not external contingencies can be identified when a particular patient is being assessed. Anxiety can be loosely arranged along a continuum according to the degree of specificity of external stimuli that precipitate the anxiety (Figure 25-1). There is now strong empirical evidence that psychological treatments based on behavioral principles such as in vivo exposure are increasingly effective toward the high-stimulus end of the spectrum (Marks, 1981). More than 90% of patients with simple animal phobias can be cured by means of this method, and two thirds of patients with agoraphobia or social phobia can be helped to overcome their

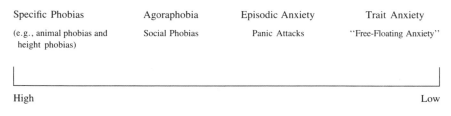

Figure 25-1. Levels of External Stimuli Leading to Anxiety

problems. These approaches can be classified according to which of the three components of anxiety—the behavior, the thoughts or cognitions, and the physiological sensations—that the therapist targets as a goal.

Methods Aimed at Changing Behavior

Exposure in vivo is the most extensively researched psychological method used in the treatment of anxiety. Its effectiveness in anxiety associated with simple phobias, agoraphobia, social phobia, and obsessive-compulsive rituals has been demonstrated in well-designed, controlled studies in a number of countries (Marks, 1981). Treatment gains include not only a decrease in avoidance behavior but also a decrease in generalized anxiety and improvement in general functioning. Follow-up studies demonstrate that gains are maintained for up to 9 years (Munby & Johnston, 1980). Despite this being a symptom-oriented treatment, no evidence of symptom substitution has been reported. Treatment is as effective in the hands of specially trained nurse therapists as when applied by psychiatrists or psychologists (Marks, Bird, & Lindley, 1978).

Methods Aimed at Inducing Cognitive Change

A cognitively oriented therapist intentionally, directly, and overtly attempts to alter perception, memory, attitude, and controllability of the patient as well as the amount of information that the patient has in stressful situations. The aim is to correct misperception, misinterpretation, incompatible attitudes, and counterproductive styles of thinking. Reduction of unpleasant affect or uncomfortable physiological sensations is not the primary target of therapy, and the emphasis is on coping with disabling symptoms rather than eliminating them altogether.

There are a greater number of studies evaluating cognitive methods in the treatment of depression than those evaluating such methods for anxiety. Nevertheless, those studies that are available show encouraging results. Jannoun, Oppenheimer, and Gelder (1982) used a time-series design to study 27 patients experiencing anxiety state who were given anxiety management training and evaluated by independent assessors after the training and again 3 months later.

They showed significant and lasting treatment effects. In another study, Woodward and Jones (1980) examined the treatment of 27 outpatients experiencing general anxiety who were selected from a hospital waiting list. A no-treatment control group was compared to a "pure cognitive restructuring" group, a "modified systematic desensitization" group, and a combined treatment group that they called "cognitive behavioral modification." All active treatments were superior to the control, and the combined treatment was significantly better than both the other active treatments.

In summary, psychological methods are well established in the treatment of conditions where anxiety is of a phobic type. As far as their use in more general forms of anxiety is concerned, psychological methods may be described as promising but for the most part unproven.

Controlled studies also show tranquilizers to be superior to placebo in the treatment of acute anxiety symptoms. The symptomatic efficacy of these drugs has been demonstrated in hundreds of individual investigations; according to a survey by Freedman (1980), in 80% to 90% of all controlled studies the effects of tranquilizers were clearly superior compared to placebo. The success rate appears to be independent of the nature of the functional symptoms. Most investigators recommended that tranquilizers not be administered for more than 6 to 12 weeks and that psychotherapy be undertaken wherever possible in the cases of disorders of longer duration (del Giudice, 1978).

Combining drug therapy and psychotherapy has certain advantages. In 13 of 16 comparative trials between psychotherapy and a combination of drug therapy and psychotherapy, combined therapy was more effective in the treatment of states of tension and anxiety as well as in neurotic disorders. Of 16 studies, 3 showed no significant differences. Of 11 comparisons between drug therapy on the one hand and combined therapy on the other hand, 6 showed the combined therapy to be superior and 5 comparisons yielded no significant differences (Luborsky, Singer, & Luborsky, 1975; Freedman, 1980).

A recent development has been the use of the so-called β-blockers in the treatment of the vegetative concomitant symptoms of states of anxiety and tension (Kelly, 1980; Suzman, 1981). Students worried about exams achieved better results with β-blockers during controlled studies than with diazepam and placebo (Freedman, 1980). Musicians and lecturers were able to combat their stage fright because the β-blockers are able to suppress peripheral arousal, and as a result the state of agitation loses a great deal of its severity while mental clarity and artistic performance are unimpaired (Neftel et al., 1982).

Methods Aimed at Peripheral Physiological Change

The relaxation response, which involves a generalized reduction in multiple physiological systems, can be achieved by a wide variety of means. These include progressive muscular relaxation, autogenic training, methods involving the induction of various fantasies, hypnosis, and meditation techniques. Several studies have demonstrated a lack of consistent differences between the various methods of inducing relaxation. For example, transcendental meditation produces similar results to those of muscular relaxation (Thomas & Abbas, 1978), as does biofeedback (Townsend, House, & Addario, 1975). Interestingly, prayer by itself was found to be significantly less effective than relaxation training (Elkins, Anchor, & Sandler, 1979). Though several different techniques have similar effects, the method of application appears to be important. Regular practice enhanced beneficial effects (Lavall'ee et al., 1976) and live relaxation was more effective than taped instructions (Beiman et al., 1978).

CONCLUSION

In the final analysis, it is the clinical judgment on the part of the primary treatment provider, whether he or she is a medical or a nonmedical therapist, that determines the treatment approach. There are many aspects to consider when attempting to provide the best treatment approach for any specific disorder with a specific individual.

REFERENCES

American Psychiatric Association. (1980). *Diagnostic and statistical manual of mental disorders* (3rd ed.). Washington, DC: Author.

Beck, A.T. (1973). *The diagonosis and management of depression.* Philadelphia: Univ. of Pennsylvania Press.

Beck, A.T., Rush, J., Shaw, B.F., & Emery, G. (1979). *Cognitive therapy of depression.* New York: Guilford Press.

Beiman, I., Israel, E., & Johnson, S.A. (1978). During training and post-training effects on live and taped extended progressive relaxation, self relaxation and electromyogram feedback. *Journal of Consulting Psychology, 46,* 314–321.

Bowlby, J. (1973). *Attachment and loss. Part 2: Separation, anxiety and anger.* London: Hogarth Press.

del Giudice, J. (1978). Clinical use of anxiolytic drugs in psychiatry. In W.G. Clark & J. del Giudice (Eds.), *Principles of psychopharmacology.* (pp. 561–571). New York: Academic Press.

Elkins, D., Anchor, K.N., & Sandler, H.M. (1979). Relaxation training and prayer behavior as tension reduction techniques. *Behavioral Engineering, 5,* 81–87.

Freedman, A.M. (1980). Psychopharmacology and psychotherapy in the treatment of anxiety. *Pharmakopsychiatry, 13,* 277–289.

Freud, S. (1917). Mourning and melancholia. In *Collected Papers* (Vol. 4, pp. 237–246). London: Hogarth Press.

Haggerty, J.J., Evans, D.L., McCarthey, C.F., & Raft, D. (1982). Psychotropic prescribing patterns of nonpsychiatric residents in a general hospital. *Hospital and Community Psychiatry, 37*(4), 357–361.

Hogarty, G.E., & Goldberg, S. (1973). Drug and sociotherapy in the aftercare of schizophrenic patients: One-year relapse rates. *Archives of General Psychiatry, 28,* 54–64.

Jannoun, L., Oppenheimer, C., & Gelder, M. (1982). Treatment for anxiety. *Behavioral Therapy, 13,* 103–111.

Kelly, D. (1980). Clinical review of beta-blockers in anxiety. *Pharmakopsychiatry, 13,* 259–266.

Ketai, R.M., & Hull, A.L. (1978). Tricyclic antidepressant prescribing habits: A comparison of family physicians and psychiatrists. *Journal of Family Practice, 7,* 1011–1014.

Klein, D.F. (1964). Delineation of two drug-responsive anxiety syndromes. *Psychopharmacologia, 5,* 397–408.

Klerman, G.L., DiMascio, A., Weissman, M., Prusoff, B., & Paykel, E.S. (1974). Treatment of depression by drugs and psychotherapy. *American Journal of Psychiatry, 131,* 186–191.

Lavall'ee, Y.J., Lamontagne, Y., Pinard, G., Annable, L., & Tetreault, L. (1976). Effects of EMG feedback, diazepam and their combination on chronic anxiety. *Journal of Psychosomatic Research, 21,* 65–71.

Lawson, G., Peterson, J.S., & Lawson, A. (1983). *Alcoholism and the family: A guide to treatment and prevention.* Rockville, MD: Aspen Publishers.

Leff, J., Kuipers, L., Berdowitz, R., Eberlein-Vries, R., & Sturgeon, D. (1982). A controlled trial of social intervention in the families of schizophrenic patients. *British Journal of Psychiatry, 141,* 121–134.

Lindemann, E. (1944). Symptomatology and management of acute grief. *American Journal of Psychiatry, 101,* 141–150.

Lipsedge, M.S., Hafioff, J., Huggins, P., Napier, L., Pearce, J., Pike, D.J., & Rich, M. (1973). The management of severe agoraphobia: A comparison of iproniazid and systematic desensitisation. *Psychopharmacologia, 32,* 67–80.

Luborsky, L., Singer, B., & Luborsky, L. (1975). Comparative studies of psychotherapies. *Archives of General Psychiatry, 32,* 995–1008.

Malm, U. (1982). The influences of group therapy on schizophrenia. *Acta Psychiatry Scandinavia, 65* (Suppl.), 1–65.

Marks, I.M. (1981). *Cure and care of neuroses.* New York: Wiley.

Marks, I.M., Bird, J., & Lindley, P. (1978). Psychiatric nurse therapy: Developments and implications. *Behavioral Psychotherapy, 6,* 25–36.

May, R.A. (1968). Anti-psychotic drugs and other forms of therapy. In D.H. Dfron, J.O. Cole, J. Levine, and J.R. Wittenborn (Eds.), *Psychopharmacology: A review of progress* (PHS Publication No. 1836, pp. 1155–1176). Washington, DC: U.S. Government Printing Office.

Mogul, K.M. (1985). Psychological considerations in the use of psychotropic drugs with women patients. *Hospital and Community Psychiatry, 36*(10), 1080–1085.

Morris, J.B., & Beck, A.T. (1974). The efficacy of antidepressant drugs. *Archives of General Psychiatry, 30,* 667–674.

Munby, M., & Johnston, D.W. (1980). Agoraphobia: The long-term follow-up of behavioral treatment. *British Journal of Psychiatry, 137,* 418–427.

Neftel, K.A., Adler, R.H., Kaeppeli, L., Rossi, M., Dolder, M., Kaeser, H.E., Bruggesser, H.H., & Vorkauf, H. (1982). Stage fright in musicians: A model illustrating the effect of beta blockers. *Psychosomatic Medicine, 44,* 461–469.

Paykel, E.S., DiMascio, A., Klerman, G.L., Prusoff, B.A., & Weissman, M.M. (1976). Maintenance therapy of depression. *Pharmacopsychiatry, 9,* 127–136.

Prien, R.F., & Caffey, E.M. (1977). Long-term maintenance drug therapy in recurrent affective illness: Current status and issues. *Diseases of the Nervous System, 38,* 981–992.

Rogers, S.C., & Clay, P.M. (1975). A statistical review of controlled trials of imipramine and placebo in the treatment of depressive illness. *British Journal of Psychiatry, 127,* 599–603.

Rose, A.J. (1983). Controversies in practice. In M.R. Trimble (Ed.), *Benzodiazepines divided* (pp. 61–65). New York: Wiley.

Rush, A.J., & Beck, A.T. (1978). Cognitive therapy of depression and suicide. *American Journal of Psychotherapy, 32,* 201–219.

Rush, A.J., Beck, A.T., Kovacs, M., Weissenburger, J., & Hollon, S.D. (1982). Comparison of the effects of cognitive therapy and pharmacotherapy on hopelessness and self-concept. *American Journal of Psychiatry, 139,* 862–866.

Schuyler, D., & Katz, M.M. (1973). *The depressive illness: A major public health problem.* Washington, DC: U.S. Government Printing Office.

Shapiro, A.D., & Morris, L.A. (1978). Placebo effects in medical and psychological therapies. In S.L. Garfield & A.E. Bergin (Eds.), *Handbook of psychotherapy and behavior change: An empirical analysis* (2nd ed.). New York: Wiley.

Spiegel, R., & Aebi, H. (1983). *Psychopharmacology: An introduction.* New York: Wiley.

Spitzer, R.L. (1976). Discussion of paper by Weissman et al. (1976). In R.L. Spitzer & D.F. Klein (Eds.), *Evaluation of psychological therapies* (p. 178). Baltimore: Johns Hopkins Univ. Press.

Suzman, M.M. (1981). Use of beta-adrenergic receptors blocking agents in psychiatry. In G.C. Palmer (Ed.), *Neuropharmacology of central nervous system and behavioral disorders* (pp. 339–391). New York: Academic Press.

Thomas, D., & Abbas, D.A. (1978). Comparison of transcendental meditation and progressive relaxation in reducing anxiety. *British Medical Journal, 2,* 1749–1752.

Townsend, R.E., House, J.F., and Addario, D. (1975). A comparison of biofeedback-meditated relaxation and group therapy in the treatment of chronic anxiety. *American Journal of Psychiatry, 132,* 598–601.

Weissman, M.M. (1978). Psychotherapy and its relevance to the pharmacotherapy of affective disorder: From ideology to evidence. In M.A. Lipton, A. DiMascio, & K.F. Killam (Eds.), *Psychopharmacology: A generation of progress* (pp. 771–778). New York: Raven.

Weissman, M.M., Klerman, G.L., Paykel, E.S., Prusoff, B., & Hanson, B. (1974). Treatment effects on the social adjustment of depressed patients. *Archives of General Psychiatry, 30,* 771–778.

Woodward, R., & Jones, R.B. (1980). Cognitive restructuring treatment. *Behavioral Research Therapy, 18,* 401–407.

Chapter 26

Collaboration between the Medical and Nonmedical Professions

Gary W. Lawson

This chapter calls attention to the working relationship between the physician and the nonmedical practitioner. Some suggestions for making the best out of this relationship, with the patient as the ultimate beneficiary, are provided, and some of the problems that have kept the nonmedical psychotherapist from working hand-in-hand with medical professionals are examined. Possible future directions are suggested for those working in the field of nonmedical psychotherapy to improve their working relationships with physicians.

PROBLEMS IN THE RELATIONSHIP

Of the present health care services in the United States, only a small proportion (2% to 3%) is directed toward outpatient mental health services. Of this small proportion, psychiatrists comprise 70%, psychologists 18%, and social workers 12%. Psychologists in particular are increasingly beginning to feel that their livelihood is being threatened as large corporations turn to self-insurance, under which their services are excluded (Berg, 1986). Where they are included as service providers, it is only under the direct supervision of a physician. Situations such as these do not improve the working relationships between professions; in fact they may cloud other areas where compromises could be reached.

There is a considerable difference between psychiatrists and other types of physicians with regard to their relationship with nonmedical psychotherapists. The psychiatrist often suffers an identity conflict within the medical profession. Psychiatrists have often been regarded by other medical professionals as ineffective practitioners, as not being ''real doctors,'' and as being unscientific. Often the media and literature characterize them negatively and question their value (Berg, 1986). This can only increase the level of tension between them and their nonmedical colleagues. The animosity goes both ways, as reflected by a common characterization of psychiatrists by psychologists: psychiatrists are "those who study medicine and don't practice it and those who practice psychology without studying it."

The reality, however, is that all mental health professions have their strengths and weaknesses and that all the helping professions have skills in common with each other. The key to the professionals working together is for each to recognize their own and others' unique qualifications. It is equally important for all to recognize the skills and information that must be shared to provide the best mental health service possible for patients. For example, it would be unfair to the patient for a nonmedical practitioner to neglect the use of medication because of a lack of information about psychopharmacology, and it would be unwise for a medical practitioner to overmedicate a patient because of a lack of reasonable psychotherapeutic skills.

If a psychotherapist is to deal adequately with patients undergoing drug therapy, it is essential that he or she be aware of the various effects of the different drugs in terms of both therapeutic and side effects. This information cannot be considered under the sole proprietorship of the medical professional. In fact, in the best of circumstances the patient will take an active role in both choosing drugs and managing side effects. The more information he or she has about psychopharmacology, the better the ultimate decisions regarding his or her mental and physical health.

During the process of determining what services will be provided and who will provide them, the patient's best interests should be the final consideration. Even where this is a goal, however, there can be problems. In a position paper of the Canadian Psychiatric Association, where such a goal was stated, the following position was taken:

> The diagnosis of a patient's condition is a mandatory prerequisite for proper treatment. The psychiatrist through his medical education and training is the only one competent to formulate a differential diagnosis and from this to develop a protocol for the investigation, rational therapy and rehabilitation of each patient. . . . The Association deplores any concerted effort by a profession to redefine its own identity by making the case for equivalence or superiority in a delineated skill and/or ability and broadening the claim to equivalence with another profession, with a striving for independent functioning being the ultimate professional goal. Patient needs must have primacy over professional aspirations; the issue is not one of equality in the performance of a number of skills, but equivalence in overall training (El-Guebaly, 1984, pp. 163–168).

There seem to be several problems with regard to this position. First is the assumption that there are enough psychiatrists to do all diagnosing and treatment planning, with little or no delay or inconvenience to patients. This is not the case.

Psychiatrists are generally in short supply, which raises the second point: it is often assumed that all psychiatrists are equally trained or that they meet some minimum level of advanced training in psychiatry that somehow prepares them better than nonmedical psychotherapists to make a differential diagnosis. However, according to Kopp (1972), because of a shortage of psychiatrists willing to work in public psychiatric facilities and state hospitals, doctors trained in non-English–speaking countries and who have no psychiatric training beyond that received during a 1-year residency may be allowed to act as psychiatrists in these institutions. Many of them go on to practice psychiatry in private practice after they have passed their medical examinations. This does little to encourage confidence in the training or ability of psychiatrists, especially since the practice of psychiatry calls for an ability to communicate at an advanced level in the language of the patient. To practice without this skill is not in the best interests of the patient.

This example is provided not to belittle the psychiatric profession but to point out some of the complexities involved in the continuing effort to clarify the roles of each mental health profession. Even within professions there are disagreements as to roles. The American Psychological Association has over 45 different divisions, and each one has a goal of defining and protecting its domain. The divisions of clinical and counseling psychology are often in conflict regarding issues of who is qualified to perform various functions. New divisions such as the Division of Family Therapy are also involved in such issues. It appears that the more the specializations are alike the more conflicts there are among them.

Different perspectives on how to approach mental health issues also cause problems. As Berg (1986) states, "Whereas the orthodoxy of medicine relies on time-tested procedures, clinical psychology is oriented toward technical innovations based on research. Consequently, the psychologist's proposals for new methods are frequently met with wary caution by the more conservative psychiatrist" (pp. 52–59). Differences in perspective are rooted in differences in training. The psychologist's academic training supports skepticism and questioning of assumptions. Differing views and theories encourage debate over ideas. This contrasts with the medical education of the physician, which emphasizes mastery of volumes of concrete facts.

Against this background of conflict and rivalry it may seem to be impossible for nonmedical practitioners ever to work hand-in-hand with their medical colleagues, particularly psychiatrists. The position that all have in common, however, is the best interests of the patient, and it is from that starting point that all can begin to resolve the issues that keep the professions at odds.

SUGGESTIONS FOR WORKING WITH MEDICAL PROFESSIONALS

The amount and type of contact that a nonmedical therapist has with a medical doctor is determined by the type of clients he or she has. A school psychologist might have little contact with medical professionals, and a therapist in a community mental health clinic might have a great deal of contact. It is hard to imagine a psychotherapist who has no contact with a medical practitioner, however. When it becomes necessary to make this contact, the following suggestions will be of benefit to the nonmedical psychotherapist.

1. The best interests of the patient must always be kept in mind. When this is the case, the therapist's relationship with the physician is likely to be a positive one. If there are conflicts or differences of opinion about treatment procedures, the physician should be reminded that the therapist only has the patient's best interests in mind.

2. The physician's time should be respected. Most physicians are busy people, and they would appreciate brevity. The therapist should therefore be prepared when discussing a case with a physician. If a prescription for a patient or some medical information is needed, that point should be made directly and specifically.

3. A professional attitude should be maintained in all relationships, whether a telephone call is being made or a letter requesting information is being sent. Again brevity, specificity, and directness are essential.

4. A signed release should always be obtained from the patient before consultations about the patient are undertaken. The physician should be informed that the release has been obtained and should be offered a copy. When writing for information, the therapist should always include a signed release from the patient in question.

5. Attempts to impress a physician with knowledge of psychopharmacology or psychology are misdirected. It is appropriate to establish a basis for professional discussion, but the therapist should not press the point.

6. The therapist's training and experience should not be underrated, nor should the abilities of the physician be overrated. Both have areas of expertise that should be respected. If the therapist is dissatisfied with one physician's advice or assistance, a second opinion should be sought.

7. If a therapist receives a physician's referral, he or she should always provide a "thank you" and follow-up information about progress with the patient.

8. Records should be kept of the contacts that the therapist makes on behalf of a patient, and the patient should be informed of the intent of the contact.

9. It should be kept in mind that some medical doctors will be easy to work with and some will not be. Doctors who are found to be especially cooperative or compatible should be retained as the therapist's main medical referral sources.

10. Since many physicians are not extensively informed as to the training of nonmedical psychotherapists, providing such information as the professional relationship develops and as time permits is an excellent way to solidify contacts.

Most of these suggestions are simply common sense, but they are worth mentioning here for review purposes or for the new therapist working for the first time on a professional basis with a medical practitioner.

IMPROVING RELATIONS FOR THE FUTURE

It is clear that when nonmedical psychotherapists and medical doctors work in coordination and harmony with one another the patient is the one who benefits the most. The following suggestions are aimed at improving the working relationship between the professions.

The place to begin is the training of each professional. The nonmedical therapist should have as part of his or her training some formal coursework about how to use the medical professional as a resource. The medical practitioner should in turn be taught as part of his or her medical training how best to take advantage of a relationship with the nonmedical psychotherapist.

From there it is a logical extension to focus on similarities and to learn to appreciate differences. For example, physicians and therapists can work together to develop prevention programs or to develop plans to promote mental health through institutions such as schools or families. Conventions, professional meetings, and professional organizations can be jointly arranged and attended; to some extent this has been accomplished through organizations such as the American Association of Orthopsychiatry, which is open to all mental health professionals. A more global view of mental health will promote working together in the best interests of those served.

REFERENCES

Berg, M. (1986). *The American Psychologist, 41*, pp. 52–59.

El-Guebaly, N. (1984). "The interaction with allied non-medical professions: The Canadian Psychiatric Association's guidelines." *Canadian Journal of Psychiatry. 29*, pp. 163–168.

Kopp, S.B. (1972). *If you meet Buddha on the road, kill him!* Palo Alto, CA: Science and Behavior Books.

Chapter 27

A Final Note on the Future

Gary W. Lawson

It should be clear by now to nonmedical therapists as well as to medical professionals that psychopharmacology does not include only the basic understanding of physiological actions of psychoactive compounds. There are many considerations when a chemical is used to alter the mind, either as a medical intervention or for recreational purposes. Many issues are as yet unresolved, including questions that relate to the human behaviors involved in drug use. What is it about the human condition that makes people want to escape into the world of drugs? What causes the conditions that call for psychotropic medications? Are there physical problems or chemical imbalances in the body that lead to psychological disorders, or are there perhaps environmental conditions that lead to chemical changes that in turn lead to behavior changes? What interventions are necessary under these circumstances?

The advances in clinical psychopharmacology over the past 20 years have been enormous, but they will seem small when compared to the advances that probably will be made in the next 20 years. For example, as this book was being written, drugs were being developed that block the intoxicating effect of alcohol even after the user is intoxicated. How will developments such as this affect society? What will change in the drinking and driving laws? Should drugs like these even be released to the public? These and many other questions will need to be answered about these and all other drugs that are currently under development or yet to be developed.

Along with these new questions, many questions still remain to be answered about the use of existing medications. For example, should antipsychotic medications continue to be prescribed when side effects such as tardive dyskinesia can result? Is it clinically wise to allow patients to remain on antianxiety medications for long periods when they are making no attempt therapeutically to resolve the issues surrounding their anxiety? And what about the drugs that society continues to abuse or use illegally? What measures should be taken to stop the abuse of drugs? Should some personal freedoms be given up in order to curb the tide of illegal drugs?

These questions will be answered, and solutions will be found for old problems as new ones arise. Nonmedical psychotherapists should play a major role in making decisions about how these issues are resolved and in helping to find solutions for problems related to psychopharmacology. In the past, nonmedical therapists have been content to let what seemed to be "medical questions" be answered by "medical authorities." The reality is that these decisions affect all mental health professionals, and behavioral scientists in all areas have valuable data to apply to the ultimate solutions for these problems. The medical practitioner as well as the psychologist, the sociologist, the social worker, the mental health counselor, and all others whose work is related to the use of drugs will need to provide important input from their special vantage points. These problems no longer can be viewed from a limited perspective. For example, asking young people to "just say no to drugs" is not enough because the problem of drug abuse is far too complicated for simple answers. Tough questions must be posed and appropriate answers developed to provide the directions necessary to make changes in society that will allow young people to grow up without the need to use drugs. What is it about society that encourages so many young people to use drugs? What can be done to make them feel wanted and to know that they are an important part of society? Until solutions to these and other problems have been found, young people cannot be expected to say no to drugs. This will take a true understanding of the relation between the physical, psychological, and sociological aspects of drug use.

In considering what can be done, we must examine the major institutions of our society. The family is the primary institution that provides the individual with a sense of worth and well-being. If the family is dysfunctional, the chances of a family member using drugs in a negative manner are increased dramatically. A major example of this is the alcoholic family. The chances for a child who grows up in an alcoholic family to become an alcoholic are twice as great as the chances for a child who grows up in a nonalcoholic family. Providing a nurturing family situation is the responsibility of the parents, but they cannot be expected to provide this if they did not grow up in a nurturing family themselves. Thus the dilemma becomes self-perpetuating. Mental health professionals must intervene in these high-risk families and provide training on how they can meet the needs of each and every family member.

Part of this training could be done in another critical institution, the schools. Schools are the places where most young people are introduced to illegal drugs. Teachers and peers often have more influence than parents on adolescents. School personnel must consider what more they can do to foster students' development of self-image and confidence as well as the skills to interact on a meaningful level with their peers. Some adolescents use drugs to reduce the anxiety associated with relating to the opposite sex. Perhaps if they were more comfortable with themselves and learned to relate in the school situation, drugs would not be so attractive in the social situation.

The electronic and printed media share some of the responsibility for the way drugs are viewed in our society. The media must continue to help dispel the image of drug use as glamorous so that teenagers are not encouraged to experiment with drugs. Furthermore, entertainment and sports figures must understand that they are role models and that they have a responsibility to set a positive example. Religious institutions must provide values and guidance based on the real world rather than dogma. It will take the entire society working together to solve its drug problems, but nonmedical psychotherapists should be in leadership roles by virtue of their knowledge of human behavior and the addiction process. Nonmedical therapists must seek positions of leadership in professional and community organizations that make the policies that ultimately reflect social values and become drug laws.

Perhaps in the not-too-distant future lawmakers will come to consider the health of the public over the money they receive from lobbyists. Smoking might be banned in all public places. Cigarette advertisements aimed at young people might be prohibited. Warning labels and instructions for proper use might be required for all potentially harmful substances, including alcohol. Children might even be taught in schools that, since they will someday have a decision to make about using drugs, there are appropriate and inappropriate ways to do so. They might also be taught the physiological consequences of abusing a substance. Knowledge is a clear part of making informed choices, and it plays an all-important role in how to deal with drug problems. Drug use and abuse are emotional issues, but the solutions that work will come through logic and reason.

Common Abbreviations Used in Neuropharmacology

A	Adrenalin (epinephrine)
Acetyl CoA	Acetyl coenzyme A
ACh	acetylcholine
AChE	acetylcholinesterase
ACTH	adrenocorticotropic hormone
ACTH$_{4-10}$	fragment of ACTH from amino acid 4 to 10
ADP	Adenosine diphosphate
ADTN	2-Amino-6,7-dihydroxy-1,2,3,4-tetrahydronaphthalene
AMP	Adenosine monophosphate
AMPT	A-Methyl-*p*-tyrosine
AOAA	Aminooxyacetic acid
APUD	Amine precursor uptake and decarboxylation
ATP	Adenosine triphosphate
ATPase	Adenosinetriphosphatase
BOL	2-Brom-LSD
Ca^{2+}	Calcium ion
cAMP	Cyclic AMP (adenosine 3′,5′-monophosphate)
CAT	Choline acetyltransferase
CDP	Chlordiazepoxide
cGMP	Cyclic GMP (guanosine 3′,5′-monophosphate)
ChE	Cholinesterase
CNS	Central nervous system
COMT	Catechol-0-methyltransferase
CRF	Corticotropin-releasing factor
CSF	Cerebrospinal fluid
DA	Dopamine
d-cAMP	Dibutyryl cyclic AMP
DBH	dopamine β-hydroxylase
5,6-DHT	5,6-Dihydroxytryptamine
5,7-DHT	5,7-Dihydroxytryptamine

$DMPH_4$	6,7-Dimethyl-5,6,7,8-tetrahydropterin
DOMA	3,4-Dihydroxymandelic acid
DOPA	Dihydroxyphenylalanine
DOPAC	Dihydroxyphenylacetic acid
DOPS	Dihydroxyphenylserine
E	Epinephrine (Adrenalin)
ECS	Electroconvulsive shock
ECT	Electroconvulsive therapy
EDTA	Ethylene diamine tetraacetic acid
EEG	Electroencephalogram
EGTA	Ethylene gycol bis-(β-aminoethyl ether) tetraacetic acid
EPSP	Excitatory postsynaptic potential
GABA	γ-Aminobutyric acid
GAD	L-Glutamate decarboxylase (glutamic acid decarboxylase)
GLC	Gas-liquid chromatography
GC/MS	Gas chromatography/mass spectroscopy
GH	Growth hormone
Glu	Glutamate
GMP	Guanosine monophosphate
GTP	Guanosine triphosphate
5-HIAA	5-Hydroxyindoleacetic acid
HIOMT	Hydroxyindole-0-methyltransferase
5-HT	5-Hydroxytryptamine (serotonin)
5-HTOH	5-Hydroxytryptophol
5-HTP	5-Hydroxytryptophan
HVA	Homovanillic acid
IAA	Indoleacetic acid
IC_{50}	Concentration for 50% inhibition
IPSP	Inhibitory postsynaptic potential
K^+	Potassium ion
K_a	Association constant
K_d	Dissociation constant
K_i	Inhibition constant
K_m	Michaelis constant
LC	Locus coeruleus
Leu	Leucine
LHRH	Luteinizing hormone releasing hormone
Li^+	Lithium ion
LPH	β-lipotropic
LSD (LSD_{25})	D-Lysergic acid diethylamide
MAO	Monoamine oxidase
MAOI	Monoamine oxidase inhibitor
5-MeO-DMT	5-Methoxy-N,N-dimethyltryptamine
Met	Methionine
Mg^{2+}	Magnesium ion

MHPG (MOPEG)	3-Methoxy-4-hydroxyphenylglycol
MTA	3-Methoxytryramine
NA	Noradrenalin (norepinephrine)
Na$^+$	Sodium ion
NAD	Nicotinamide-adenine dinucleotide
NE	Norepinephrine (noradrenalin)
NEFA	Nonesterfied fatty acids
NM	Normetanephrine
6-OHDA	6-Hydroxydopamine
PCPA	*P*-Chlorophenylalanine
PEA	Phenethylamine
PGE$_1$	Prostaglandin E$_1$
Phe	Phenylalanine
PRL	Prolactin
PTZ	Pentylenetetrazol
REM	Rapid eye movement (sleep)
SAM	*S*-Adenosylmethionine
sd	Standard deviation
sem	Standard error of the mean
SP	Substance P
SRIF	Somatotropin release inhibiting factor
$t_{1/2}$	Half-life
T$_3$	*L*-triiodothyronine
T$_4$	Thyroxine
TBZ	Tetrabenazine
TCA	Tricarboxylic acid
Δ⁹-THC	Δ^9-tetrahydrocannabinol
TLC	Thin-layer chromotography
TRH	Thyrotropin releasing hormone
Trp	Tryptophan
TSH	Thyroid stimulating hormone (thyrotropin)
Tyr	Tyrosine
VMA	3-Methoxy-4-hydroxymandelic acid
V_{max}	Maximum velocity

Weights, Measures, and Prescription Abbreviations

METRIC SYSTEM

1 kilogram	=	1000 grams (g)
1 gram	=	1000 milligrams (mg)
1 milligram	=	1000 micrograms (μg)
1 liter	=	1000 milliliters (ml)
1 ml	=	1 cubic centimeter (cc)

EQUIVALENT WEIGHTS AND MEASURES

1 gram	=	15.4 grains
1 grain	=	65 mg
1 ounce	=	28.35 g
1 kilogram	=	2.20 lb
1 pound	=	454 g
1 pint	=	473 ml
1 fluid ounce	=	30 ml
1 teaspoon	=	5 ml
1 tablespoon	=	15 ml
1 teacup	=	120 ml
98.6°F	=	37.0°C

Conversion Equation for Celcius and Fahrenheit Scales

$$(°C) = \tfrac{5}{9}\,[(°F) - 32]$$

PRESCRIPTION ABBREVIATIONS

Latin Abbreviation	Meaning
ā.ā.	of each
a.c.	before meals
p.c.	after meals
ad. lib.	freely as desired
aq.	water
b.i.d.	twice a day
t.i.d.	three times daily
q.i.d.	four times daily
c̄	with
q̄	every
q̄.h.	every hour
h.s.	at bedtime
stat	immediately
p.r.n.	as needed, or when required
non.rep.	do not repeat
o.d.	right eye
o.s.	left eye

TYPES OF MEDICATION

Latin Abbreviation	Meaning
amp.	ampule
cap.	capsule
elx.	elixir
ext.	extract
soln.	solution
spt.	spirit
supp.	suppository
syr.	syrup
tinc.	tincture
tab.	tablet
ung.	ointment

Appendix C

Some Questions and Answers

Gary W. Lawson

The questions below are ones frequently asked by psychology students and other mental health workers during courses on psychopharmacology.

1. What should a psychologist or nonmedical psychotherapist know about psychopharmacology, and why?

The answer to this question depends on the type of work in which the therapist is involved. Obviously someone with a specialization in chemical dependency needs to know a great deal about drugs of abuse, physical addiction, drug effects on the body, and so on. Therapists who see patients of all types, however, still need a working knowledge in many areas of psychopharmacology. At a minimum they need to know what conditions respond to medication and the medications most often used for these conditions. They need to know the positive and negative effects of these drugs and what to expect from a patient who is taking one of these medications. Even though nonmedical therapists do not prescribe drugs, they are often in the position of having to make a decision regarding a medical referral. This decision in itself can often determine whether or not the patient is ultimately medicated. The more the therapist knows about the issues in psychopharmacology, the better equipped he or she is to make decisions of this nature.

2. How can it be determined that the psychiatrist to whom a patient is referred is a good one?

It may not be necessary to refer a patient to a psychiatrist if the therapist can work with the patient's regular physician. In cases of nondebilitating psychological problems, such as mild depression or anxiety, the general practitioner may be able to provide the medical backup that is needed, allowing the nonmedical professional to continue to be the primary therapist. The physician then functions only as a monitor for the medication on the basis of the therapist's feedback. If a psychiatrist is called for and the therapist does not know of one, he or she can ask the advice of a local physician. Just as it is a mistake to assume that all psychologists or nonmedical psychotherapists are professionally competent, it is also a

319

mistake to assume that all psychiatrists are competent. It is important to remember that in the United States foreign-trained physicians are not allowed to practice medicine until they have demonstrated competence both in English and in medicine. In the absence of such proven competence, however, they are allowed to work as resident psychiatrists in state mental institutions. Further, many states allow medical doctors to work as psychiatrists regardless of their training or lack of training in the field. For the nonmedical practitioner, it is a good idea to identify one or two local board-certified psychiatrists to work with and refer to on a regular basis. A potential referral source should be questioned about his or her training or philosophy. The nonmedical therapist has a responsibility to his or her patients to make the best referral possible.

3. How can it be determined whether psychotherapy is to be the sole treatment method or whether a patient should be referred for medication?

A clear diagnosis based on the best information available is the first step in making this decision. The second consideration is the goal that both the therapist and the patient have for therapy. A history of whether drugs have been used in the past and if they worked is also useful and something many nonmedical psychotherapists forget to ask about. Finally, a consultation with a medical practitioner could provide the information on which to base the final decision. The choices are of course psychotherapy alone, medication alone, or psychotherapy in combination with medication. It is reasonable to first choose the one that has the best prognosis given the diagnosis, but the potential negative reaction to any choice must also be considered. Many medications have side effects that may be as bad as the symptom, and in some cases patients may be better off without psychotherapy when it forces them to deal with issues they do not have the ego strength to deal with. Choosing both medication and psychotherapy can give patients mixed messages about who must take ultimate responsibility for their getting better. In the final analysis, it is good clinical judgment based on accurate information that leads to a proper decision. Information about issues in pharmacology are an important part of that decision-making process.

4. How can it be determined whether a patient is an alcoholic or just a problem drinker? Is there a difference?

There is a great deal of controversy in the field concerning this issue, especially regarding what it means in terms of treatment. Problem drinkers can be distinguished from alcoholics on the basis of whether they can ever return to drinking for an extended period of time without reverting to their previous behavior patterns. If the problem drinker is given a reasonable chance to stop drinking with assistance and support from a therapist and significant others, he or she can probably return to occasional drinking. In contrast, no matter what alcoholics do they cannot drink alcohol without considerable problems in their lives, and they are best advised by the therapist not to try drinking alcohol in any form. If the therapist is uncertain about specific patients who want to try to drink without problems, the therapist can allow them to do so but make a "contract" with them that if they do not succeed in a reasonable time they will give up alcohol. These contracts are better negotiated with the patient's entire family rather than the patient alone.

5. Should a patient ever be encouraged not to take a prescribed medication?

If in the process of an interview with a patient the therapist discovers that he or she is experiencing problems with medication, such as extreme side effects or adverse reactions, or if the patient is continuing medication prescribed by two physicians, the therapist should take action at once. First, a release of information should be obtained from the patient and the primary physician contacted by phone to discuss these concerns. There are times when patients go to several doctors and neglect to tell one doctor about the medication that was prescribed by another doctor. They may take both medications even though there is a great potential for danger when the drugs are mixed. A nonmedical psychotherapist could generate many legal problems by telling a patient to take or not to take medication, but if a patient has a problem or a potential problem with a medication it is always advisable to consult a physician.

6. Should psychologists lobby for the right to prescribe drugs?

This is a political issue that is currently being debated. Members of the medical community will probably fight such a move, and they have a powerful lobby. Psychologists at present are not trained to prescribe medication, but with some special training (perhaps a year's internship and a year of coursework beyond the 20 years of training it takes to become a psychologist) there is no reason to believe that this would be a move that would be harmful to the public. In some states a physician's assistant can write prescriptions under the supervision of a physician. There are moves in other professions, nursing and pharmacy for example, to gain this right on a limited basis. As health maintenance organizations exert more influence over the administration of health care, there will probably be many changes in health care. Perhaps psychologists prescribing psychotropic medications on a limited basis will be among those changes.

7. What is the best way to deal with patients who use illegal drugs for recreation?

This is an issue that individual therapists need to address according to their own values. The use of chemical substances to alter the mind has been a practice throughout recorded history. Some people experience physiological as well as legal problems as a result of the use of mind-altering substances, and others do not. It is one of the therapist's responsibilities to make sure that patients know the risk of any activity that they choose to engage in, including the use of illegal drugs. One major problem to point out is that illegal drugs may not be what they are sold as and are often adulterated with other harmful substances. The physical and psychological changes that occur may not be consistent between people or over time, and in most cases the process of physical or psychological addiction can occur before the user realizes it. If the use of mind-altering substances of any kind is causing problems that the patient is denying, that patient should be confronted, perhaps with an intervention that involves family members and significant others.

8. When so many of the problems brought to physicians are psychological or emotional in nature, why is it that more of them do not refer patients to nonmedical mental health workers or psychotherapists?

Part of this problem is due to the lack of consistency in training, philosophy, and approach to mental health problems among nonmedical mental health practitioners. There are many professions that work with the psychologically or emotionally disturbed. Further, each state seems to have its own idea of what credentials these individuals need. Even though there have been attempts to standardize training programs, there are vast differences between programs. As a result, medical doctors are reluctant to make referrals because they are not sure of the probable outcome. Another reason is that medical doctors have been trained, in many cases, to be the final authority and to deal with problems themselves whenever possible. Most nonmedical psychotherapists would not think of practicing medicine with a psychotherapy patient, but the reverse is not always the case, so that what a medical doctor passes off as friendly advice may become an attempt at psychotherapy.

9. Should nonmedical psychotherapists routinely ask patients about their drug use or any medications they may be taking?

Any information about the use of medications or illicit drugs can be valuable in making clinical decisions about a patient. Therapists should not depend on patients to provide such information voluntarily. It only takes a few minutes to ask some routine questions that will provide this information. Questions that should be part of a routine intake interview include the following: Are you on any medication? Do you use any drugs recreationally? How much alcohol, coffee, or tobacco products do you use? Do you think you have a problem with any drugs?

10. Should the goal of psychotherapy be to get patients off of psychotropic drugs?

The ideal situation is when all people lead ''normal,'' happy, and functional lives without the use of any medications. This is especially true with psychotropic medications, which all have what could be considered some negative side effects. The final consideration, however, is the quality of life for the patient and his or her family. In some cases the only way to maintain the optimum quality of life is through the continued use of medication by the patient. This does not mean that once a patient is medicated the job of the therapist is over. Many patients want to learn to function without medication, and still others need help learning to live with the side effects of the drugs they are taking. Drugs themselves are neither good nor bad; it is how they are used that is important.

Suggested Readings

To enhance and expand the information provided in this book, the references listed below may be consulted. Books are presented by subject, and each listing includes a summary of the book's contents.

ADDICTION

Lenters, W. (1985). *The freedom we crave: Addiction the human condition*. Grand Rapids, MI: Wm. B. Eerdmans.

Lenters examines how people develop addictive patterns of living to cope with stress and offers a step-by-step recovery program.

Meyer, R. (Ed.). (1986). *Psychopathology and addictive disorders*. New York: Guilford.

This is a scholarly, well-written book that covers psychiatric disorders among alcohol and drug abusers in terms of antisocial personality disorders as risk factors and the development of personality disorders as a result of drug abuse.

Milby, J.B. (1981). *Addictive behavior and its treatment*. New York: Springer.

This is a relatively short book that presents a mostly behavioral approach to the treatment of addiction.

Orford, J. (1985). *Excessive appetites: A psychological view of addictions*. New York: Wiley.

This book covers most addictions, including addiction to sex, gambling, and food. It contains some valuable information to help the reader understand the addiction process.

Shaffer, E., & Burglass, M. (Eds.). (1981). *Classic contributions in the addictions*. New York: Brunner/Mazel.

This book is a collection of articles that are research oriented; it is not suggested for a reader with only a casual interest in addiction.

ALCOHOLISM (GENERAL)

Estes, N.J., & Heinemann, M.E. (Eds.). (1977). *Alcoholism: Development, consequences, and interventions*. St. Louis, MO: C.V. Mosby.

This is one of the early books on alcoholism. It has several chapters that would be of more interest to a nurse than a psychotherapist. There are several newer editions that have come out since the one listed above.

Goodwin, D.W. (1981). *Alcoholism: The facts*. New York: Oxford Univ. Press.

This book is written by a psychiatrist for nonpsychiatrists to facilitate their understanding of alcoholism; it is short and easy to read.

Kinney, J., & Leaton, G. (1987). *Loosening the grip: A handbook of alcohol information*. St. Louis, MO: C.V. Mosby.

This book is appropriate for high school students and college freshmen who want a brief background on alcoholism. It includes cartoon pictures and is written at the eighth-grade reading level. It is popular in alcohol treatment programs.

Pattison, E.M., & Kaufman, E. (1982). *Encyclopedic handbook of alcoholism*. New York: Gardner.

This book is a large and comprehensive reference on alcoholism.

Royce, J.E. (1981). *Alcohol problems and alcoholism: A comprehensive survey*. New York: The Free Press.

Dr. Royce was the first person to offer a university course on alcoholism. His book, although conventional, is an excellent introduction.

Vaillant, G.E. (1983). *The natural history of alcoholism*. Cambridge, MA: Harvard Univ. Press.

Although this book may become a classic, the author has been taken to task already about some of his conclusions. The book should be read together with the article about the book in the *American Psychologist:* Zucker, R., & Gomberg, E.S.L. (1986). Etiology of alcoholism reconsidered: The case for a biopsychosocial process. *American Psychologist, 41*(7).

Ward, D.E. (Ed.). (1980). *Alcoholism: Introduction to theory and treatment*. Dubuque, IA: Kendall Hunt.

This is an excellent text for a beginning course on alcoholism. It is now in its third edition.

ALCOHOLISM TREATMENT

Bratter, T.E., & Forrest, G.G. (1985). *Alcoholism and substance abuse: Strategies for clinical intervention*. New York: The Free Press.

This is one of the better texts on treatment of chemical dependency.

Cain, A.H. (1964). *The cured alcoholic: New concepts in alcoholism treatment and research*. New York: John Day.

Although this book is no longer in print, it is included here because it is perhaps one of the best books ever written on alcoholism.

Edwards, G., & Grant, M. (Eds.). (1980). *Alcoholism treatment in transition*. Baltimore: University Park Press.

This paperback brings up some issues worth discussing and makes a good reader for an alcoholism treatment course.

Forrest, G.G. (1978). *The diagnosis and treatment of alcoholism*. Springfield, IL: Charles C Thomas.

This text covers the basics of alcoholism treatment.

Lawson, G., Ellis, D.C., & Rivers, C.P. (1984). *Essentials of chemical dependency counseling*. Rockville, MD: Aspen Publishers.

This is one of the few books on chemical dependency counseling. It is written at the basic level for the beginning counselor and is an excellent text for a chemical dependency counseling course.

Mendelson, J.H., & Mello, N.K. (Eds.). (1979). *The diagnosis and treatment of alcoholism*. New York: McGraw-Hill.

This is a clinically oriented book that presents some excellent ideas regarding diagnosis and treatment of alcoholism.

Polich, M.J., Armor, D.J., & Braiker, M.B. (1981). *The course of alcoholism: Four years after treatment*. New York: Wiley.

This is an account of the famous Rand report. It follows a group of men who went through traditional treatment for alcoholism and examines them at 18 months and then again at 4 years.

FAMILY THERAPY

Bepko, C., & Krestan, J. (1985). *The responsibility trap: A blueprint for treating the alcoholic family*. New York: The Free Press.

This is one of the new books available on treating families; because family therapy seems to be the ideal way to treat the problem, this book is highly recommended.

Bernard, C.P. (1981). *Families, alcoholism and therapy*. Springfield, IL: Charles C Thomas.

This small paperback contains some interesting material. It was one of the first books to look at family issues in addiction.

Davis, D.I. (1987). *Alcoholism treatment: An integrative family and individual approach*. New York: Gardner.

This book was written for the practitioner and contains many case examples and sample interviews.

Kaufman, E. (1975). *Substance abuse and family therapy*. Orlando, FL: Grune & Stratton.

This book is psychoanalytically oriented and written by a psychiatrist.

Kaufman, E., & Kaufmann, P. (Eds.). (1979). *Family therapy of drug and alcohol abuse*. New York: Gardner.

This is one of the first books to attempt to explain the role of family therapy in the treatment of substance abuse.

Lawson, G., Peterson, J., & Lawson, A. (1984). *Alcoholism and the family: A guide to treatment and prevention*. Rockville, MD: Aspen Publishers.

This book presents a model of treatment and prevention based on the role that the family plays in the risk each member has of becoming alcoholic. It is intended to provide a basic understanding of families and alcoholism. It prescribes family therapy as the major treatment for alcoholism.

CONTROLLED DRINKING

Heather, N., & Robinson, I. (1981). *Controlled drinking*. New York: Methuen.

This book makes a strong case, on the basis of research, for controlled drinking as a treatment goal for some people with drinking problems. It lists 163 studies on controlled drinking and presents the outcomes for most of them.

Vogler, R.E., & Bartz, W.R. (1982). *A better way to drink: Moderation and control of problem drinking*. Oakland, CA: New Harbinger Publications.

This book offers a prescription for learning to control problem drinking. It is a good book to give to patients who have this goal.

DRUGS

Blum, K. (Ed.). (1984). *Handbook of abusable drugs*. New York: Gardner.

This is a 721-page book that covers many areas, including some general sociopharmacologic aspects of substance abuse and basic pharmacologic considerations and principles.

Dusek, D., & Girdano, D.A. (1980). *Drugs: A factual account*. Reading, MA: Addison-Wesley.

This book was written as a beginning text for basic college freshman courses on drugs.

Jones-Witters, P., & Witters, W. (1983). *Drugs and society: A biological perspective*. Monterey, CA: Wadsworth.

This is another book appropriate for beginning courses on drugs.

Julien, R.M. (1981). *A primer of drug action*. New York: Freeman.

This book was written for beginning courses on drugs.

Liska, K. (1981). *Drugs and the human body*. New York: Macmillan.

This book was written for beginning courses on drugs.

Ray, O., & Ksir, C. (1987). *Drugs, society and human behavior*. St. Louis, MO: C.V. Mosby.

This is an updated edition of a classic beginning text. It has been used in many drug courses at several universities.

Rucker, W.B., & Rucker, M.E. (1987). *Drugs, society and behavior*. Guilford, CT: Dushkin Publishing.

This is a fine collection of popular articles on drugs. It is an excellent reader for a course on drugs in American society.

PRESCRIPTION DRUGS

Bassuk, E.L., & Schoonover, S.C. (1978). *The practitioner's guide to psychoactive drugs*. New York: Plenum.

This book is designed as a quick reference for the mental health and medical professional who prescribes psychoactive drugs frequently.

Griffith, W.H. (1983). *Drugs: Side effects, warnings and vital data for safe use*. Tucson, AZ: HP Books.

This is an easy-to-use consumer drug book. It includes warnings and precautions, possible adverse reactions, dosage and usage information, and interaction and overdose information.

Honingfeld, G., & Howard, A. (1978). *Psychiatric drugs: A desk reference*. New York: Academic Press.

This book is a handy guide to psychiatric drugs.

Long, J.W. (1982). *The essential guide to prescription drugs*. New York: Harper & Row.

This book is another useful guide to prescription drugs.

Physicians' desk reference (41st ed.). (1987). Oradell, NJ: Medical Economics Co.

This book contains all the information that is published about prescription drugs in the inserts that drug manufacturers provide with their drugs. This is the major reference source on prescription drugs.

Shader, R. (Ed.). (1977). *Manual of psychiatric therapeutics: Practical psychopharmacology and psychiatry*. Boston: Little, Brown & Co.

This is a basic manual used mainly by psychiatrists that provides information about psychiatric disorders and drugs used to treat them.

PSYCHOPHARMACOLOGY

Cook, T., Ferris, S., & Bartus, R. (Eds.). (1983). *Assessment in geriatric psychopharmacology*. New Canaan, CT: Mark Powley Associates.

This book presents a practical guide to the assessment instruments that represent the current state of the art in geriatric psychopharmacology.

Green, R.A., & Costain, D.W. (1981). *Pharmacology and biochemistry of psychiatric disorders*. New York: Wiley.

The aim of this book is to provide an overview of the current state of knowledge of the pharmacology and biochemistry of psychiatric disorders.

Radcliffe, A., Rush, P., Sites, C., & Cruse, J. (1985). *Pharmer's almanac: Pharmacology of drugs*. Denver, CO: M.A.C.

This book is designed to help teach nonmedically-trained professionals about the drugs on which people become dependent or to which they become addicted. It is written in simple terms and makes a complex topic understandable.

Sanger, D.J., & Blackman, D.E. (Eds.). (1984). *Aspects of psychopharmacology*. New York: Methuen.

This book reviews research on the effects of the psychoactive drugs in experimental, social, and therapeutic settings.

Spiegel, R., & Aebi, H.J. (1984). *Psychopharmacology: An introduction*. New York: Wiley.

This book is directed toward students of psychology and medicine and members of other professions who deal with clients and patients who take psychopharmaceutical agents.

Swonger, A., & Constantine, L.L. (1976). *Drugs and therapy: A psychotherapist's handbook of psychotropic drugs*. Boston: Little, Brown & Co.

This book is somewhat outdated. It is included here because it was one of the original books written for nonmedical therapists. Written to provide a broad awareness of physiological and pharmacological influences on psychological processes, it is still an excellent book.

Wiener, J.M. (Ed.). (1985). *Diagnosis and psychopharmacology of childhood and adolescent disorders*. New York: Wiley.

This book brings together the work of leading investigators and clinical practitioners in a comprehensive review of the latest clinical and theoretical information about the use of psychoactive medication in childhood psychiatric and behavioral disorders.

Glossary

A-bomb Marijuana cigarette dusted with opium or heroin.

Abortifacient Drug or substance capable of inducing abortion.

Absorbent Agent that takes up water or fluid and increases in bulk; see also Adsorbent.

Absorption Process whereby a drug gains entry into the main circulation.

Abstinence Discontinuance and avoidance of further use of a drug.

Abstinence syndrome Physiological and psychological symptoms that result from abrupt withdrawal from depressants; intense manifestation of the stress reaction.

Abuse To use improperly.

Acapulco gold Marijuana of gold color and high potency, said to be grown around Acapulco, Mexico.

Accused Defendant; an individual who is facing a criminal proceeding based on charges brought against him or her.

Acetaldehyde Toxic breakdown product of ethyl alcohol.

Acetylcholine Neurotransmitter in the parasympathetic nervous system; abbreviated Ach or ACh.

Acid LSD (lysergic acid diethylamide).

Acid freak User of LSD whose behavior is bizarrely affected.

Acidhead Chronic user of LSD.

Acidosis Condition of reduced alkali (bicarbonate) reserve in the blood and other body fluids, with or without an actual decrease in the blood pH. If untreated, this condition can be lethal.

Acid rock Kind of music (loud, frenetic, electronic, and fast-moving).

Active ingredient Specific chemical in a plant or drug responsible for the drug action ascribed to the entire plant.

Acupuncture Method of analgesia in which needles are inserted in the skin at special points and a stimulus applied by twirling, vibration, or an electrical charge.

Acute Of short duration and severe.

Acute effect Immediate, short-term response to a single dosage of a drug; compare to Chronic effect.

Addiction Defined in 1957 by the World Health Organization as a state of periodic or chronic intoxication produced by the repeated consumption of a drug. Its characteristics include (1) an overpowering desire or compulsion to continue taking the drug and to obtain it by any means; (2) a tendency to increase the dosage; (3) a psychic (psychological) and generally a physical dependence on the effects of the drug; and (4) an effect detrimental to the individual and to society. See also Drug dependence and Psychological dependence.

Addiction (physical) Drug-induced change in a person such that he or she requires the continued presence of the drug to function normally and to prevent the occurrence of a withdrawal syndrome.

Additive effects Enhancement of the effect of one chemical by the presence of another. The effect is doubled or equal to the combined amount of the two chemicals.

A-delta fiber Type of nerve fiber that transmits impulses rapidly and leads to the sensation of sharp, pricking pain; see also C-fiber.

Administration, drug Procedure through which a drug gains entrance into the body (oral administration of tablets or liquids, inhalation of powders, injection of sterile liquids, and so on).

Adrenal medulla Innermost portion of the adrenal glands that produces sympathetic hormones (i.e., adrenalin or epinephrine and noradrenalin or norepinephrine).

Adrenergic Of or pertaining to the sympathetic nervous system and the synthesis, storage, and release of sympathomimetic substances.

Adrenergic blocker Drug acting at sympathetic nerve endings to reduce the effective concentration of norepinephrine; examples are guanethidine and methyldopamine. Different drugs can block the alpha, beta-1, or beta-2 functions selectively.

Adrenergic receptors Those components of a cell that are responsive to adrenergic substances and are directly involved with the initial action of such substances.

α-Adrenergic receptors That part of the dual adrenergic receptive mechanism that is specifically blocked by either phenoxybenzamine or phentolamine, which are specific α-adrenergic blockers.

β-Adrenergic receptors That part of the dual adrenergic receptive mechanism specifically blocked by dichloroisoproterenol or propanolol effects.

The "alpha effects" are blocked by an α-adrenergic blocker, and the "beta effects" are blocked by a β-adrenergic blocker, so that if both α- and β-adrenergic blockers are administered and then an adrenergic substance is administered, there will be no effect of the adrenergic substance on the organism.

Adsorbent Agent that binds chemical substances to its surface, such as charcoal; compare to Absorbent.

Adulterant Cheap substitute mixed with a pure drug; an example is heroin diluted with quinine.

Adverse reaction Reaction of an organism to a drug that is different from the desired reaction and is determined to be detrimental to the organism.

Affect Mood, feelings, or emotions.

Affective (nerve transmission) Messages coming into the brain.

Affinity Attraction between ligand and receptor, quantified in terms of the affinity constant.

Agnosia Loss of the ability to recognize sensory stimuli.

Agonist Drug that mimics the action of a normally present biological compound such as neurotransmitter or hormone.

A-Head Habitual user (possibly exclusively) of amphetamines.

Akathisia Side effect of major tranquilizers that causes restlessness and possibly the inability to sit or lie down quietly or to sleep.

Akinesia Absence (or reduction) of voluntary muscular movement.

A la canoña Abrupt withdrawal from heroin without medication or treatment (Puerto Rican slang).

Albuminuria Presence of protein, chiefly albumin, in the urine; usually indicative of disease but sometimes results from a temporary dysfunction of the kidneys (as opposed to a truly pathologic condition).

Alcohol (ethyl alcohol, ethanol) Widely used sedative-hypnotic drug.

Alcohol dehydrogenase Liver enzyme involved in the reaction that converts alcohol to acetaldehyde.

Alkaline phosphatase test Test that measures the blood level of the enzyme alkaline phosphatase and thereby determines the potential presence or absence of certain disease states.

Alkaloid Any member of a diverse group of organic compounds containing a nitrogen atom in a ring structure; examples are morphine, nicotine, and cocaine. The basic molecule is unstable and is usually prepared in the more stable salt form.

Alkyl A prefix referring to a radical derived from an open-chain hydrocarbon, often referred to as an aliphatic molecule.

Allergenic reaction Hypersensitivity to a drug or other substance due to an unwanted immune system response.

All lit up Under the influence of a drug.

Alpha receptor Postjunctional receptor site that responds primarily to norepinephrine.

Ambulatory Able to walk; that is, not confined to a bed or wheelchair.

Ames Small glass vials of amyl nitrite (also known as pearls or snappers).

Amine Substance having an NH_2 group in its chemical structure.

Amino acid Organic acid in which one of the hydrogen atoms is replaced by an NH_2 group; small amine molecules combine to form proteins.

Amphetamine Behavioral stimulant.

Amytal Barbiturate of intermediate action.

Anabolic steroid Steroid hormone that promotes general body growth (anabolism); examples are testosterone or one of the synthetic androgens.

Anabolism Metabolism (body functioning) in which tissues or chemicals are built up from simpler substances.

Analeptic Drug that stimulates the central nervous system.

Analgesic Drug that produces relief from pain without loss of consciousness; examples are the opiates and phenacetin.

Anaphylactic shock Serious, often fatal allergic reaction occurring in a previously sensitized person, starting within minutes after administration of a foreign serum or certain drug such as typhoid vaccine or penicillin.

Androgen Class of chemical compounds, some of which are synthetic, that are similar to testosterone in action (also called masculinizing hormone).

Anesthesia Condition in which pain or other sensation is partially or totally lost but consciousness is not.

Anesthetic Drug that causes loss of sensation or feeling, especially pain, by its depressant effect on the nervous system.

Angel dust PCP (phencyclidine).

Angel off To arrest the buyers from a drug dealer who is being watched.

Angina pectoris Severe chest pain caused by inadequate blood supply to the heart muscle brought on by exertion or excitement.

Anorexia State of not feeling hungry; a blocked hunger center caused by some drugs and psychological factors.

Anorexiant Anoretic; drug that causes loss of appetite.

Antabuse syndrome Accumulation of the toxic metabolite of alcohol, acetaldehyde, due to Antabuse or a genetic deficiency, which causes unpleasant symptoms: intense throbbing in the head and neck, a pulsating headache, difficulty in breathing, nausea, copious vomiting, sweating, thirst, and chest pain.

Antagonist Drug that blocks or interferes with the action of a normally present biological compound, such as a neurotransmitter or hormone, or of another drug.

Anthropometry Measurement of the size, weight, and proportions of the body.

Antianxiety agent Sedative-hypnotic compound used at subhypnotic dosages.

Antibiotic Drug produced by a microorganism and having the ability to inhibit the growth of or to kill other microorganisms.

Antibody Specific protein molecule synthesized by the immune response system as a defense against invading antigens.

Anticholinergic Cholinergic blocking agent. An example is atropine, which prevents acetylcholine from stimulating the cholinergic receptor.

Anticholinergic effects Antagonistic to the action of parasympathetic or other cholinergic nerve fibers.

Anticoagulant Substance that slows the rate of blood-clot formation.

Antidepressant Group of drugs used to elevate mood in severely depressed persons; an example is Tofranil.

Antigen Substance that stimulates production of antibodies; an example is penicillin.

Antihistamine Drug that prevents or antagonizes the action of histamine; examples are chlorpheniramine and isoproterenol.

Antihypertensive Drug used to reduce hypertension (high blood pressure).

Anti-inflammatory Drug that reduces inflammation; an example is cortisone.

Antimetabolite Drug with a structure so similar to that of a natural metabolite that it can inhibit or block the utilization of the natural metabolite by preferentially occupying the receptor site.

Antimuscarinic Anticholinergic drug that affects the muscarinic (not the nicotinic) type of receptor; an example is belladonna.

Antinociceptive Having the action of reducing or abolishing painful stimuli.

Antipsychotic (neuroleptic) Drugs that produce an effect of emotional quieting and relative indifference to one's surroundings.

Antipyretic Drug that reduces fever; an example is aspirin.

Anywhere Possessing illegal drugs.

Aphrodisiac Substance that produces a sexually enhancing effect in a person who does not expect this result.

Aplastic anemia Condition in which there is a reduction of circulating red blood cells in the bloodstream because of a lack of regeneration or destruction of the bone marrow by certain chemical agents (benzine or arsenic) or physical factors (radiation).

APUD (amine precursor uptake and decarboxylation) cells Cells derived from the ectoblast.

Around the turn Having passed through the worst part of withdrawal.

Arraignment First step in the criminal process, when the accused is formally charged with an offense.

Arrythmias Loss of normal heart rhythm or heart beat or irregularities that can be lethal.

Arteriosclerosis Thickening, hardening, and loss of elasticity of arteries.

Artillery Apparatus used for injecting drugs.

Aryl Prefix referring to a radical derived from benzene, often referred to as an aromatic molecule.

Ascending reticular activating system (ARAS) Network of neurons in the brainstem thought to function in arousal mechanisms.

Ataxia Loss of muscular coordination.

Autistic Mentally introverted, self-centered condition in which reality is excluded. Autistic children have little affect and show either no emotional response or a very inappropriate response.

Autonomic nervous system Motor system consisting of the nerves that control heart muscle, glands, and smooth muscle. It has two major divisions: the sympathetic (thoracolumbar) and the parasympathetic (craniosacral).

Autopsy Postmortem operation.

Autoreceptor Receptor situated on the presynaptic nerve ending that is sensitive to the transmitter released by the neuron. Also called presynaptic receptors.

Autosome Chromosome not determinant of sexual differentiation. Autosomal dominance: inheritance of non–sex-linked genetic factors where the gene needs to be present on only one chromosome.

Axon Extension from a neuron; it usually carries impulses away from the cell body and may have an insulating myelin sheath.

Baby Marijuana.

Backwards Tranquilizers (to bring one back from LSD or amphetamines).

Bador Hallucinogenic seed from the morning glory plant (Aztec slang).

Bad trip Unpleasant experience with a drug (usually a hallucinogen).

Bag "Measured" amount of a street drug (usually heroin) indicated by the price.

Bagman Drug dealer.

Bail Money or other security posted to ensure the appearance of the defendant throughout court proceedings.

Bale Pound of marijuana.

Bam Amphetamine injected or taken orally.

Bamboo Opium pipe.

Banana smoking Previous fad; the inner fibrous peelings of the banana were smoked for their elating effects (mellow yellow), although psychotropic activity has not been proven.

Bang To inject drugs intravenously or to get a thrill from injection.

Bank bandit pills Barbiturates or other sedative pills.

Bar Solid block of marijuana stuck together with honey or sugar water (also called a brick).

Barbiturate Class of chemically related sedative-hypnotic compounds, all of which share a characteristic six-membered ring structure.

Barbs Barbiturates.

Basal ganglia Interconnected structures in the forebrain that direct involuntary muscle function not under conscious control, including maintenance of muscle tone and posture; dopamine is probably the neurotransmitter involved.

Basal metabolic rate (BMR) Rate at which the body uses oxygen for energy required to maintain homeostasis; measured in the quietly resting person, at least 12 hours after the latest meal, to obtain the lowest essential level.

B-bombs Benzedrine inhalers (removed from the market in 1949).

B.C. (BCP) Birth control pills.

Beast LSD-25 (Harlem slang).

Beat To cheat or rob someone of money or goods (also, beat the system).

Bee Box or bag of marijuana.

Behavioral stereotypy Getting "hung up" in a meaningless repetition of a simple activity for hours at a time; characteristic of amphetamine abuse and paranoid schizophrenia.

Behavioral tolerance Learning of control over some drug effects over a period of time; thought to be a subtype of pharmacodynamic tolerance.

Belly habit Opiate addiction.

Benny Benzedrine.

Benny jag "High" on Benzedrine.

Bent (High, stoned, plastered, ripped) Intoxicated from drugs.

Benzodiazepine Chemical class of sedative-hypnotic drugs that includes drugs similar to diazepam, lorazepam, and chlordiazepoxide.

Bernice Cocaine.

Beta blocker Drug capable of competing with β-adrenergic receptor-stimulating agents for available receptor sites.

Beta receptor Postjunctional receptor site that responds primarily to epinephrine; divided into beta-1 and beta-2 types on the basis of the response to sympathomimetic drugs.

Bhang From India; the marijuana plant and the drink made with the plant used to produce psychotropic effects.

Big bags $5 to $10 bags of heroin.

Big bloke Cocaine.

Big chief Mescaline.

Big "D" LSD-25.

Big John Police.

Big man Distributor of wholesale illegal drugs to other dealers.

Big supplier Same as Big man.

Bindle Small folded paper containing heroin.

Bingle Dope dealer.

Biofeedback Use of a signal, such as muscle tension or brain waves, to control a normally involuntary physiological process.

Biological half-life Amount of time required to remove half the original amount of a drug from the body.

Biopharmaceutical metabolism How the body processes a drug.

Biotransformation Process of metabolism of drugs in the body, usually in the liver.

Biphasic drug Type of drug whose half-life is marked by two distinctly different rates of clearance from the blood.

Bipolar illness Affective illness where both depression and mania occur.

Black beauties Biamphetamine capsules.

Black gunion Thick, potent, dark, and gummy marijuana.

Blackout Temporary loss of memory.

Black pills Pellets of opium heated over a flame and smoked.

Black Russian Dark-colored, very potent hashish.

Blank Container of white powder that was falsely sold as heroin (also called dummy).

Blast To smoke a drug.

Blast party   Party held to smoke marijuana.

Blockbusters   White and yellow striped barbiturate pills.

Blood alcohol concentration   Percentage of alcohol per unit volume of blood (0.15% alcohol in the blood constitutes intoxication in most states).

Blood-brain barrier   Selective filtering system that permits ready passage of oxygen, glucose, and other nutrients into neurons but largely excludes proteins, ionized molecules, and non-fat–soluble substances.

Blood-placenta barrier   Selective filtering system involving the placenta, the organ that interfaces between the mother's and the fetus' blood supply; the placenta excludes transfer of some water-soluble substances to the fetus. Most lipid-soluble drugs and many water-soluble drugs penetrate this barrier and enter the fetus' blood.

Blotter acid   LSD on porous paper.

Blow   To smoke marijuana, to inhale cocaine or heroin through the nose, or to miss a vein while trying to inject drugs intravenously.

Blow snow   To inhale cocaine through the nose.

Blow your mind   To alter one's consciousness drastically (possibly with drugs).

Blow your mind roulette   Game played with barbiturate and amphetamine pills.

Blue acid   LSD.

Bluebirds   Amytal sodium capsules.

Blue devils   Amytal.

Blue heavens   Same as Bluebirds.

Blue velvets   Combination of terpin hydrate elixir, codeine, and tripelennamine.

BMR   See Basal metabolic rate.

Body drugs   Drugs that produce physical dependence.

Body trip   Drug experience that seems physical rather than mental (that is, one is "sped up" or "slowed down" physically, or possibly sexually aroused).

Bogue   Withdrawal from drugs that produce physical dependence.

Bolsa   Bag of heroin.

Bombed out (high, ripped, stoned, blasted)   Intoxicated from drugs.

Bong   Water pipe used to smoke marijuana.

Boo   Marijuana.

Booting   Technique of injecting heroin a little at a time in order to prolong the initial pleasurable sensation.

Bouncing powder   Cocaine.

Bound drugs   Association of drugs with plasma proteins (also applying to tryptophan). The combination of ligand with receptor is known as specific binding, and the combination of ligand with nonreceptor material is known as nonspecific binding.

Bradykinin   One of a group of naturally present peptides that acts on blood vessels, smooth muscles, and nociceptors; its function is presently unknown.

Brain syndrome, organic   Pattern of behavior induced when neurons are either reversibly depressed or irreversibly destroyed. Behavior is characterized by clouded sensorium; disorientation; shallow and labile affect; and impaired memory, intellectual function, insight, and judgment.

Brain tickles   Amphetamines or barbiturates.

Bread   Money.

Brompton's cocktail (or mixture)   An alcoholic solution of an opioid (usually heroin or morphine) and cocaine, amphetamine, or a phenothiazine tranquilizer; used to control severe pain in terminal cancer patients.

Bronchitis   Inflammation of the bronchial tubes in the lungs, causing difficulty in breathing.

Brownies   Amphetamines, especially Dexedrine capsules.

Buccal cavity   Space between the inside of the cheek and the teeth; a good area for drug absorption.

Bufotenine   Psychoactive drug found in cohoba snuff, the skin and parotid gland of the toad, and in small amounts in the mushroom *Amanita muscaria.*

Bum bend   "Bad trip"; unpleasant experience with a drug.

Bum kicks   Troubled, worried, or depressed.

Bummer   "Bad trip"; unpleasant experience with a drug.

Bundle   Package of twenty-five $5 bags of heroin stacked together.

Burese Cocaine.

Burned To have obtained false drugs.

Burned out Sclerosis of veins from puncturing.

Burning Smoking marijuana.

Bursitis Painful inflammation of the fluid-filled sac between a tendon and a bone, such as in the shoulder or elbow.

Bush Marijuana.

Businessman's trip Dimethyltriptamine (DMT); so called because of its short duration of action.

Bust To arrest or to be arrested by the police.

Button Surface growth of the peyote cactus; peyote.

Buzz Moderate ''high'' from any drug without hallucinations.

Buzz, rolling Moderate ''high'' from a drug that continues after the intake of the drug has stopped.

C Cocaine.

Caapi Hallucinogenic tea made from the vine banisteriopsis.

Ca-Ca Shit; counterfeit or very poor quality drugs (Puerto Rican slang).

Caffeine Behavioral and general cellular stimulant found in coffee, tea, cola drinks, and chocolate.

Calorie Unit used to measure the heat energy available in a food.

Canadian black Variety of marijuana grown in Canada.

Candy Drugs.

Candy man Drug dealer.

Cannabis Genus of plants of which marijuana (*Cannabis sativa*) is a species.

Cap Capsule of a drug.

Carcinogen Agent or factor that causes cancer.

Carcinogenesis Originating or producing a cancer.

Carcinoid syndrome Medical condition with a 5-hydroxyindole–secreting tumor, usually located in the gastrointestinal system.

Cardiac dysrhythmia Disturbance of the normal synchronized rhythm of the heartbeat, so that the heart does not pump blood; it is fatal if not reversed.

Cardiac palpitations Abnormally rapid or violent fluttering or throbbing pulsation of the heart.

Carry To have drugs on one's person (also, Hold).

Cartwheels Amphetamine tablets (also called Crossroads).

Catalase system One pathway of ethanol metabolism involving hydrogen peroxide.

Catalepsy State of rigidity with either resistance, alteration, or ready adoption of a new imposed posture. Often used to refer to animalistic behavior.

Catalyst Substance that increases the rate of a chemical reaction.

Catatonia Clinical symptom which may be either a marked reduction or an increase in mobility or an alternation between the two. May also describe automatism or stereotyped movements.

Catechol 1,2-Dihydrobenzene. Catecholamines are a group of compounds containing the catechol structure; see also Monoamines.

Catecholamines Neurotransmitters in the body having the dihydroxyphenethylamine chemical structure. Examples are epinephrine, norepinephrine, and dopamine.

Catnip Strong-smelling herb sometimes sold as marijuana to unsuspecting buyers.

Centrilobular necrosis Disease of the liver in which one or more cells near the center of a liver lobule are irreversibly destroyed, especially as in the case of exposure to substances such as chloroform, carbon tetrachloride, and naphthalenes.

Cerebellar dysfunction Abnormality manifested by lack of control of some or all voluntary muscular actions (walking, moving the arms, and so forth).

Cerebellum Part of the brainstem; concerned especially with the coordination of muscles and bodily equilibrium.

Cerebral dysfunction Abnormality of that part of the brain concerned with processing and interpreting outside impulses and forming modes of action concerning them (hence thought); therefore, some abnormality of the thought processes that can have thousands of manifestations.

Cerebrospinal fluid　Fluid bathing the brain and spinal cord that is also contained in the cerebral ventricles. Drawn for sampling by lumbar puncture or, more rarely, from the ventricles.

Cerebrum (cerebral cortex)　Convoluted layer of gray matter that forms the largest part of the brain in humans. The highest neural center for coordination and interpretation of external and internal stimuli, it contains sensory, motor, and association areas.

C-fiber　Type of nerve fiber that transmits slowly and gives rise to the sensation of dull, diffuse, or burning pain.

Chalk　Amphetamine tablets.

Charas　Resin exuded by the flowering tops of female hemp (cannabis) plants in India; it is very potent (also called hashish).

Charge　That offense for which the defendant is accused or indicted.

Charles　Cocaine.

Charlie　One dollar.

Chasing the bag　Hustling for heroin, or physically dependent on heroin.

Chasing the dragon　Inhaling the fumes of a heroin and barbiturate mixture that has been placed in tinfoil and heated over a flame.

Chelation　Chemical reaction in which a metallic ion is sequestered and therefore inactivated.

Chemical　Substance capable of altering body function.

Chief　LSD-25.

Chill　To ignore or refuse to deal with someone who is requesting drugs.

Chipper　Controlled, nonaddicted heroin user.

Chipping　Using heroin irregularly to avoid physical dependence.

Chlordiazepoxide (Librium)　A benzodiazepine (sedative-hypnotic drug).

Chlorinated　Addition of a chlorine atom to a basic molecule.

Chlorpromaxine (Thorazine)　A phenothiazine (antipsychotic drug).

Cholinergic　Nerves that use acetylcholine as their synaptic transmitter.

Cholinergic effects　Effects similar to those induced by acetylcholine. These are the type seen with stimulation of the parasympathetic nervous system.

Cholinoceptive site　Postjunctional receptor for acetylcholine; also affected by the agonists muscarine and nicotine.

Chorea　Repetitive, involuntary jerky movements.

Chota　Informer; "rat" (Puerto Rican slang).

Christmas trees　Dexamyl.

Chronic　Of long duration.

Chronic effect　Long-term response to repeated dosages of drugs.

Cibas　Glutethimide.

Circadian rhythm　Of or pertaining to events that occur at approximately 24-hour intervals.

Circling　Behavior elicited by amphetamines or dopamine agonists in animals produced by a unilateral lesion of the nigrostriatal pathway.

Cirrhosis　Chronic liver disease marked by scarring of liver tissue and eventually liver failure.

Classical pharmacology　Study of the effects of certain drugs on test subjects or laboratory animals under controlled conditions.

Clean　Free from suspicion; not being in possession of narcotics; or marijuana with seeds and stems removed.

Clearance　Measure of the rate of elimination of a drug from the body.

Climacteric　Sum of all the physiological changes that occur as part of the natural aging process as the pituitary-gonad relation diminishes in men and women.

Clomiphene (Clomid)　Ovulation-inducing agent thought to act by blocking the inhibitory (negative-feedback) effects that estrogens exert on the hypothalamus.

CNS　Central nervous system; that is, the brain and spinal cord.

Coast　Euphoric "nodding" state induced by a heroin injection.

Coasting Somnolent, "nodding" state of heroin use after recent injection of the drug.

Cocaine Behavioral stimulant.

Cocktail Tobacco cigarette used to smoke the end of a marijuana cigarette; made by removing a bit of tobacco from the tobacco cigarette.

Codeine Sedative and pain-relieving agent found in opium, structurally related to morphine but less potent, and constituting approximately 0.5% of the opium extract.

Co-factor Compound or ion facilitating an enzyme reaction but not itself involved in the reaction.

Cognitive Pertaining to all actions of the mind involved in thinking, perceiving, and remembering.

Coke Cocaine.

Coke head Habitual user of cocaine, possibly exclusively.

Cold turkey Abrupt withdrawal from drugs that have produced physical dependence with no medication or treatment.

Collar To arrest.

Combination pill (oral contraceptive) Medication containing a fixed proportion of synthetic progestin and estrogen.

Come down Gradual loss of effect of a drug on the consciousness.

Compartments Areas of drug or neurotransmitter distribution having different kinetic characteristics.

Competitive inhibition Inhibition that is dependent on the concentration of inhibitor and substrate.

Complex Combination of a molecule of a drug, hormone, or neurotransmitter with a particular protein in the blood or in association with a cell. Some complexes function as transport units; in others, the protein changes shape because of the interaction, initiating a metabolic change.

Complex drug action Drug action manifested by more than one mechanism, effect, dosage, or biochemical metabolism.

Condition Legally binding requirement attached to or made part of a grant, privilege, requisite, or requirement.

Confabulation Fabrication invented to fill gaps in memory.

Congener Nonalcoholic constituents in alcoholic beverages derived from the fermentation process, storage, the original plant material, or added substances.

Conjugation In metabolism of chemicals, the combination (usually in the liver) of a chemical with glucuronic acid or sulfuric acid to form a more water-soluble compound for excretion.

Conjunctival infection Reddened, irritated appearance of the whites of the eyes, such as caused by smoking marijuana.

Connect To find a source of drugs or to buy drugs.

Contact Drug supplier or dealer.

Contact habit Experiencing the effects of physical dependence on a drug by constantly associating with those who use it and are dependent.

Continuance Postponement of an action that is pending in a court.

Contraceptive Any means that prevents pregnancy, including substances or devices that prevent ovulation, fertilization, or implantation.

Controlled substance Drug or chemical regulated under the federal Controlled Substances Act of 1970. Its manufacture, distribution, and sale are subject to federal control or punishment. The key criterion for controlling a substance is its potential for abuse and dependence.

Convulsion Involuntary, violent, and irregular series of contractions of the skeletal muscles.

Cook To heat a mixture of heroin and water until the heroin is dissolved.

Cooker Small metal container in which heroin and water are heated (such as a spoon).

Cop To connect or score; to buy narcotics.

Cop a super rush To inhale more smoke (someone blows on the lit end of a marijuana cigarette while the smoker inhales).

Copilot One who stays with a person who has taken a powerful drug (usually LSD) to help or comfort that person if necessary.

Corpus luteum   Yellow mass in an ovary found at the site of expulsion of the egg. In pregnancy, it secretes estrogen and progesterone.

Corpus striatum   Area of the brain; part of the basal ganglia consisting of the caudate nucleus and putamen.

Corrine   Cocaine.

Counterirritant   Preparation containing an irritant applied to the skin to stimulate sensory receptors, increase blood flow, and induce a sensation of warmth (oil of mustard); may have an analgesic action (methyl salicylate).

Courage pills   Barbiturates or other sedative pills.

Crap   Low-quality drugs of any type, but usually heroin or marijuana.

Crash   To go to sleep or to bed; to come down after using a stimulant.

Creep   Person using heroin who does not engage in risky activities to pay for the drugs.

Cross dependence   Condition in which one drug can prevent the withdrawal symptoms associated with physical dependence on a different drug.

Crossroads   Amphetamine tablets.

Cross tolerance   Condition in which tolerance of one drug results in a lessened response to another drug.

Crutch   Anything used to hold the last bit of a marijuana cigarette so that it can be smoked.

Crystal   PCP (phencyclidine) or methamphetamine.

CSF   Cerebrospinal fluid.

Cube   Cube of sugar containing LSD.

Cumulative effect   Strong, often intense, effect of the last of a series of drug dosages, the preceding dosages of which had a moderate, mild, or even negligible effect.

Cut   To dilute a drug with another substance to increase the quantity for sale.

Cyclazocine   Long-acting narcotic antagonist.

Cyclic hydrocarbon   Chemicals composed of hydrogen and carbon that exist in ring form.

Cytoplasm   Fluid and structures within a cell wall and surrounding the cell nucleus.

D   Doriden (glutethimide).

Dabble   To use drugs irregularly.

Dagga   Marijuana (South Africa).

Datura   Jimson weed; found in Mexico, United States, India, and South America. It has psychotropic properties.

DAWN (Drug Abuse Warning Network)   Federal program designed to identify drugs currently abused and the patterns of abuse in selected metropolitan areas from medical records of emergency room patients and morgues.

DEA (Drug Enforcement Administration)   Division of the U.S. Department of Justice.

Deadly nightshade   Belladonna.

Deal   To buy or sell drugs.

Dealer   Seller or "pusher" of drugs.

Dealer's band   Rubber band around the wrist that secures packets of drugs (usually heroin), so that if the wrist is flipped violently the drugs will fall into the hand.

Deck   Folded paper or glassine envelope containing drugs (usually heroin or cocaine).

Deeda   LSD-25.

Defendant   The accused.

Delerium   Condition characterized by mental excitement, confusion, disordered speech, and often hallucinations.

Delerium tremens (DT's "rum fits")   Syndrome of tremulousness with hallucinations, psychomotor agitation, confusion and disorientation, sleep disorders, and other associated discomforts lasting for several days after alcohol withdrawal.

Delusion   Belief held without any supportive evidence, usually but not necessarily false.

Dementia   Mental deterioration due to organic or emotional causes.

Dendrite   Thin, cellular extension from a neuron; serves as a reception area (postsynaptic) for signals coming to the neuron from other neurons.

Dependency   Psychic or physical state resulting from the interaction between a living organism and a psychoactive drug characterized by behavioral and other responses that always include a compulsion to take the drug on a continuous or periodic basis in order to experience its psychic effects and sometimes to avoid the discomfort of abstaining from it.

Depersonalization Subjective experience that the body is unreal or changed in some way.

Depressant Any of several drugs that sedate by acting on the central nervous system; medical uses include the treatment of anxiety, tension, and high blood pressure.

Derealization State of being characterized by a person losing awareness of tangible and measurable reality on which laws are based. The person may feel that he or she is dead or in another universe.

Desensitization (1) Adaptation of a receptor neuron to reduce the function of the nervous system. (2) Psychological treatment designed to reduce anxiety to specific situations by controlled exposure to them.

Detention State of being detained or held in custody to ensure future court appearances; usually takes place in jail.

Detoxification Biological process by which toxins (poisons), drugs, and hormones are modified into less toxic, or more readily excretable, substances, usually in the liver; see also Biotransformation.

Dexie Dexedrine (an amphetamine).

Diabetes mellitus Serious disorder in which carbohydrates are improperly metabolized, leading typically to excessively high blood sugar levels.

Diazepam (Valium) A benzodiazepine (antianxiety drug).

Dicarbamates Class of chemically related sedative-hypnotic agents of which meprobamate (Equanil, Miltown) is an example.

Diencephalon Anterior part of brain stem including hypothalamus, thalamus, and posterior pituitary.

Diethylstilbesterol (DES) Synthetic compound with estrogenic activity; carcinogenic in animals; sometimes used as a ''morning after'' birth control method.

Diisopropyl fluorophosphate (DFP) Irreversible acetylcholine esterase (AChE) inhibitor.

Dilation Increase in the inner diameter of blood vessels or organs.

Dime Ten dollars.

Dirty Person or place that contains illegal drugs.

Discretion Reasonable exercise of power or right to act in an official capacity.

Discretionary decision maker Prosecutor or judge (or both) during criminal proceedings.

Disinhibition Physiologic state within the central nervous system characterized by decreased activity of inhibitory synapses, which results in a net excess of excitatory activity.

Dissociation constant Measure of the tendency of compounds to separate. In ligand binding studies it is a measure of the attraction between ligand and receptor; the reciprocal of the affinity constant.

Distribution Pattern of specific organs or areas of the body in which a drug spreads or concentrates.

Disulfiram ethanol reaction Group of symptoms that are seen as a result of blocking the metabolism of acetaldehyde.

Diuresis Urine excretion in excess of the usual amount.

Diuretic Drug used to increase the excretion of water by the kidneys, with a concurrent loss of sodium.

Dizygotic twins Twins who have developed from two ova and therefore have different genetic characteristics.

Djamba Marijuana (Brazil).

Djomba Marijuana (Central Africa).

DMT Dimethoxymethylamphetamine (also called STP).

DMT (N, N-Dimethyltryptamine) Fast-acting hallucinogenic drug with a short duration of action or effect.

Do To use drugs.

Dogie Heroin.

Dol Unit of pain intensity based on a sequence of just-noticeable-difference steps in stimulus intensity.

Dollies Dolophine pills.

Dolls Barbiturate or amphetamine pills.

Dolophine Methadone; synthetic opiate slightly more potent than morphine and with much longer duration of action.

Dopamine   Catecholaminergic transmitter substance and immediate precursor of norepinephrine. Involved in inhibitory motor regulation and motivational-emotional functions.

Dopamine hypothesis   Hypothesis that schizophrenia is related to an increased amount of brain dopamine, based on evidence that drugs that block dopamine receptors reduce schizophrenic symptoms.

Dope   Any drug that will produce a change in mental state (including alcohol).

Dope fiend   Term ironically and defiantly applied to themselves by those physically dependent on drugs.

Dosage   Determination of the proper amount of a given remedy (a drug or other treatment modality).

Dose   The quantity of a drug or other remedy to be taken or applied at one time or in fractional amounts within a given period.

Dose-effect relationship   Relationship between the quantity of a drug being administered and the amount of the observed effect. This relationship is such that there are usually one or more points at which, for a given quantity of drug, there is a maximum observed effect such that, if more or less of the same drug were administered, the effect would be less per unit of the drug administered.

Double-blind, placebo-controlled study   Study in which the intensity and character of response to a drug depend on the amount administered and individual variability; see also Effective dose.

Double trouble   Tuinal (a barbiturate).

Downers   Barbiturates, tranquilizers, alcohol; any depressant.

Down trip   Depression or boring experience.

Dragged   To be frightened or hysterical after using a drug (usually marijuana).

Dreamer   Morphine.

Dried out   Detoxified, no longer physically dependent on a drug or drugs.

Drivers; truckdrivers   Amphetamines.

Drop   To swallow a pill, capsule, or tablet.

Dropper   Medicine dropper used as a syringe for injecting drugs.

Drug   Substance with potential use as medicine in treatment of disease.

Drug antagonist   Any means (usually another drug) of neutralizing, preventing the action of, or destroying the effects of a certain other drug.

Drug disposition tolerance   State in which enzyme systems in the liver increase their capacity to metabolize a drug so that the body disposes of the drug faster.

Drug hunger   Common manifestation of psychologic drug dependence in which the subject has a drive or craving for a particular drug or for the past, subjectively pleasurable effects of a particular drug.

Drug interaction   State characterized by modification of the effects of one drug by prior or concurrent administration of another drug. (This interaction can be either advantageous or adverse, depending on the drugs used and the effect desired.)

Drug metabolism   Sum total of all bodily processing of a drug, including uptake, biotransformation, distribution throughout the body, storage, and excretion of the drug or its by-products.

Drug misuse   Use of any drug (legal or illegal) for a medical or recreational purpose when other alternatives are available, practical, or warranted, or when drug use endangers either the user or others with whom he or she may interact.

Drug receptor complex   Those components of a cell that are directly involved with the initial action of a drug.

Drug tolerance   State of progressively decreased responsiveness to a drug.

Duby   Marijuana.

Dummy   Counterfeit heroin or cocaine.

Dusting   Putting a drug on another substance to be smoked (an example is opium-dusted marijuana).

Dynamite   Very potent version of any drug (dynamite dope), or cocaine and heroin taken in combination.

Dyskinesia   Impairment of voluntary movements.

Dysphasia   Impairment of language.

Dysphoria Mental uneasiness, restlessness, or anxiety.

Dyspraxia Impairment of the ability to perform coordinated movements.

Edema See Oedema.

EEG (Electroencephalogram) Recording of the small electrical currents (brain waves) generated by groups of neurons in the several lobes of the brain.

Effective dose (ED$_{50}$) Amount of a drug that produces the desired effect in 50% of the test animals or subjects.

Eighth One-eighth ounce of a drug, usually heroin or cocaine.

Electric Containing either marijuana or a hallucinogenic drug.

Electric Kool-Aid Liquid beverage made with Kool-Aid to which a hallucinogenic drug has been added.

Electrocardiograph Instrument for measuring the potential of the electric currents that traverse the heart and initiate its beat. It is used to measure the quality and quantity of the heart beat and in many cases to ascertain whether the heart is functioning properly.

Electrolytic lesions Destruction of specific neuronal pathways by passage of electricity between electrodes inserted into the brain.

Elephant tranquilizer PCP (phencyclidine).

Embalao Strongly addicted, ''strung out'' (Puerto Rican slang).

Embolization Obstruction of a blood vessel by a transported piece of matter, such as a blood clot, vegetation, bacteria, or other foreign matter.

Embryo Developing creature in the uterus during the first trimester of pregnancy. Embryonic tissue is more susceptible to teratogenic effects than is fetal tissue.

Emphysema Disease in which the lungs are inelastic, causing oxygen and carbon dioxide exchange to be impaired; heart action is often impaired as well.

Enchaioui Man who has centered his life around marijuana (Arabic slang).

End bulb or presynaptic terminal Part of the axon of the neuron where neurotransmitters are released.

Endocrine system All the glands that secrete hormones.

Endogenous Coming from within.

Endogenous paranoid schizophrenic reaction State of mind such that the person experiencing it, through no overt external stimuli, will manifest the symptoms of paranoid schizophrenia (that is, ambivalence, autism, loose associations, and flat or labile affect) with an overriding fear that he or she is in grave danger from an external force that may or may not be identifiable.

Endometrium Inner membrane (or lining) of the uterus.

Endorphins Naturally occurring proteins with endogenous morphine-like activity.

Enkephalin Naturally occurring protein with morphine-like activity.

Enteral drug Drug that is taken orally.

Enzyme Biological chemical, protein in nature and produced by living cells, that can influence the rate of body processes. Enzymes can act independently of the cells that produce them.

Enzyme induction Increased production of drug-metabolizing enzymes in the liver stimulated by certain drugs, such that use of these drugs increases the rate at which the body can metabolize them. It is one mechanism by which pharmacological tolerance is produced.

Enzyme inhibition Process by which certain enzymes are rendered less active by the administration of certain drugs or disease states.

Epena Hallucinogenic snuff made from the bark of trees and used by South American natives in Brazil.

Ergotism Poisoning by toxic substances containing the fungus *Claviceps purpurea* (from which the drug LSD is purified). The symptoms are lameness and necrosis of the extremities resulting from contraction of the peripheral vascular bed.

Ergotropic That which incites to activity; hyperaroused (compare with Trophotropic).

Esrar Marijuana (Turkish).

Estrogen Body hormone secreted primarily from the ovaries of females in response to stimulation by follicle-stimulating hormone (FSH) from the pituitary gland.

Ethanol   Ethyl alcohol, or the beverage type of alcohol.

Etorphine   Potent narcotic analgesic.

Euphoria   Extreme sense of physical and emotional well-being referred to by drug users as the "high."

Excipient ingredient   Substance (usually without drug action) added to medications to give form, consistency, flavor, and other properties.

Excretion   Process by which a drug and its metabolic products are eliminated from the body.

Expectorant   Compounds that enhance the removal of respiratory tract fluids by coughing; an example is Ipecac.

Experience   LSD-type "trip."

Explorer's club   Illicit circle of LSD users.

Extrapyramidal   Motor control not involving pyramidal tracts, having its origin in the basal ganglia.

Eye openers   Amphetamines.

F-40's   Secobarbital.

Factory   Place in which drugs are made, diluted, or cleaned for sale.

Falling out   Dozing off or going to sleep under the influence of a drug.

Fatty   Thickly rolled marijuana cigarette.

FDA   U.S. Food and Drug Administration.

Feds   Federal Bureau of Narcotics agents.

Fermentation   Biochemical process in which yeast converts sugar to alcohol.

Fetal alcohol syndrome   Associated group of symptoms such as mental retardation, impairment of growth, and facial deformities caused by prenatal exposure to alcohol.

Fetus   Developing creature in the uterus during the second and third trimesters of pregnancy.

Finding   Court decision based on issue of fact.

Five cent paper $5 bag of heroin.

Five dollar bag   Bag of heroin sold for $5 and containing five grains of from 0% to 80% pure heroin.

Fives   Tablets containing 5 mg of a drug.

Fix   To inject a drug, usually heroin, amphetamines, or cocaine, intravenously (also, to fix up).

Flake   Cocaine.

Flash   Sudden rush of euphoria after injection of speed or heroin.

Flashback   Spontaneous recurrence of an experience identical to a chemical effect but in the absence of any chemical.

Flea powder   False or inferior drugs.

Flight of ideas   Rapid succession of thoughts without logical connections.

Flit out   State of fear and loss of control produced by a drug or some external stimulus.

Floating (high, stoned, ripped)   Intoxicated from drugs.

Flower power   Power of love rather than force.

Fluorinated   Addition of a fluorine atom to a basic molecule.

Flush   Sudden onset of euphoria from a drug (usually injected).

Flying (high, stoned, etc.)   Intoxicated from drugs.

Flying saucers   Variety of morning glory plant, the seeds of which are hallucinogenic.

Footballs   Diamphetamine pills; or dilaudid, a synthetic opiate.

Formication (cocaine bugs)   Sensation of insects crawling underneath the skin, caused by stimulants such as cocaine and amphetamine.

Forwards   Amphetamine pills.

Freak   Person whose lifestyle, behavior, appearance, or ideas determine that the person is different, usually in an unacceptable way, from the rest of society; or a person who prefers a particular drug or behavior (speed freak, acid freak, television freak).

Freaking freely   Spontaneous, random behavior, usually produced by hallucinogenics.

Freak out   Panic reaction from the effects of a drug or experience.

Free   Form of compound not bound.

Free-basing   Conversion of the stable salt from an alkaloid, such as cocaine, into the less chemically stable but more biologically potent basic form "freed" of the ionic salt; also, using a drug in this form.

Freon   Liquid fluorocarbons used mainly as refrigerants, coolants, or aerosol propellants.

Frisco speedball Heroin, cocaine, and LSD mixed.

Fruit salad Game in which each participant takes one pill from every bottle in the medicine cabinet.

FSH (follicle-stimulating hormone) Gonadotropin from the pituitary gland; it directs the ovary to mature follicles in preparation for ovulation and the testes to continue spermatogenesis.

Full moon Large peyote chunk greater than four inches in diameter.

Funny cigarette Marijuana cigarette.

Fuzz (pigs, cops, the man, turds, narcs) Police, especially narcotics officers.

Gage Marijuana.

Galactorrhea Excessive or spontaneous flow of milk when not physiologically appropriate, such as a side effect of a drug.

Gammon One microgram (one millionth of one gram) of LSD.

Ganga Marijuana of high potency.

Ganglia Groups of nerve cell bodies outside the central nervous system, such as along the spinal cord.

Gangster Marijuana.

Gangster pills Barbiturates of high potency.

Gas chromatography Separation of volatile compounds by injection into a gas stream that is percolated over a stationary phase, which may be either a solid or a liquid (the latter is spread as a thin film over an inert solid). The separated compounds then pass into a suitable detector.

Gassing Sniffing the fumes from gasoline.

Gastritis Inflammation of the stomach, causing damage to the blood vessels and erosion of stomach tissue; the beginning of a peptic ulcer.

G.B. Goofball, barbiturates.

Gee head Person physically dependent on paregoric.

Get down To use heroin.

Ghanja Active constituent of marijuana in highly concentrated form.

Ghost LSD.

Giggle weed Marijuana.

Girl Cocaine.

GI tract Gastrointestinal tract, consisting of the stomach and intestines.

Glaucoma Disease of the eye characterized by increased intraocular pressure that results in defects in the field of vision and eventually in potential total blindness.

Glial cells Supporting cells within the central nervous system, thought not to be directly involved in neurotransmission.

Globetrotter Person who goes to various drug dealers looking for the best drugs.

Globus pallidus Specific nucleus within the basal ganglia.

Glow (high, stoned, etc.) Intoxicated from drugs.

Glucose Blood sugar; also called dextrose.

Glycoside Plant product consisting of an organic molecule combined with a sugar. Some very important drugs are glycosides.

Going down Going well.

Going high Continuing state of intoxication from drugs, not necessitating more drugs.

Gold dust Cocaine.

Golden leaf Acapulco gold marijuana.

Gonad Sex gland (an ovary or testis).

Gonadotropin Hormone secreted by the pituitary gland that stimulates the function of the gonads.

Goods Any kind of drugs.

Good stuff Best drugs of any kind.

Goofball Barbiturate pill.

Goofer Doriden.

Gorilla pills Barbiturates or other sedative pills.

Gout Metabolic disease (sometimes induced by alcoholism) characterized by recurrent attacks of arthritis, especially of the great toe.

Graduation Successful completion of the conditions set by a treatment program, marked by a ceremony similar to graduation.

Grand mal Major seizure disorder with tonic and clonic muscular movements and loss of consciousness.

Granulomatous reaction Any one of a rather large group of distinctive focal reactions characterized by formation, as a result of inflammation due to biologic, chemical, or physical agents, of a gross granule-like appearance (appearance at some time of large mononuclear phagocytes) that persists in the tissue as slow smoldering reactions or inflammations.

Grass   Marijuana.

Grasshopper   One who uses marijuana.

GRAS substance   Drug or food additive generally regarded as safe because of its long use by the population without any apparent deleterious effects.

Gravy   Mixture of blood from a vein and heroin that is reheated because it has coagulated.

Greasy junkie   Passive, indolent person who is physically dependent on heroin but who will make no great effort to obtain money for drugs.

Grefa   Marijuana.

Ground control   One who helps or talks to a person under the influence of a hallucinogenic drug in order for that person to have a good experience.

Guide   One who helps or guides another person who is under the influence of a hallucinogenic drug through the experience.

Guru   Same as Guide.

Gynecomastia   Development of the breasts when physiologically inappropriate, such as in men.

H   Heroin.

Habituation   As defined in 1957 by the World Health Organization, a condition resulting from the repeated consumption of a drug, which includes these characteristics: (1) a desire (but not compulsion) to continue taking the drug for the sense of improved well-being that it engenders; (2) little or no tendency to increase the dosage; (3) some degree of psychic dependence and hence no abstinence syndrome; (4) primarily a detrimental effect, if any, on the user.

Half-life   Amount of time it takes for the body to eliminate 50% of drug molecules from the blood stream.

Half-load   Fifteen packages of heroin, wrapped together for resale.

Hallucinations   Perceptions with no external reality.

Hallucinogens   Any of several drugs, popularly called psychedelics, that produce sensations such as distortions of time, space, sound, and color and other bizarre effects. Although they are pharmacologically nonnarcotic, some of these drugs have been regulated under federal narcotic laws (Schedule 1).

Haloperidol (Haldol)   Antipsychotic drug chemically classified as a butyrophenone.

Hand to hand   Transfer of drugs at the point of sale.

Hapten   Substance that does not stimulate antibody formation itself but that will combine with a carrier antigen to stimulate antibody formation.

Haraz   Policeman or cop (Puerto Rican slang).

Hard stuff   Derivatives of opium, especially heroin, cocaine, and sometimes hallucinogens, depending on the person using them.

Harmine   Psychedelic agent obtained from the seeds of *Peganum harmala*.

Harry   Heroin.

Hash   Pure resinous extract from the marijuana plant.

Hashish   Extract of the hemp plant (*Cannabis sativum*) with a higher concentration of tetrahydrocannabinol than marijuana.

Hawk   LSD-25.

Hay   Marijuana.

H-caps   Gelatin capsules of heroin.

HDL (high-density lipoprotein)   Currently considered by some authorities as a key substance in the prevention of hardening of the arteries.

Head   Heavy abuser.

Head drugs   Those that appear to affect the mind and not the body (hallucinogens mostly, but sometimes amphetamines and marijuana).

Head shop   Store specializing in the paraphernalia of drug use.

Hearts   Amphetamine tablets so shaped.

Heat (fuzz, pigs, cops)   Police.

Heavenly dust   Cocaine.

Heavenly blue   Variety of morning glory seeds that have hallucinogenic properties.

Hematuria   Any condition in which the urine contains blood or red blood cells.

Hemp   Marijuana.

Henry   Heroin.

Hep Hepatitis.

Hepatic cirrhosis Disease of the liver of many causes, characterized by degeneration, fatty infiltration, atrophy, and inflammation, that gives rise to a deformity that interferes with liver function and circulation of the blood and bile.

Her Cocaine.

Herb Marijuana.

Heroin Semisynthetic opiate produced by a chemical modification of morphine.

HGH Human growth hormone.

Him Heroin.

Histamine Biochemical substance (in the amine class) stored in mast cells and released in response to tissue injury, including allergic reactions; histamine has no known functional role, but it may be a neurotransmitter.

Histochemistry Study of the composition of cells by means of chemical techniques. Fluorescence histochemistry involves reacting the monoamine neurotransmitters with chemicals to produce a fluorescent derivative that can be mapped.

Hit To inject (any drug) intravenously.

Hold To possess drugs.

Homeostasis Maintenance of a stable biochemical environment within the body's cells and the fluid bathing the cells in response to constant internal and external fluctuations, such as variations in nutrient supply and demands on organs (especially the liver and kidney) to metabolize and excrete natural and foreign substances.

Hookah Pipe for smoking marijuana.

Hop Opium.

Hophead Person physically dependent upon heroin or opium.

Hormone Biochemical substance produced and secreted by an endocrine gland that brings about an adjustment in or development of a target tissue.

Horse Heroin.

Hot-shot Injection that is supposed to be heroin but is usually poison.

Hungry croaker Doctor who, for money, will prescribe drugs to a person who is physically dependent on them.

Hustling Prostitution, stealing, or otherwise getting money for drugs.

Hydrolysis Chemical reaction that results in the breaking down of a large molecule into smaller molecules and water.

Hydroxylation In the metabolism of a chemical, the addition of an -OH (hydroxyl) group to a chemical to render it more water soluble for urinary excretion.

Hyperbaric Increased pressure (for example, hyperbaric oxygen is increased oxygen pressure).

Hypercholesterolemia Abnormally high level of cholesterol in the blood.

Hyperglycemia Abnormally high level of glucose in the blood.

Hyperkinesis Hyperactivity; a behavioral disorder in which the person, usually a child, is abnormally and uncontrollably active.

Hyperpyrexia Abnormally elevated body temperature, as from a fever or activation of the sympathetic nervous system due to a drug such as amphetamine.

Hypertension Blood pressure elevated beyond normal values for age and sex; classified as mild, moderate, or severe.

Hypnotic Central nervous system depressant that induces sleep.

Hypochondriasis Excessive concern about health.

Hypodermic Under, or inserted under, the skin (as in hypodermic injection).

Hypoglycemia Abnormally low level of glucose in the blood.

Hypophysis Pituitary. Hypophysectomy is the removal of the pituitary.

Hypotension Low blood pressure.

Hypothalamus Region of the forebrain below the thalamus that is the major central control of the autonomic nervous system and is important in the regulation of blood pressure and heart rate and maintenance of body temperature, metabolism, and the endocrine system.

Hypothermia Low body temperature.

Hypothyroidism Inadequate secretion of the thyroid gland's hormone; causes slowed reflexes, impaired metabolism, and psychological disturbances.

Iatrogenic disease Disorder caused by the treatment process.

Ibotinic acid Psychedelic agent found in the mushroom *Amanita muscaria*.

Ice cream habit Infrequent or moderate use of drugs producing physical dependence.

Ideas of reference Ideas that normal events have relevance to or are commenting on oneself.

Idiosyncratic Peculiar or unexpected.

Idiot pills Barbiturates or other sedative pills.

Immunofluorescence Fluorescent histochemistry in which antibodies are used to identify compounds under investigation.

Implantation Process in which a fertilized human egg burrows into the uterine lining to obtain nutrients and exchange waste; marks the beginning of pregnancy.

Impotence Condition in which the affected man is unable to achieve and maintain an erection.

IND (Investigational New Drug) number FDA assigned code number used during human clinical tests of a new drug before granting permission to market it.

Indian hay Marijuana.

Indoles 2,3-Benzopyrrole, indolamines; a group of compounds containing the indole structure; see also Monoamines.

Infarct Areas of tissue death due to reduced blood supply.

Inflammation Defensive body process characterized by redness, heat, pain, and swelling and caused by injury to tissue.

Inhalant Volatile substance that is introduced into the body through the lungs.

Inhibitory center Part of the brain that controls the quality and quantity of inhibitions to particular actions or thought patterns of an organism.

Initial response First response, subjective or objective, to the administration of a particular drug.

Injection Dosage form in which the drug is administered; that is, intravenously (IV), intramuscularly (IM), intraperitoneally (IP, into the abdominal cavity), or subcutaneously (SC, under the skin).

Inositol Vitamin in the B complex found as an adulterant in street cocaine.

Into Using or paying special attention to something.

In transit On an LSD trip.

Intrauterine Device (IUD) Foreign object placed into the uterus for contraceptive purposes.

Ion channel Channel concerned with the passage of ions across a cell membrane.

Ionized Existing in a more water-soluble form.

Ionophoresis Administration of compounds through micropipettes that are released by an electric current.

Isomerism (1) Structural chemistry: the possession of two or more compounds of the same molecular formula but different structures. (2) Stereochemistry: two or more compounds having the same molecular and structural formulas but different spatial configurations.

Jag Intoxication.

Jammed up Having taken an overdose of a drug.

Jay Short for "joint" or marijuana cigarette.

Jerk off Injecting a little heroin at a time in order to prolong the initial euphoria.

Joint Marijuana cigarette.

Jolly beans Amphetamine pills.

Jones Heroin withdrawal.

Joy juice Chloral hydrate, appetizers, or tonics.

Joy-pop; skin-pop To inject drugs under the skin.

Juanita Marijuana.

Judgment Court's determination.

Juice Liquor.

Junk Narcotics.

Junkie A person who uses narcotics regularly; usually addicted.

K_I Concentration of an inhibitor required to displace 50% of a bound ligand (or drug) to its receptor site ($K_I = 1 + F/k_d$).

Kava Mild psychotropic beverage drunk by the people of New Guinea.

Ketamine Psychedelic surgical anesthetic.

Key (or ki) Kilogram; an amount of a drug (usually marijuana, cocaine, or heroin).

Khat Shrub native to Africa and Arabia; the leaves and twigs are chewed, brewed like tea, or fermented with honey. Causes a stimulatory, euphoric effect and a particular type of drug dependence.

Kick To withdraw from physical dependence on drugs.

Kicks Pleasure or pleasurable experience.

Kick the habit on the elevator Easy withdrawal from a drug by a person who is only minimally physically dependent on it.

Kilo Same as Key.

Kilter Marijuana.

King Kong pills Barbiturates or other sedative pills.

Korsakoff's psychosis Nervous system disorder resulting in memory failure, confabulation, and sometimes hallucinations and agitation.

KW (Killer weed or marijuana) Substance sprinkled on leaves to be smoked.

L LSD-25.

LAAM (1-α-acetylmethodol) Long-acting narcotic analgesic.

Lacrimation Secretion and discharge of tears.

Lady snow Cocaine.

LD$_{50}$ Quantity of a chemical that is lethal to 50% of a test population.

Leapers Amphetamines.

Left-handed cigarette Marijuana cigarette.

Legend drug Drug that bears on its label the warning "Caution: Federal law prohibits dispensing without a prescription."

Lemonade (shit, blank, crap, garbage) Poor quality drugs.

LH (luteinizing hormone) Gonadotropin from the pituitary gland that directs the testes to secrete testosterone and the ovaries to form the corpus luteum.

Libido Sexual drive or desire.

Lid Street measure of marijuana (about 1 ounce).

Lid poppers Amphetamines.

Life Characteristic pattern of the life of one whose existence revolves around use of drugs.

Life events Experiences that are part of normal life but are stressful and thought to be involved in the precipitation of psychiatric disorders.

Life expectancy at birth Number of years a newborn infant can expect to live, figured according to the levels of mortality prevailing in the year of its birth.

Ligand Compound that specifically binds to a receptor.

Light stuff Marijuana or other non-dependence–producing hallucinogenic drugs.

Limbic system Neurons in the hippocampus, amygdala, and other structures integrating the cerebral cortex with the hypothalamus; concerned with emotion and motivation; probably uses dopamine as the neurotransmitter.

Line Vein used to inject drugs.

Lipid Fat-soluble molecule.

Lipophilic Drug or other substance that is more soluble in lipid (fat) than in water.

β-Lipotropin A 91–amino acid protein containing amino acid sequences that has morphine-like activity.

Lithium An alkali metal effective in the treatment of mania and depression.

Liver induction See Enzyme induction.

Load Some 25 to 30 packets of heroin stacked and held together with a rubber band for delivery.

Loco Marijuana.

Look-alike Inert or less potent chemical that is intentionally prepared to look like a well-known form of a more powerful, expensive, or less-available chemical. The look-alikes in use in any community depend on availability and local use patterns (e.g., diazepam for methaqualone or secobarbital).

LSD-25 d-Lysergic acid diethylamide tartrate 25.

Lumbar puncture Sampling of cerebrospinal fluid by insertion of a hypodermic needle through the lumbar region of the spine into the space surrounding the spinal cord and nerves.

Lush Heavy drinker or alcoholic.

Lysergic acid diethylamide (LSD) Semisynthetic psychedelic drug.

M Morphine.

Main effect Drug's desired effect; no known drug has only a main effect.

Mainline Large vein used to inject drugs, usually heroin or amphetamines.

Maintaining Keeping a certain level of drug habit.

Majoon Hashish produced in the Middle East.

Making a croaker for a reader Bribing a doctor to write an illegal prescription for drugs.

Man Police.

Mandrake European herb whose roots may resemble the human form; contains hallucinogenic belladonna compounds.

Manic depressive Mental disorder characterized by alternating extremes of excitement and depression.

Manicure Marijuana of high grade; or to remove the stems and seeds from the marijuana plant.

Mannitol Mannite; a white, powdery type of sugar found as an adulterant in street cocaine and heroin.

MAOI (monoamine oxidase inhibitor) Drug that inhibits the activity of the enzyme monoamine oxidase.

Margin of safety Dosage range between an ineffective (threshold) amount and a lethal amount of a drug.

Marijuana Mixture of the crushed leaves, flowers, and small branches of both male and female individuals of the hemp plant.

Mary Morphine.

Maryann Marijuana.

Mass fragmentography Quantitative analysis of compounds by measurement of specific fragments by means of mass spectrometry.

Mass spectrometry Analysis of the chemical structure of a compound by measurement of the molecular weight of fragments of it. Fragments are formed by bombardment of the molecule by ions.

Matchbox Small one-penny matchbox full of marijuana for sale.

MDA (methyldiethylamine) Synthetic derivation of amphetamine.

Medial forebrain bundle Group of nerve fibers connecting the forebrain, midbrain, and hypothalamus; location of the pleasure (reward) center; probably uses norepinephrine as a neurotransmitter.

Meditation State of constant and continuous flow of awareness of one chosen object, created by maintaining a thought-free state of mind.

Medulla oblongata Area of the brain lying below the pons.

Mellow out To forget tensions and worries.

Mellow yellow Inner fibrous layer of banana peels that are scraped and smoked; thought (but not proved) to have psychotropic effects.

Membrane Thin layer of tissue (often made up of fat and protein complexes) separating one structure from another.

Menopause Cessation of menstrual cycles; part of the female climacteric.

Meperidine (Demerol) Synthetically produced opiate narcotic.

Meprobamate (Equanil) Sedative-hypnotic agent frequently used as an antianxiety drug.

Mesc (mescal, mescaline) Hallucinogenic drug made from peyote cactus.

Mesencephalon Area of the brain, also known as the midbrain, that contains the tegmentum and substantia nigra.

Mesolimbic forebrain Area of the brain containing the nucleus accumbens, olfactory tubercle, and projections to the cortex.

Metabolism (of drugs) All the chemical and physical reactions that the body carries out to prepare a drug for excretion.

Metabolite Any substance produced by the body as a result of normal functioning.

Meth Methamphetamine.

Methamphetamine A powerful amphetamine (also Methadrine and Desoxyn).

Meth freak One who uses methamphetamines habitually, and possibly exclusively.

Methylphenidate (Ritalin) Central nervous system stimulant chemically and pharmacologically related to amphetamine.

Mexican brown Grade of marijuana.

Mexican locoweed Marijuana.

Mexican mushroom Hallucinogenic mushroom containing psilocybin.

Microdot Tiny tablet of LSD.

Microsomal ethanol oxidizing system (MEOS) One pathway of ethanol metabolism; it is inducible and may be partially responsible for tolerance to alcohol.

Microsomes Protein structures in the cytoplasm involved in metabolism.

Midbrain Component of the brain between the brainstem and the forebrain; it has tracts from the spinal cord and medulla oblongata to the higher cortical centers and has relays that control vision and hearing.

Migraine Syndrome characterized by localized headache and often accompanied by nausea, vomiting, and sensory disturbances.

Mike One microgram (one millionth of one gram) of a drug, usually LSD.

Milk sugar (mannite) A substance used to dilute drugs that come in powdered form (such as heroin).

Milligram One thousandth of one gram.

Miltown Meprobamate (a tranquilizer).

Mind detergent LSD-25.

Mind trippers People who use drugs to explore their minds.

Minimal effective dose Amount of a particular drug less than which will not produce the desired effect.

Minor tranquilizer Any sedative-hypnotic drug promoted primarily for use in the treatment of anxiety.

Miosis Constriction of the pupils of the eyes; compare to Mydriasis.

Miss Emma Morphine.

Mitochondria Rod-shaped subcellular organelles involved in metabolism.

M.J. Marijuana.

Mojo Heroin, cocaine, or morphine.

Monkey Physical addiction to a drug, usually heroin.

Monkey dust PCP (phencyclidine).

Monoamine Generic name for the catecholamine or indolamine neurotransmitters.

Monozygotic Twins who have developed from a single ovum and therefore have the same genetic characteristics.

Moon Peyote cactus top, or cake or bulk hashish.

Morbidity Characterized by disease; state of being physically or mentally diseased.

Morning after pill Drug taken shortly after sexual intercourse to prevent implantation of a fertilized ovum, thus preventing pregnancy.

Morning shot Wake-up injection, usually of heroin.

Morph Morphine.

Morphine Major sedative and pain-relieving drug found in opium, being approximately 10% of the crude opium exudate.

Mortality ratio Number obtained by dividing the death rate in one group of people, such as drug users, by a matched group of people who do not use that drug in order to estimate what contribution to the death rate is made by the drug.

Mota Marijuana.

Mother Drug dealer.

Mu Marijuana.

Mucarinic Having a mucarine-like action; that is, producing effects that resemble postganglionic parasympathetic stimulation.

Mucous membrane Lining of passages and cavities in communication with the air (mouth and lungs, vagina, glans penis, rectum, and nasal passages).

Muscarine Drug extracted from the mushroom *Amanita muscaria* that directly stimulates acetylcholine receptors.

Muscarinic cholinoceptive site Postjunctional receptor for acetylcholine; also affected by muscarine.

Muscimol Psychedelic agent found in the mushroom *Amanita muscaria*.

Mutagen Agent that causes mutations (that is, permanent changes in genetic material).

Mutagenesis Origin or production of a mutation in an organism.

Mydriasis Unusual dilation of the pupil of the eye.

Myristicin Psychedelic agent obtained from nutmeg and mace.

Nab Same as Bust.

NAD (nicotinamide-adenine dinucle-otide) Energy cofactor necessary for many of the chemical reactions in the body to occur.

Nail Hypodermic needle used for injecting drugs.

Nalline Nalorphine hydrochloride; a semisynthetic derivative of morphine.

Naltrexone Long-acting narcotic antagonist.

Narc Federal narcotics officer.

Narcolepsy Condition in which a person falls asleep spontaneously and without warning.

Narcotic Medically, any drug that produces sleep or stupor and also relieves pain; legally, any drug regulated under the Harrison Act and other federal narcotics laws.

Narcotic analgesic Any natural or synthetic drug with pharmacologic actions similar to those of morphine (also called opioid).

Natch Not using drugs; natural.

NDA New Drug Application required by the FDA.

Needle park Place used for injecting drugs.

Nembies Nembutal; a barbiturate.

Nemish Nembutal capsules.

Nerve block Method of analgesia in which a nerve-destroying agent is injected close to the troublesome area or nerve.

Nervous system One of the two major systems of the body that control homeostasis. The nervous system receives and interprets stimuli and transmits impulses to effector organs.

Neuralgia Sharp, paroxysmal pain along the path followed by a nerve.

Neurohumor Chemical substance liberated in the tissues by a nerve impulse.

Neuroleptics Major tranquilizing drugs used to treat psychotic episodes.

Neuromodulator Compound postulated to regulate the action of a neurotransmitter; the term is particularly used to describe certain peptides.

Neuromuscular block Interruption of the transmission of nerve impulses to muscles by preventing the action of the transmitter at the receptor on the muscle surface.

Neuroregulator Compounds that have not been shown to fulfill all the criteria of a neurotransmitter.

Neurotic Psychiatric conditions in which contact with reality and insight are maintained; the term is often used loosely and ambiguously.

Neurotransmitter Chemical released from the end of one nerve to carry the nerve impulse across the synapse to the next nerve.

NIAAA (National Institute for Alcohol Abuse and Alcoholism) One of the federal National Institutes of Health in Washington, DC.

Nickel Five dollars.

Nickel bag Five dollars worth of drugs.

Nicotine Behavioral stimulant found in tobacco.

Nicotine effects Of or pertaining to cholinergic receptor theory.

Nicotinic cholinoceptive site Postjunctional receptor for acetylcholine; also affected by nicotine.

NIDA National Institute on Drug Abuse.

Nigrostriatal pathway Neural projection from cell bodies in the substantia nigra to the straitum.

NIMH National Institute of Mental Health.

Nitrites Class of compounds derived from nitrous acid that act as potent vasodilators.

Nociceptor Sensory receptor that transmits a pain signal when sufficiently stimulated.

Nodding Drowsy, dreamy, dozing state that follows injection of heroin; characterized by the head lolling forward and slowly jerking back up.

Nominal scale Rating scale that involves only the identification and not the quantification of characteristics that are not hierarchical (e.g., freezing and not freezing).

Norepinephrine (NE) Neurotransmitter in the sympathetic nervous system.

Nuclear schizophrenia Term referring to the core clinical symptomatology of schizophrenia rather than associated or social factors.

Nucleic acids Family of substances of high molecular weight found in chromosomes, mitochondria, and viruses. Nucleic acids are important constituents of cellular physiology and are thought to be the ultimate carriers of genetic inheritance or physical characteristics of cells.

Nucleus Spherical body in a cell that controls cell growth, metabolism, and reproduction.

Nystagmus Oscillation of the eyeballs.

O Opium.

O.D. Overdose.

Oedema Swelling due the presence of excess fluid in the intercellular spaces of the body (American spelling: edema).

Offender Individual convicted of committing an offense.

Ololiuqui Aztec name for morning glory seeds.

On Using drugs.

On the needle Injecting drugs.

On the street Out of jail.

On the tip Just short of the elated state of a "high."

Operant pain Learned pain behavior that may respond to behavioral modification.

Opiate Opium and its derivatives (morphine, heroin, codeine, and methadone).

Opiate narcotic Drug that has both sedative and analgesic actions.

Opioid Any synthetic narcotic analgesic that has opiate-like pharmacology but is not derived from opium.

Opium Crude resinous exudate from the opium poppy.

Oral contraceptive (the pill) Oral synthetic progestin or a combination of oral progestin and estrogen used to prevent pregnancy.

Oranges Dexedrine tablets.

Ordinal scale Rating scale that involves the allocation of characteristics to categories that have a hierarchical relationship (e.g., hot, warm, and cold).

Orphan drugs Those used in the treatment of rare diseases; drug manufacturers are reluctant to produce such drugs because they are not profitable.

OTC Over the counter.

Outfit Equipment used for injecting drugs.

Outpatient Patient who comes to a hospital or clinic for treatment but who does not occupy a bed.

Overdose Drug intake in excess of the specified quantity.

Overjolt Overdose.

Over the counter (OTC) Pharmaceutical substance that can be purchased without a prescription (for example, aspirin); claims for the effectiveness of such a substance are regulated to some extent by the FDA.

Ovulation Process by which egg, or female germ cells, are released from the ovary.

Oxytocic Drug that stimulates the uterus to contract.

O One ounce.

P Peyote.

Pad Room or house; may imply place for taking drugs.

Pain Perception of a sensation as extremely uncomfortable physically; a signal of possible damage to the body. Subclassified as visceral (nonskeletal) or somatic (skeletal muscle and bone) and sharp (carried by A-delta fibers) or dull (carried by C-fibers).

Pain gate Hypothetical system in the spinal cord thought to account for varying perception of pain by modulating signals ascending into the brain. The gate can be "closed" by acupuncture and hypnosis, which may work by activating higher centers to send inhibitory signals back down the spinal cord.

Pain threshold Level at which a stimulus is first recognized as unpleasant.

Pain tolerance Level of painful stimulation at which the person says he or she cannot bear more; psychological factors are important in determining pain tolerance.

Palpitations Unduly rapid beating of the heart that is noticed by the subject.

Panama red Type of marijuana.

Panic Anxiety about a shortage of drugs on the market.

Paper Paper for writing prescriptions; or cigarette (rolling) papers.

Paper chromatography Separation of compounds by placing a dried mixture on a filter paper and allowing a solvent to move across the paper by capillary action. Separation of compounds up the paper depends on their relative solubility in the solvent.

Parachlorophenylalanine (PCPA)   Drug that blocks serotonin synthesis and produces a deficiency of that neurotransmitter.

Paranoia   State of having delusions, commonly but not necessarily of a persecutory nature.

Paranoic psychosis   State of mind such that a person is so frightened of being harmed by some external force that he or she experiences an inability to continue with some previous normal function.

Paranoid delusions of grandeur   Thoughts or perceptions of oneself or one's plans that are greatly exaggerated and have as their stimulating basis a fear of some external force.

Parasympathetic nervous system   Part of the autonomic nervous system that opposes the effects of the sympathetic nervous system. Generally, it tends to stimulate digestive secretions, slowing of the heart, and dilation of blood vessels. It is often referred to as the "feed and breed" system.

Parasympatholytic   Agent that annuls or antagonizes the effects of parasympathetic nerve action.

Parasympathomimetic   Denoting stimulation of parasympathetic nerve action.

Parenteral   Taking a drug other than orally (for example, by injection, topically, and so on).

Parkinson's disease   Progressive degenerative disease of the nervous system's motor control center in the basal ganglia, causing muscular tremors, stiffness, and difficulty in moving.

Particulate   Usually, that fraction of a tissue homogenate that contains the subcellular particles.

Passivity feelings   Feelings of being under the control or will of an outside agency.

Peachies   Benzedrine in tablet form.

Pearls   Amyl nitrite.

Pellets   LSD capsules.

Pelvic inflammatory disease (PID)   Inflammation of the pelvic organs through infection of the urethra or the vagina with gonorrhea or by various organisms.

Penetrance   In genetics, the degree to which a genetically inherited characteristic is expressed.

People   Police.

Pep pills   Amphetamines.

Peptide   Biochemical polymer of two or more amino acids linked between the amine group ($-NH_2$) of one and the carboxyl group (-COOH) of the next amino acid; a chain of more than 100 amino acids is usually called a protein.

Perceptual distorter   Chemical that has the ability to cause altered states of perception, thought, and feeling.

Performance   Measurement of the fulfillment of contractual agreement or the obligations of a conditionally granted privilege.

Peripheral nervous system   All the neurons located outside the brain and spinal cord.

Peristalsis   Wavelike contractions of the gastrointestinal tract by which the contents are propelled along.

Periventricular system   Group of neurons in the hypothalamus and thalamus; location of the punishment (avoidance) center; probably uses acetylcholine as a neurotransmitter.

Permissive theory   Theory that proposes that affective disorders are related to insufficient serotonin. Depression occurs when serotonin levels are low and norepinephrine levels are low; mania results when serotonin levels are low and norepinephrine levels are high.

Perseveration   Persistent reference to a theme, persistent use of a word or phrase, or persistent behavior that is out of context.

Peyote   Small grey-green cactus from which the hallucinogenic drug mescaline is derived.

PG   Paregoric.

pH   Artificial scale from 1 to 14 used to express the acidity or alkalinity of water solutions.

Phagocyte   Type of white blood cell that attacks and engulfs foreign objects such as bacteria and sperm. Once inside the phagocyte, the foreign objects are broken down by enzymes.

Phantom pain   Pain experienced by some amputees "in" the missing limb.

Pharmacodynamics   Study of the actions of drugs on the living organism.

Pharmacogenetics   Study of genetically determined variations in responses to drugs in humans or laboratory animals.

Pharmacology Branch of basic science that deals with the actions on biological systems, usually human, of chemicals used in medicine for diagnostic and therapeutic purposes.

Pharmacology, behavioral Study of the alteration of behavior by certain drugs.

Pharmacology, biochemical Study of the mechanism and metabolism by which certain drugs manifest their effects.

Pharmacology, classical Study of the effects of certain drugs on test subjects or laboratory animals under controlled conditions.

Pharynx Anatomic portion that connects the mouth and nasal passages with the esophagus.

Phencyclidine (Sernyl) Psychedelic surgical anesthetic.

Phenos Phenobarbital.

Phenothiazine Class of compounds useful in the treatment of psychosis.

Phobia Persistent, abnormal fear of some situation or object.

Phospholipid Lipid containing phosphorus.

Physical dependence Physiological adaptation of the body to the presence of a drug. In effect, the body develops a continuing need for the drug.

Physostigmine Acetylchole esterase (AChE) inhibitor.

Picked up To have smoked marijuana.

Picrotoxin Convulsant drug.

Piece Measure or part of a quantity of a drug.

Pill Barbiturate or amphetamine pill.

Pill head A person who uses barbiturates or amphetamines to excess.

Piloerection Hair standing up, as during the skin's response to cold.

Pin Very thin marijuana cigarette.

Pineal gland Small gland in the midline of the brain. In many animals it responds to diurnal changes in light. This gland is the site of synthesis of metatonin (5-methoxy-*N*-acetyl serotonin).

Pink ladies Same as Pinks.

Pinks Seconal; a barbiturate.

Pinned Constricted (as in "The pupils of his eyes are *pinned* after he injects heroin").

Pituitary gland Important endocrine gland situated at the base of the hypothalamus and directed by it; secretes (among many other hormones) the gonadotropins.

Placebo Inert substance, such as a sugar tablet or an injection of sterile water, given as if it were a real medication; also, an ineffective dosage of an active drug.

Placental barrier Lipid membranes that impede transfer of many substances from the blood into the placenta.

Plant Stash or cache of drugs; hiding place for drugs.

Plasma Blood from which the formed elements (red blood cells, white blood cells, and platelets) have been removed.

Platelets Normal constituents of the blood that are smaller than red cells and are essential to the process of blood clotting.

Polydipsia Excessive drinking.

Polydrug abuse Simultaneous abuse of more than one psychoactive or other substance.

Polypharmacy Prescribing more than one drug concurrently.

Pons Area of the hindbrain beneath the cerebellum.

Pop To swallow a pill or to inject heroin subcutaneously.

Popped "Busted," or arrested by the police.

Poppers Small vials of amyl nitrite that are broken and inhaled.

Pore Place in a cell membrane involved in the transport of a substance across the membrane barrier.

Postganglionic nerve endings Those nerve endings denoting autonomic fibers of the second order arising from the cells in the peripheral autonomic ganglia.

Postjunctional receptor site Receptor for a neurotransmitter on the receiving neuron.

Postmortem operation Autopsy.

Pot Marijuana.

Potency Absolute amount of a drug required to produce a given pharmacological effect.

Potlikker Tea brewed with marijuana seeds and stems.

Potsville Using marijuana.

Precursor   In a metabolic sequence of reactions, a compound that gives rise to the next compound; for example, choline is the precursor for the neurotransmitter acetylcholine.

Prescription drug   Pharmaceutical substance whose prescription order is regulated by law to a licensed person, such as a physician.

Pressor   Substance that elevates blood pressure (for example, tyramine).

Presynaptic   Events or structures proximal to the synapse.

Pretrial release   Release on bail or in lieu of bail, subject to specified conditions, between court appearances as an alternative to pretrial detention. Either money bail or conditions are no more severe than is necessary to ensure the accused's appearance in court.

Priapism   Uncomfortable, prolonged penile erection caused by a pathological condition or a drug such as spanish fly.

Primo   Very good drug, usually marijuana.

Probation   Court release without imprisonment, subject to the accused's compliance with court-imposed conditions.

Process schizophrenia   Term referring to core clinical symptomatology of schizophrenia rather than associated or social factors.

Progesterone   Hormone secreted from the ovaries in response to stimulation by luteinizing hormone (LH) from the pituitary gland.

Progestin   Class of chemical compounds, some of which are synthetic and administered orally, that are similar to ovarian progesterone in action; used in oral contraceptive pills, injectable contraceptives, and medicated intrauterine devices.

Prolactin   Hormone from the pituitary gland that acts on the breasts to stimulate secretion of milk.

Prophylactic   Warding off disease.

Prostate   One of the secondary male sex organs; a three-lobed organ near the urinary bladder whose secretions make up much of the volume of the ejaculate.

Protein   Class of substances found in all areas of nature that are composed of amino acids bound together through peptide linkages.

Protein binding   The adhesion of drugs and hormones to carrier proteins to circulate in blood; the proportion of bound to unbound (free) proteins varies with the drug's structure.

Pseudohallucinations   Similar to delusions; the perception of an object that already exists as something other than what it is (for example, a perception of a brown desk as a multicolored miniature rocket).

Pseudoparkinsonism   Extrapyramidal side effect of the neuroleptics (e.g., phenothiazine, haloperidol, and thiothixene). Resembles true parkinsonism and is characterized by akinesia, tremor, muscle rigidity, and shuffling gait.

Psilocybin   Psychedelic drug obtained from the Mexican mushroom *Psilocybe mexicana*.

Psychedelic   Mind-manifesting; group of drugs producing a mental state of great calm and intensely pleasurable perception.

Psychedelic drug   Any drug with the ability to alter sensory perception.

Psychoactive (psychotropic) drug   One that affects mood or consciousness; may be a prescription (Valium) or a nonprescription (marijuana) drug.

Psychoadjuvant   Remedy or drug added to the main type or mode of psychotherapy to assist, aid, or increase the efficacy of the main mode of psychotherapy.

Psychodynamic tolerance   State in which a drug's target tissue, such as the brain, has adapted to the drug gradually, over a period of weeks to months, by an unknown mechanism so that the same concentration of drug produces a decreased response.

Psychological addiction   See Psychological dependence.

Psychological dependence, primary   Attachment to drug use that arises from a drug's ability to satisfy some emotional or personality need; see also Habituation.

Psychological dependence, secondary   Taking a drug to avoid the withdrawal symptoms once physical dependence has developed.

Psychosis   Major mental derangement; the deeper, more far-reaching, and prolonged behavioral disorders. (Compare to "insanity," which is a social and legal term referring to a mental derangement.)

Psychotogen Drug that produces psychotic manifestations.

Psychotomimetic Mimicking a psychosis; compounds capable of producing hallucinations, sensory illusions, and bizarre thoughts.

Psychotoxic Drugs, including therapeutic and abused, that can produce (1) a psychosis (psychotogenic drugs), (2) a mood change, or (3) anxiety. The psychotogenic drugs (amphetamines, LSD, or marijuana) can produce euphoria in low dosages but in higher dosages can produce a psychotic state.

Psychotropic Affecting the mind in some way.

Psychotropic drug Drug that acts on psychic mood behavior or experience.

Pulmonary edema Perceptible accumulation of excessive clear watery fluid in the tissues of the lungs, pulmonary arteries, and bronchi.

Pulmonary hypertension High arterial blood pressure in the pulmonary circuit (the circuit of the pulmonary arteries, pulmonary veins, and both sides of the heart). It can cause pulmonary edema and can be lethal.

Pulmonary talc granulomatosis A granulomatous inflammation of the lungs caused by the inhalation of talc granules. It can interfere with respiration and lead to respiratory failure and death if untreated or with continued use.

Purple hearts Luminal tablets, or a combination of barbiturates and amphetamines.

Pusher Drug dealer; one who sells drugs.

Putamen Area of the brain that includes the corpus straitum.

Putting the bean Begging for narcotics.

Quantitative analysis Determination of the amount as well as the nature of each of the elements that composes a compound being investigated.

Quarter bag Bag of drugs that sells for $25.

Quasi medical Having the characteristics of medical use but not accepted in usual modern medical practice.

Quill Folded matchbook cover used to inhale a drug through the nose.

Quinine White alkaloid with a bitter taste, found as an adulterant in street heroin.

Radioactive tag Chemical or drug used in research that bears a radioactive atom (tag), thereby permitting an investigator to follow its behavior and ultimate fate in the body.

Radioimmunoassay Assay technique that uses an antibody to the compound to be measured. The displacement of a fixed concentration of the radiolabeled compound provides a measure of the amount of unlabeled compound present.

Radiolabeled compound Compound synthesized to contain one or more radioactive atoms in particular parts of the molecule.

Rainbow Tuinal capsule.

Rainy day woman Marijuana cigarette.

Rap To talk.

Rat An informer; one who gives information to the police.

Reader Prescription for drugs.

Receptor Special protein on the membrane or in the cytoplasm of a target cell with which a drug, a neurotransmitter, or a hormone interacts.

Receptor blocker Archaic and rather misleading phrase denoting a receptor antagonist.

Receptor site Portion of a cell that participates in drug-cell interactions to initiate a drug action.

Recidivism Return or relapse to a type of behavior, such as drug taking.

Red and blues Tuinal capsules.

Red birds Seconal capsules.

Red devils Seconal capsules.

Red dirt marijuana Marijuana that grows wild.

Reds Seconal capsules.

Reefer Marijuana cigarette.

Reflex action Automatic response to a stimulus during which a nerve impulse from a receptor passes to a nerve center, such as the spinal cord, and then outward to an effector without reaching the level of conscious action.

Reliability Measure of the similarity of scores produced by rating instruments when used under slightly different conditions (e.g., test-retest reliability, interrater reliability). See also Sensitivity and Specificity.

REM (rapid eye movement) sleep Stage of sleep during which REM occurs; this stage is associated with dreaming.

REM rebound Excessive REM sleep that occurs, along with nightmares, when a person has been denied REM sleep for long periods of time.

Reserpine An antipsychotic drug.

Reservoir Any system, fluid, organ, or part of the body that can bind and hold a drug for an extended period of time, thus preventing its rapid elimination from the body.

Respondent pain Pain with a definite physical cause.

Reticular activating system Network of nerve fibers located in the central portion of the brainstem with neural connections to the cerebral cortex. Its function is to arouse the cortex and maintain a state of consciousness; it is suppressed by most general anesthetics.

Retrospective study Collecting information from people after they have contracted a disease in an attempt to discover what caused it.

Re-uptake Process of active transport of neurotransmitters from extracellular fluid (synapse) to the cytoplasmic mobile pool (presynaptic terminal).

Reversed tolerance State produced by a particular drug, process, or individual, such that lower dosages of the same drug produce the same amount and quality of the desired or observed effect that previously was observed only with higher dosages.

Rhinophyma Painless increase in the size of the lower part of the nose.

Rhinorrhea Persistent discharge of thin nasal mucus.

Rig Hypodermic equipment.

Righteous bush Marijuana.

Ripped (stoned, high, floating, etc.) Intoxicated from drugs.

Risk-benefit ratio Comparison of the value of a drug in treating or preventing morbidity with the hazards of its use, leading to a conclusion to use the drug or to find an alternative.

Roach Marijuana cigarette butt.

Roach holder Matchbook cover, toothpick, hairpin, or other device used to hold the last bit of a marijuana cigarette so that it can be smoked (also called roach clip).

Root Marijuana cigarette.

Rope Marijuana.

Roses Benzedrine tablets.

Rubefaction Condition of inducing increased blood flow and a redness to the skin without blistering, such as by a counterirritant drug.

Run Period of time in which a person uses a particular drug successively, without stopping (especially, a speed run); also, to make a trip to purchase a particular kind of drug.

Rush Initial onset or feeling of euphoria after taking a drug.

Sacred mushrooms Mushrooms containing psilocybin, a hallucinogen.

Salt shot Injection, intravenously, of salt and water into the vein of someone who has overdosed on heroin; believed to revive the person, but actually it does not.

Sam Narcotic agent of the federal government.

Scag Heroin.

Scars Needle marks that cause scars on the body.

Schedule I substances Drugs that have no accepted medical usage in the United States and that have a high abuse potential (for example, heroin, LSD, marijuana, and psilocybin).

Schedule II substances Drugs considered to have a high abuse potential with severe psychological or physical dependence liability (for example, amphetamine, methaqualone, and morphine). The physician must write the prescription in ink or type it and sign it, and it cannot be refilled.

Schedule III substances Drugs considered to have less abuse potential than Schedule II substances, including compounds with limited quantities of certain narcotic drugs, and non-narcotic drugs (for example, glutethimide and nalorphine). The prescription may be written or given orally to the pharmacist, and it can be refilled if specified.

Schedule IV substances Drugs considered to have less abuse potential than Schedule III substances (for example, phenobarbital and Valium).

Schedule V substances Drugs that have an abuse potential less than that of Schedule IV substances and that consist of preparations containing limited quantities of certain narcotic drugs for antitussive (cough) and antidiarrheal purposes (for example, Robitussin and Lomotil). These may be dispensed (subject to state law) without a prescription by a pharmacist, who is required to maintain a record book of these purchases.

Schizophrenia-like psychosis Psychosis-like state resembling the named disease schizophrenia (the subject is ambivalent and autistic and has loose association, a labile or flat affect, and nebulous ego boundaries).

Schlook Puff of a marijuana cigarette.

Schmack Usually heroin; but can refer to cocaine or any drug.

Schmeck Heroin.

Scissors Marijuana.

Scoff To eat; food.

Scoop Folded matchbook cover used to inhale drugs (cocaine or heroin) through the nose.

Score, to To connect; to buy drugs successfully.

Scratch Physically dependent on drugs.

Scrip Drug prescription.

Seccy Seconal capsules.

Secondary sex organs Prostate and seminal vesicles.

Sedative Psychoactive drug that decreases excitability and anxiety as part of its general depressant action; high dosages may be hypnotic (sleep inducing).

Seed Marijuana cigarette butt.

Seizure Uncontrolled or paroxysmal brain activity that may be expressed through the motor system.

Seminal vesicles Secondary male sex organs; a pair of sacs located on both sides of the urinary bladder that contribute substances and fluid to the ejaculate.

Seminiferous tubules Those tubules from the testicles that carry the semen and sperm.

Sensitivity Measure of the ability of a rating instrument to identify all those items of relevance in a study population.

Sensitizing contact Contact with a drug or substance that triggers the "immune system" such that any further contact with the same substance will result in an allergic or hypersensitive reaction.

Serial sevens Mental dexterity test during which the subject is given a two-digit number and then told to add or subtract 7 from that number many times in succession as rapidly as possible, stating each new number aloud. The speed and accuracy with which the subject produces the answers gives the test administrator a good estimation of the intactness of the subject's thinking processes.

Serotonin (5-hydroxytryptamine, 5-HT) Synaptic transmitter in the brain and the peripheral nervous system.

Serum Fluid formed from blood as a result of clotting.

Set Psychological makeup or behavior of a drug user. For example, if a good result is expected from a given situation, that result is more likely to occur.

Setting Physical surroundings in which a drug is taken. A pleasant environment is often important in determining the effects of a hallucinogen.

Shelf-life Period of storage time during which a drug is expected to remain stable and effective. The "shelf" can refer to the drugstore or to the home medicine cabinet.

Shooting gallery Place where people gather in a group to inject heroin, most of whom are physically dependent on the drug.

Shoot up To inject drugs, usually heroin.

Sick Heroin withdrawal symptoms.

Side effect Any drug-induced effect that accompanies the primary effect for which the drug is administered.

Sitter Person who is experienced in the use of LSD and aids someone else through the experience.

Sizzle Drugs carried on the person.

Skid bag Bag containing highly diluted heroin.

Skin Cigarette paper used to roll marijuana cigarettes.

Skin popping To inject heroin subcutaneously, not intravenously.

Sleep walker   Person who is physically dependent on heroin.

Smack   Heroin, or one who uses heroin.

Snappers   Glass vials of amyl nitrite.

Sniffing   Inhaling heroin or cocaine through the nose.

Snop   Marijuana.

Snort   To inhale heroin or cocaine through the nose.

Snow   Cocaine crystals.

Sociopathic   The characteristic of being poorly adjusted to society because of quarrelsome, rebellious, aggressive, or immoral attitudes.

Solution   Dosage form in which a drug is dissolved in a liquid.

Solvent   Substance (usually liquid) that is capable of dissolving another substance.

Source   Supplier of drugs.

Spaced (high, stoned, ripped, etc.)   Intoxicated from drugs.

Spanish fly   Preparation of the irritating substance cantharide from blister beetles; used as an aphrodisiac; produces an inflammation of the lining of the urinary bladder and the urethra in both males and females.

Sparkle plenties   Amphetamines.

Specificity   (1) Measuring of the ability of a rating instrument to identify only those items of relevance in a study population. (2) Characteristics of receptors or enzymes to recognize defined chemical structures.

Speed   Amphetamines, methamphetamine, or Methedrine.

Speedball   Injected mixture of heroin and cocaine.

Spermatogenesis   Production of sperm or male gametes; one of the functions of the testes.

Spermicidal jelly   Contraceptive agent in the form of a gel with a chemical ingredient to kill sperm.

Spider angiomas   Star-shaped swelling due to dilation of the blood vessels.

Spike   Hypodermic needle.

Splash   Amphetamines.

Spliff   Large marijuana cigarette.

Split   To go, run away, leave.

Splits   Tranquilizers.

Spoon   Usually $\frac{1}{16}$ of 1 ounce of heroin.

Square   Nonuser of drugs.

Star-dust   Cocaine

Stash   Hiding place for drugs.

Status epilepticus   Condition in which major seizures follow one after another with little or no intermission.

Steady state   Situation that exists when the rate of elimination of a drug equals the rate of its intake.

Stereotaxic surgery   Method of producing accurately placed lesions in the brain, often by electrocoagulation or by implantation of radioactive pellets.

Stereotypy   Persistent repetition of particular movements.

Stick   Marijuana cigarette.

Stimulant   Any of several drugs that act on the central nervous system to produce excitation, alertness, and wakefulness. Medical uses include the treatment of hyperkinesis and narcolepsy.

Stone (stoned)   Intoxicated from drugs.

Stone addict   One who is physically dependent on drugs of a very potent nature.

Stool (stoolie)   Informer or "rat."

STP (z,5-dimethoxy-4-methylamphetamine, DOM)   very long-acting (36 to 72 hours) hallucinogenic drug.

Straight   Not using drugs; not intoxicated with drugs or under their influence.

Straight-chain hydrocarbons   Chemicals composed of hydrogen and carbon that do not contain branched or cyclic compounds.

Straitum   See Corpus straitum.

Street, out on the   Out searching for drugs.

Strung out   Addicted.

Strychnine   A convulsant drug.

Stuff   Heroin.

Subcutaneous   Under the skin.

Sublingual   Under the tongue.

Subsensitivity   (1) Pharmacological: decreased response to a fixed concentration of a drug; shift of the dose-response curve to the right.

(2) Behavioral: decreased behavioral response to a fixed dosage of a drug.

Substance P Peptide found in nerves that transmit pain signals; may be a pain neurotransmitter.

Success Compliance with and completion of the conditions of a treatment program, often celebrated by graduation.

Superpot Very potent marijuana.

Supersensitivity (1) Pharmacological: increased response to a fixed concentration of a drug; shift of the dose-response curve to the left. (2) Behavioral: increased behavioral response to a fixed dosage of a drug.

Suppository Dosage form of a drug that is placed in a bodily orifice such as the anus or vagina.

Suspension Dosage form in which particles of an insoluble drug are suspended in a liquid.

Sweet Lucy Marijuana.

Swingman Drug dealer or pusher.

Sympathetic (adrenergic) Relating to nerve fibers that liberate adrenalin-like substances.

Sympathetic nervous system Portion of the autonomic nervous system that usually opposes the parasympathetic nervous system. It is sometimes referred to as the ''fight-or-flight'' system, and among other effects it dilates respiratory passages, increases blood flow to vital organs, and decreases gastrointestinal activity.

Sympatholytic Agent that annuls or inhibits the effects of adrenergic stimulation.

Sympathomimetic Denoting stimulation of adrenergic nerve action.

Symptom re-emergence After discontinuation of administration of a chemical, the re-occurrence of disorders or symptoms that had been treated by that chemical.

Synapse Place where a nerve impulse is transmitted from one neuron to another.

Synaptic cleft Space between the terminal process of one neuron and the receptor site of another.

Synaptic vehicle Membrane-enclosed package of neurotransmitters found in the end bulb of the axon.

Synaptosomes Pinched-off and resealed nerve endings formed by careful homogenization of brain tissue in isotonic saline.

Syndrome All the signs and symptoms associated with a disease.

Synergism Unpredictable enhancement of the effect of one chemical by the presence of another. The effect is more than expected from the combined amount of the two chemicals.

Synesthesia Occurrence of one type of stimulation evoking the sensation of another; for example, the hearing of a sound resulting in the sensation of visualizating a color.

Tabs Tablets.

Tachycardia Rapid heartbeat, such as from stress or stimulant drugs.

Tachyphylaxis Rapid production of immunity to effects.

Tall Intoxicated on drugs.

Tapita Bottle cap used for melting heroin.

Tardive dyskinesia Long-term side effect of major tranquilizers in which, after years of treatment, the person has difficulty controlling voluntary movement, especially of the lips and tongue.

Target tissue Glands or cells in the body to which a drug binds and thus exerts its pharmacological effect.

Taste Small amount of a drug.

Tea Marijuana.

Tea bag Smoking marijuana.

Tea head One who regularly uses marijuana.

Tecata Heroin.

Ten-cent pistol Heroin bag that actually contains poison.

Teratogen Agent or factor that causes physical defects in a developing embryo.

Termination Prematurely ended treatment, usually due to the individual's failure to comply with program rules and conditions.

Testosterone Sex hormone from the testes that maintains libido and male characteristics such as body and facial hair and musculature; it is a naturally occurring compound in the class of androgens.

Tetrahydroisoquinolines Alkaloids chemically related to morphine that affect addictive behavior in some laboratory animals.

Texas tea Marijuana.

Thalamus Portion of the forebrain where sensations such as pain are interpreted and relayed to appropriate areas of the cerebral cortex; important in emotional responses associated with feelings of pleasantness and unpleasantness.

THC (tetrahydrocannabinol) Active ingredient in marijuana and hashish that causes psychogenic reactions.

Therapeutic Curative or healing.

Therapeutic index Ratio between the dosage of a drug needed to produce a therapeutic effect (taken as unity) and the dosage of a drug that is toxic.

Threshold dosage Least amount of a drug that shows any therapeutic value.

Thromboembolism Obstruction of a blood vessel by a thrombus (blood clot) that has broken loose and moved from its site of formation.

Thrombosis Formation or presence of a blood clot (thrombus).

Thrusters Amphetamine pills.

Thumb Flat marijuana cigarette.

Thyroid gland Endocrine gland situated in the neck that secretes thyroid hormone, which regulates many aspects of metabolism including maintenance of reproductive function.

Ticket LSD-25.

Tin Small amount of opium.

Tingle Rush or "high" feeling.

TMA Synthetic hallucinogen of greater potency than mescaline.

Toak (toke) To puff a marijuana cigarette; also, such a puff (i.e., "take a toke").

Toke pipes Short-stemmed pipes in which marijuana is smoked.

Tolerance Condition in which a person must keep increasing the dosage of a drug to maintain the same effect. Tolerance develops with the barbiturates, amphetamines and related compounds, and opiates.

Tooies Tuinal capsules.

Topi Peyote cactus that contains mescaline as the hallucinogen.

Topical Dosage form in which a drug is applied to an external body surface.

Torn up (ripped, stoned, floating, etc.) Intoxicated from drugs.

Toss out To feign withdrawal symptoms to a doctor in order to obtain a prescription for the drug.

Toxicity Degree of poisonousness; any substance in excessive amounts can act as a poison or toxin. With drugs, the margin between the dosage that produces beneficial effects and the dosage that produces toxic or poisonous effects varies with the drug and the person receiving it. See also Lethal dosage.

Toxicology Study of the noxious or poisonous effects of certain drugs, agents, or processes.

Toxin Literally, poison; any noxious or poisonous substance that is an integral part of a cell or tissue, is an extracellular product, represents a combination of these two situations, or is formed or elaborated during metabolism and growth of certain microorganisms as well as some of the higher plant and animal species; or a drug or metabolic product of a drug.

Tracked up Having needle marks or scars on the body from previously injected drugs.

Tracks Needle marks or scars from injecting drugs.

Tranquilizers (major) Drugs used to relieve symptoms of severe psychosis (for example, Thorazine).

Tranquilizers (minor) Psychoactive drugs with sedative and antianxiety effects; also used as anticonvulsants and muscle relaxants (an example is Valium).

Travel agent Drug dealer who supplies LSD (for a trip).

Trip An experience with LSD or other hallucinogens.

Trophotropic That which characterizes a tranquil, restorative, nourishing state; hypoaroused; compare to Ergotropic.

Tryptaminergic Neuron that uses 5-hydroxytryptamine (serotonin) as a neurotransmitter.

T's and blues   Mixture of pentazocine (a narcotic analgesic) and tripelennamine (pyribenzamine, an antihistamine); used as a heroin substitute.

Tuberoinfundibular system   System connecting the hypothalamus with the pituitary.

Turned off   Withdrawn from drugs.

Turned on   Intoxicated from drugs.

Twenty-five   LSD-25.

Twist   Marijuana.

Twisted   Suffering withdrawal symptoms.

Tying up   Putting something around the upper arm so that the veins will stand out more clearly in the lower arm, thus facilitating injection.

Uncle   Federal narcotics officer.

Up (high, stoned, etc.)   Intoxicated from drugs.

Upper   Amphetamine pill.

Up-regulation   Adaptation, usually of a receptor, to increase the function of the system.

Up-tight   Tense, worried, or anxious.

Urinalysis   Chemical testing of a sample of an individual's urine that reveals recent use of heroin (up to 24 hours); can be used to test for recent use of other drugs.

USAN   United States Adopted Name.

Using   Taking drugs of any type.

Uterus   Womb.

Validity   Overall assessment of the sensitivity and specificity of a rating instrument.

Vascular sclerosis   Hardening of the arteries and, potentially, narrowing of the bore of the arteries.

Vas deferens   Duct that runs from a testis and joins with other ducts to open into the urethra.

Vasocongestion   Engorgement of blood vessels; more blood flows into than out of particular tissues.

Vasoconstriction   Reduction in the diameter of blood vessels by constriction of the circular muscles in their walls.

Vasodilatation   Increase in the diameter of blood vessels, causing increased volume of blood flow in that vessel.

Vasomotor system   System of nerves and chemicals that cause either dilation or constriction of the blood vessels.

Vasopressor agent   See Pressor agent.

Ventral tegmental area   Area of the midbrain dorsal to the substantia nigra.

Ventricles   Cavities within the brain that contain cerebrospinal fluid.

Ventricular fibrillation   Fine, very rapid twitching movements of the muscles of the largest chambers of the heart. This replaces normal heart contractions; if it persists, it is fatal because the heart is not contracting as a unit and there is little, if any, movement of the blood in the vessels.

Vipe   Marijuana.

Viper   Marijuana smoker.

Volatile   Capable of being easily vaporized at normal temperatures or pressures.

Volume of distribution   Apparent volume of the body through which a drug is distributed were it present throughout at the concentration found in plasma.

Voyager   Marijuana smoker.

Wake-up   Person who is physically dependent on a heroin injection in the morning.

Waste   To destroy or kill (someone).

Wasted   Very intoxicated.

Weed   Marijuana.

Weeding out   Smoking marijuana.

Wernicke's syndrome   Mental disorder marked by memory loss, disorientation, and confabulation.

White cross   X-scored tablet containing 15 to 20 mg of methamphetamine.

White lady   Heroin.

White light   Enlightening experience gained by using hallucinogenic drugs under special circumstances.

Whites   Benzedrine pills.

White stuff   Heroin.

Window pane   LSD in small squares of coated plastic or stiffened gel.

Winging   Physical withdrawal symptoms from drug dependence.

Wings   First intravenous injection.

Wired   Highly stimulated, usually under the influence of a stimulant.

Withdrawal Signs and symptoms seen after decrease or cessation of a drug on which the user has become physically dependent.

Woman years Measure used to rate effectiveness of contraceptives; it equals the number of women using the method multiplied by the number of years used.

Works Equipment for dilution and injection of drugs.

Wrap Innocent-looking covering for drugs.

Xanthine Biochemical substance in the alkaloid family with stimulant properties; an example is caffeine.

Yellow jackets Nembutal capsules.

Yen Withdrawal symptoms from physical dependence on drugs.

Yoga Physical discipline by which a person attains unity with the Supreme Being or the Absolute.

Zonked (high, stoned, ripped, etc.) Intoxicated from drugs.

Index

363

About the Authors

GARY W. LAWSON, PH.D., is Associate Dean of the School of Human Behavior, United States International University, San Diego, California. He is a professor of clinical psychology and marriage and family. He has worked in the field of substance abuse for seventeen years and is a licensed clinical psychologist in California, Nebraska, and Illinois. His other books include *Alcoholism and the Family: A Guide to Treatment and Prevention; Essentials of Chemical Dependency Counseling and Treatment;* and *Treatment and Prevention of Substance Abuse in Specific Populations.* Dr. Lawson has lectured on addiction both nationally and internationally.

CRAIG A. COOPERRIDER, PH.D., is a clinical psychologist for Pioneer Mental Health Center in Seward, Nebraska. He has served as Director of Training and Staff Development and been a counselor for Nebraska Rehabilitation Services. Dr. Cooperrider has over 10 years of experience in the mental health and rehabilitation fields. He has presented numerous courses and workshops in the areas of counseling, mental health, psychopharmacology, parenting, and personal growth for various agencies and colleges.

About the Contributors

ROBERT B. COHEN, PH.D., is a postdoctoral fellow in clinical psychology at Mercy Hospital in San Diego, California, and is a registered psychological assistant in private practice. Dr. Cohen specializes in working with children, adolescents, young adults, and families. He received his B.A. from the University of Rhode Island, his M.A. from Loyola College, and his Ph.D. from United States International University. He has done research in the area of personal space and for his doctoral dissertation he developed a text to assess the risk of alcoholism. Dr. Cohen has been working in the mental health field for 10 years.

ANN LAWSON, M.A., M.F.C.C., is Director of the Addiction Counselor Training Program at United States International University. She is a licensed marriage, family and child counselor and a doctoral candidate in psychology. She has worked in the mental health field for ten years, the last six of which have been in the field of chemical dependency. Before coming to USUI, she was the creator and director of the Children of Alcoholic Families Program at the Lincoln Child Guidance Center, Lincoln, Nebraska. Her other publications include *Alcoholism and the Family: A Guide to Treatment and Prevention,* and "Treatment of Geriatric Substance Abuse" in *Treatment and Prevention of Substance Abuse in Specific Populations.* She is a consultant to drug and alcohol prevention programs and has presented at many national and regional conventions and workshops.

GARY R. LEWIS, M.A., R.N., is in private practice as a clinical nurse specialist and psychological assistant. He has 6 years of experience in the field of chemical dependency, which includes a variety of situations and both inpatient and outpatient treatment. Mr. Lewis is currently a doctoral candidate in clinical psychology with a subspeciality in chemical dependency at the United States International University.

JOHN MCCAIG, M.A., is currently practicing as a school psychologist with the Child Guidance Clinic of Greater Winnipeg. Mr. McCaig has a graduate degree in educational psychology and cross-cultural studies and is completing his Ph.D. in general psychology at USIU.

MICHAEL J. NANKO, PH.D., is a health psychologist and corporate director of geriatrics for United Western Medical Centers, a nonprofit acute care hospital system in Orange County, California. Dr. Nanko has published articles and presented at conferences research related to the psychology of belief, states of consciousness, health behavior, and experimental parapsychology. He is also the originator of the Student Health and Assessment Program for Education (SHAPE), which has received national attention as a model program for schools. SHAPE teaches students to take more responsibility for and control of their health-related behaviors.

M. GENE ONDRUSEK, PH.D., is a clinical psychologist and pharmacologist in private practice in San Diego, California. Prior to this, he was both a pre- and postdoctoral fellow with the National Institute on Drug Abuse, with specialty areas in neurochemistry and clinical psychopharmacology. He has appointments on the faculty of both the California School of Professional Psychology and San Diego State University. Dr. Ondrusek specializes in behavioral medicine and the treatment of addictive disorders and serves as a consultant to industry on employee assistance programs.

DELIA THRASHER, M.A., is a doctoral student at United States International University and a doctoral intern at St. Lawrence Hospital, Mental Health Services, in Lansing, Michigan. Her primary interests are working in sports psychology and with children. Her publications include "Chemical Dependency and Treatment of the Professional Athlete" in *Treatment and Prevention of Substance Abuse in Specific Populations*.

JERRY WILLIAMS, PH.D., is a clinical neuropsychologist at Rehabilitation Psychology Associates in Farmington Hills, Michigan. His primary interests are working with closed-head-injury patients, environmental psychology, and psychopharmacology.

THOMAS J. YOUNG, PH.D., is an assistant professor of criminal justice at Kearney State College. He received his Ph.D. in psychological and cultural studies from the University of Nebraska-Lincoln and has completed two years of postdoctoral study in developmental psychology at the University of Kansas. He has published articles on psychopharmacology and substance abuse among special populations.